Paediatric Nursing in Australia
Principles for practice

Paediatric Nursing in Australia: Principles for practice equips students with the essential skills and knowledge to become paediatric, child and youth health nurses across a variety of clinical and community settings. It prepares students for critical thinking and problem-solving within this field by emphasising contemporary issues impacting on the health of children and young people and their families.

Written by a team of experienced paediatric nurses, the content is based on themes that align with Australian standards for practice and expectations of paediatric nursing: communication, family involvement and evidence-based practice. Comprehensive yet concise, the text examines the integration of theoretical and clinical components of nursing knowledge. To enhance learning each chapter features illustrative case studies, reflection points and learning activities.

An essential resource for nursing students, this text is well grounded in current care delivery and professional issues for care of the child to prepare future nurses for evidence-based practice in paediatric settings throughout Australia.

Additional resources are available online at
www.cambridge.edu.au/academic/paediatricnursing.

Paediatric Nursing in Australia
Principles for practice

Jennifer Fraser   Donna Waters
Elizabeth Forster   Nicola Brown

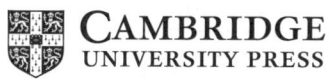

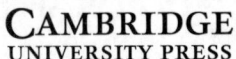

477 Williamstown Road, Port Melbourne, VIC 3207, Australia

Cambridge University Press is part of the University of Cambridge.

It furthers the University's mission by disseminating knowledge in the pursuit of education, learning and research at the highest international levels of excellence.

www.cambridge.org
Information on this title: www.cambridge.org/9781107685000

© Cambridge University Press 2014

This publication is copyright. Subject to statutory exception and to the provisions of relevant collective licensing agreements, no reproduction of any part may take place without the written permission of Cambridge University Press.

First published 2014

Cover designed by Anne-Marie Reeves
Typeset by Aptara Corp.
Printed in Australia by Ligare Pty Ltd

A catalogue record for this publication is available from the British Library

A Cataloguing-in-Publication entry is available from the catalogue
of the National Library of Australia at www.nla.gov.au

ISBN 978-1-107-68500-0 Paperback

Additional resources for this publication at www.cambridge.edu.au/academic/paediatricnursing

Reproduction and communication for educational purposes

The Australian *Copyright Act 1968* (the Act) allows a maximum of one chapter or 10% of the pages of this work, whichever is the greater, to be reproduced and/or communicated by any educational institution for its educational purposes provided that the educational institution (or the body that administers it) has given a remuneration notice to Copyright Agency Limited (CAL) under the Act.

For details of the CAL licence for educational institutions contact:

Copyright Agency Limited
Level 15, 233 Castlereagh Street
Sydney NSW 2000
Telephone: (02) 9394 7600
Facsimile: (02) 9394 7601
E-mail: info@copyright.com.au

Cambridge University Press has no responsibility for the persistence or accuracy of URLs for external or third-party internet websites referred to in this publication and does not guarantee that any content on such websites is, or will remain, accurate or appropriate.

The book has been printed on paper certified by the Programme for the Endorsement of Forest Certification (PEFC). PEFC is committed to sustainable forest management through third party forest certification of responsibly managed forests.

Cover image: 'The Games Children Play' tapestry was commissioned by the Royal Children's Hospital Foundation and Auxiliaries in 2009, with the kind support of Max and Lorraine Beck and their family, and realised by the Australian Tapestry Workshop. The original artist was Robert Ingpen and the weavers were Sue Batten, John Dicks and Emma Sulzer.

Figure 9.1: ©Shutterstock.com/Alila Medical Media

Every effort has been make in preparing this book to provide accurate and up-to-date information that is in accord with accepted standards and practice at the time of publication. Although case histories are drawn from actual cases, every effort has been made to disguise the identities of the individuals involved. Nevertheless, the authors, editors and publishers can make no warranties that the information contained herein is totally free from error, not least because clinical standards are constantly changing through research and regulation. The authors, editors and publishers therefore disclaim all liability for direct or consequential damages resulting from the use of material contained in this book. Readers are strongly advised to pay careful attention to information provided by the manufacturer of any drugs or equipment that they plan to use.

This book is dedicated to our dear friend and mentor, Professor Sue Nagy, an outstanding nurse educator, influential academic and passionate advocate for children, young people and their families.

Contents

	Preface	**xiii**
	PART 1: THE AUSTRALIAN CONTEXT OF PAEDIATRIC NURSING	**1**
1	**Australia's children and young people**	**3**
	Donna Waters	
	Introduction	3
	Australia's children and young people	4
	The health of Australia's children and young people	10
	Emerging health priorities	18
	Applying new knowledge to practice	23
	Summary	24
	Learning activities	25
	Further reading	26
	References	26
2	**Child rights in Australia**	**29**
	Jennifer Fraser and Helen Stasa	
	Introduction	29
	International legislation	30
	Australian legislation	33
	Practice implications	35
	Summary	44
	Learning activities	45
	Further reading	45
	References	46
3	**Psychosocial development and response to illness**	**49**
	Jennifer Fraser and Robyn Rosina	
	Introduction	49
	The psychosocial development of children and young people experiencing disruptions to health	50
	Trust versus mistrust: Infancy (first year of life) and the sick infant	51
	Autonomy versus shame and doubt: Infancy (second year of life) and the sick toddler	55
	Initiative versus guilt: Early childhood – the preschool years (3–5 years)	56
	Industry versus inferiority: Middle and late childhood (infants and primary school – 6 years to puberty)	60

Identity versus identity confusion: Adolescence (10–20 years) 65
Intimacy versus isolation: Early adulthood (twenties and thirties)
and the sick young adult 69
Summary 72
Learning activities 73
Further reading 73
References 74

4   Research in the paediatric setting   77
Donna Waters

Introduction 77
What is research? 79
What is evidence-based practice? 80
Researching with children and young people 84
Human research and ethics 84
Core principles of research ethics 87
Research monitoring and participation 96
Applying new knowledge to practice 101
Summary 102
Learning activity 103
Further reading 104
References 105

PART 2: EVIDENCE-BASED PAEDIATRIC NURSING CARE   107

5   Recognising and responding to the sick child   109
Elizabeth Forster and Loretta Scaini

Introduction 109
Structured assessment of the paediatric patient 111
Recognition of clinical deterioration using a Primary
   Assessment Framework 114
Paediatric neurological assessment tools 125
Responding to the sick child 127
Parental presence during resuscitation 133
Summary 135
Learning activity 136
Further reading 137
References 138

6   End-of-life and palliative care in Australian paediatric care settings   141
Elizabeth Forster

Introduction 141
Pain 143

	Fatigue	147
	Dyspnoea	149
	Gastrointestinal disturbances	150
	Anxiety	152
	Communication with children and adolescents	153
	Communication and the family in paediatric end-of-life care	154
	Summary	156
	Learning activities	157
	Further reading	157
	References	158

7 Mental health and illness in childhood and adolescence — 162
Jennifer Fraser, Lindsay Smith and Julia Taylor

Introduction	162
Mental health problems and mental disorders	163
What mental disorders affect Australian children?	165
Attention Deficit Hyperactivity Disorder	166
Autism Spectrum Disorder	169
Externalising disorders: Conduct disorders	171
Risk and protective factors	173
Internalising disorders: Anxiety and depression	174
Promoting mental health in children and young people	176
Summary	184
Learning activity	185
Further reading	185
References	185

8 Evidence-based nursing assessments and interventions: The acutely ill child — 189
Nicola Brown

Introduction	189
Fever in children	190
Dehydration	193
Gastroenteritis	195
Intravenous therapy	196
Acute otitis media (AOM)	199
Pain assessment	200
Acute respiratory illness	202
Summary	206
Learning activities	206
Further reading	207
References	207

9	**Evidence-based nursing assessments and interventions: The acutely ill young person**	**212**

Nicola Brown

    Introduction 212
    Key issues for young people during hospitalisation 213
    Injuries 214
    Abdominal pain 220
    Preoperative care 222
    Postoperative care 223
    Alcohol poisoning 224
    Summary 225
    Learning activities 226
    Further reading 226
    References 227

10	**Evidence-based nursing assessments and interventions: The child and young person with a chronic illness**	**229**

Donna Waters and Helen Stasa

    Introduction 229
    Chronic conditions 232
    Congenital, chromosomal and genetic disorders 241
    Transition to adult care 246
    Summary 251
    Learning activities 253
    Further reading 254
    References 255

11	**Evidence-based nursing assessments and interventions: The family**	**259**

Ibi Patane and Elizabeth Forster

    Introduction 259
    Families in contemporary Australian society 259
    Family Partnership Model 260
    Family-centred care 261
    Family assessment 263
    Summary 274
    Learning activities 275
    Further reading 275
    References 275

12	**Evidence-based care of children with complex medical needs**	**279**

Nicola Brown

    Introduction 279
    Types of conditions associated with complex medical needs 280

Families and children with complex medical needs ... 283
Nursing assessment and interventions ... 286
Summary ... 290
Learning activity ... 290
Further reading ... 291
References ... 291

Index   **295**

Preface

I am delighted to have the opportunity to present the first edition of an Australian paediatric nursing text, *Paediatric Nursing in Australia: Principles for practice*. As its title indicates, the aim is to provide a valuable primary resource for paediatric nurses and students of nursing who are working in paediatric settings across Australia. With its strong Australian focus, the book integrates key elements of paediatric nursing practice, communication, family involvement and evidence-based practice throughout each of two parts. Part 1 sets the context within which paediatric nurses and students of nursing can expect to practise in Australia. Child health, child illness and child injury within Australian communities are presented from an epidemiological perspective. This includes details of national health trends for children and young people in Australia, and provides comparisons with international trends. Part 2 shifts the focus to become more specific about the paediatric nurse's role, including nursing assessment, nursing care and nursing interventions in paediatric settings. Each chapter provides at least one case study to encourage reflection and critical analysis of practice. Engagement of crucial concepts into paediatric nursing practice is anticipated by using this approach.

Part 1, The Australian Context of Paediatric Nursing, comprises four chapters. Chapter 1 sets the context of health and illness in Australia for children up to age 18. Future challenges for Australia as a healthy nation – such as childhood overweight and obesity – are analysed. Chapter 3 builds on this to examine the basis for understanding the way in which children and young people's rights – including the right to be protected from all forms of violence and neglect – are upheld in Australia, and in particular within the health-care system. In Chapter 3, attention is given to the responses of children, young people and their families to experiences of illness – both acute and chronic. Cultural practices and their potential implications for care provided to children, young people and their families are considered. In particular, the ways in which Aboriginal and Torres Strait Islander children experience the health-care system are explored, and extra reading in this topic is recommended. Chapter 4 is dedicated to the conduct of research within the paediatric setting and the implementation of evidence-based interventions.

Part 2, Evidence-based Paediatric Nursing Care, consists of eight chapters. This part is more specific about the paediatric nurse's role, including nursing assessment, nursing care and nursing interventions in paediatric settings.

For the cover of this book, we have chosen a beautiful work designed by Robert Ingpen, whose body of illustrative and fine art work has been acknowledged through the Hans Christian Andersen Award for children's book illustration in 1986 and an honorary doctorate from RMIT in 2005. He was made a member of the Order of Australia in 2007. 'The Games Children Play' was commissioned by the Royal Children's Hospital Foundation, Melbourne as a tribute to Dame Elisabeth Murdoch's 75-year relationship with the hospital. This gorgeous tapestry was woven by three Royal Children's Hospital weavers: Sue Batten, John Dicks and Emma Sulzer, in 2009, and can be viewed at the Royal Children's Hospital, where it is displayed for all to enjoy.

I am most grateful to my co-authors, Donna Waters, Elizabeth Forster and Nikki Brown, and thank them for their hard work, vision and commitment to making this book such a potentially valuable contribution to the field. Their wealth of practice experience in paediatric nursing settings across a range of Australian contexts, ongoing research and leadership in teaching have combined to create a relevant and creative text. We are indebted to the team of enthusiastic contributing authors whose specialist expertise is highly regarded. These contributions should not be overlooked in a text such as this. We thank Helen Stasa, Robyn Rosina, Lindsay Smith, Julia Taylor, Loretta Scaini and Ibi Patane very much for their time and outstanding effort.

Jennifer Fraser

Part 1

The Australian Context of Paediatric Nursing

This section of the text sets the context within which student nurses can expect to practise paediatric nursing in Australia. It presents child health, child illness and child injury within Australian communities from an epidemiological perspective, and includes details of national health trends for children and young people in Australia, in comparison with international trends.

1 Australia's children and young people

Donna Waters

Learning objectives

In this chapter you will:

- Be introduced to the demographic profile of children and young people living in Australia
- Gain a sense of the current health and wellbeing of Australia's children and young people, and how their health is currently measured
- Develop an understanding of existing and emerging threats to the health and wellbeing of Australia's children and young people in the global context
- Reflect on your knowledge of the health and wellbeing of Australia's children and young people and how you might use this knowledge in your work as a nurse

Introduction

As you read more widely about the health and wellbeing of children and young people, you will become aware of many different definitions and descriptors for age groups within this population. The Australian Bureau of Statistics (ABS), for example, defines children as those aged under 15 years of age and young people as being 15–24 years of age. In Australia, legal adulthood is established at 18 years of age, and the ABS defines young adults as being in the age range 18–34 years.

In this text, infants, children, adolescents and young people approaching adulthood (up to 18 years of age) collectively constitute the group defined as Australia's children and young people. We will use the age 0–4 years to describe the period of **infancy** and **early childhood**, 5–12 years as **childhood** and 13–18 years as **adolescence**.

This chapter examines the health of children and young people living and growing up in Australia. Population characteristics,

Infancy The period from birth to 1 year of age
Early childhood The period from 1 year to the fifth birthday
Childhood The period from 5 years to the thirteenth birthday
Adolescence The period from 13–18 years of age

challenges facing children's growth and development, and emerging health and social trends among young people are discussed in a global context. The role of the paediatric nurse is not only shaped by emerging physical threats such as childhood obesity, injury and chronic illness, but also by behavioural, developmental and mental threats resulting from rapid social and environmental change affecting children and young people all over the world. We invite you to consider the idea that the health and welfare of the children and young people of Australia is as much determined by the context of the past as it will be by the context of the future.

Australia – the 'lucky country'?

Case study 1.1

According to the major indices of a successful society, Australia ranks as one of the best places to live in the world. The population of this somewhat isolated continent – the sixth-largest land-mass in the world – enjoys health, housing, nutrition, income, civil rights and a strongly performing economy. A comparatively small total population of 23 million people clusters towards the moderate climates and highly urbanised areas of the east coast, with more than 11 million Australians settled in the largest cities of Melbourne, Sydney and Brisbane.

Aboriginal Australians inhabited the continent for tens of thousands of years before colonisation by the British in 1788. After centuries of discrimination and exploitation, Aboriginal and Torres Strait Islander peoples now make up less than 3 per cent of Australia's population.

While the government formally apologised to Aboriginal Australians in 2008 for years of discrimination and injustice, Aboriginal Australians continue to experience high rates of illness, unemployment and imprisonment.

Australia's current political orientation is towards Asia, but a rich and complex immigration history has woven itself into the fabric of a country that is now home to people from over 140 countries. With the gradual dismantling of the White Australia policy in the years following World War II, the 1950s saw the arrival of mainly European migrants seeking to build a better life for their families, especially their children. In 2012, the majority of permanent migrants to Australia were from the United Kingdom, the People's Republic of China, India, the Philippines and Vietnam.

Australia's children and young people

Indicator measurement

Before we take a look at the many reports about the current and future state of the health of children and young people in Australia, we need to provide a quick update on some demographic and statistical terminology. The importance of using a common international language for the measurement and tracking of health indicators cannot be over-stated. In Australia, government agencies routinely collect data on the health and wellbeing of the population. The best known of these agencies are the Australian Bureau of Statistics (ABS) and the Australian Institute of Health and Welfare (AIHW). In addition to collecting and analysing a wide range of demographic and statistical data, the ABS produces information papers, media releases and feature articles for the Commonwealth government.

These health data organisations take the standardisation and recording of indicators very seriously, and routinely publish companion documents or large appendices outlining the rationale for their choice of a unit of measurement (e.g. average over 1 year); define numerators and denominators for **rate**-based calculations; and report centiles, summary statistics (mean and median) and measures of spread or variation (standard deviation) to facilitate comparison with other data. While rate-based statistics are mostly used to describe population-level data, a range of 'clinical' indicators are also used in Australian hospitals for measuring trends and variations in the quality and safety of health care (ACHS, 2012).

Rates Used to describe health trends over time — for example, a mortality (or death) rate is a measure of the number of deaths from a particular cause (the numerator) as a proportion of all deaths from any cause (the denominator) over a defined period of time (usually one year).

The routine measurement of standard internationally recognised indicators of health and wellbeing over time is extremely useful because health indicators can:

- offer a snapshot of the health of a community or group at a single point in time
- enable long-term tracking of specific populations or groups
- monitor upward and/or downward movements or trends
- measure the impact of specific health interventions such as health-promotion strategies
- use past information to predict (or model) what might happen in the future
- facilitate international comparisons (benchmarking).

In addition to the routine collection of Australian health data, health indicators also enable us to compare the health and wellbeing of Australian children and young people with other children growing up in countries similar to ours.

It is very common for government reports to compare statistics for Australia against those of other **Organization for Economic Cooperation and Development (OECD)** countries. For example, it is of note that, in 2008, Australia had the second highest percentage of children living in jobless families of all OECD countries (AIHW, 2008).

Table 1.1 defines indicator measures for some of the common key national indicators (or headline indicators) we use for describing the health and welfare of children and young people in Australia.

Note that this table illustrates our first example of how different definitions and descriptors are used for reporting on health trends within age groups. The AIHW *Children's headline indicators* report (AIHW, 2011a) describes the health and wellbeing of Australia's children using 12 indicators for children 0–12 years of age. A report published the following year (*A picture of Australia's children 2012*) reports on similar indicators, but this time children are those aged 0–14 years (AIHW, 2012). An earlier report, *Making progress: The health, development and wellbeing of Australia's children and young people* (AIHW, 2008) focused on children and young people up to 20 years of age. It is important to look at the age group included in each study before attempting to compare results across studies.

> **Organization for Economic Cooperation and Development (OECD)**
> A group of member countries that for the past 50 years have shared the mission of improving the economic and social wellbeing of people around the world. Starting with developed countries in Europe, the United States and Canada, there are now 34 member countries spanning the globe, including Australia and New Zealand. Various common indicators are collected across the OECD countries. It is common to see data for an individual country compared with the combined or average indicator for all OECD countries

Mothers and babies

If you were born in Australia in 2012, you were one of 12.28 births per 1000 population and are slightly more likely to be male (1.06 males to 1.00 females born). With only 2.9 **neonatal** deaths per 1000 live births per year (4.1 per 1000 infants), and a stable maternal mortality rate of fewer than seven deaths per 100 000 per year, it is expected that you have survived your birth with an intact family. You are likely to have access to nutritious food, will grow normally and generally be healthy. Living in a culturally diverse, stable and democratic society, you will attend school and live a long life (81.9 years). Being born in Australia in 2012, you contributed to a population growth of 1.2 per cent per year and joined the 5.93 migrants per 1000 population who arrived that year.

> **Neonatal** The period from birth to 28 days of age

TABLE 1.1 *Key national health indicators for children and young people*

OUTCOME	INDICATOR	HOW IT IS MEASURED (PER YEAR)
Mortality	Death rate for infants less than 1 year of age (infant mortality)	Rate per 1000
	Sudden Infant Death Syndrome (SIDS)	Rate per 100 000
	Death rate for children 1–14 years	Rate per 100 000
Morbidity	Proportion of all children (0–14 years) diagnosed with asthma	Percentage of all children with asthma 0–14 years
	New cases of type 1 diabetes among children 0–14 years	Rate per 100 000
	New cases of cancer among children 0–14 years	Rate per 100 000
Disability	Proportion of children aged 0–14 years with severe or profound core activity limitations	Percentage of all children 0–14 years
Injuries	Age-specific death rates from all injuries for children 0–14 years	Rate per 100 000
Overweight and obesity	Proportion of children whose BMI is above international cut-off point for 'overweight' or 'obese', adjusted for age and sex	Percentage of all children

Source: Adapted from AIHW (2011a).

Further, as a baby born in Australia today, it is likely that:

- your mother is 30 years of age or older (in 1991, the average age of women having their first baby was 27.9; in 2010, it was 30)
- you weighed between 3361 and 3377 grams at birth (although 6.2 per cent of you weighed less than 2500 grams and were considered to be of low birth weight
- you were delivered vaginally in a hospital following a spontaneous labour (although 32.6 per cent were born following a caesarean section and 18.4 per cent of your mothers elected to have this procedure without first going into labour
- you were conceived naturally, but 3.6 per cent of your parents will have received some form of assisted reproductive technology (Li et al., 2012)
- half of you (46 per cent) were exclusively breastfed for up to four months of age, falling to 14 per cent at six months
- approximately 92 per cent of you will be fully immunised at 1 year of age.

Children and young people

At the most recent population census in 2011, the total number of children under 15 years of age living in Australia was 4.21 million, comprising

18.9 per cent of the population. By 2015, the projected number of young people entering adulthood (turning 18 years of age) is estimated to be 153 766 males and 146 255 females, a ratio of 105.12 males to every 100 females (ABS, 2008a).

The overall number of children in Australia doubled between 1925 and 1995 (an increase of 2.4 million). Most of this growth occurred after World War II, when there was not only a rise in the birth rate, but high levels of migration of young couples with children to Australia. A small increase in fertility also occurred between the mid-1980s and mid-1990s, when the Baby Boomer generation reached child-bearing age. Since then, fertility rates have generally been below the level required to replace the Australian population.

Despite these small increases in the total number of children, a reduced fertility rate combined with increased life expectancy and lower migration all add up to proportionally fewer children in the Australian population at the current time. As in other developed countries, the trend is for the proportion of people aged 65 years and over to increase by 2.8 percentage points (from 13.6 per cent to 16.4 per cent between 2010 and 2015), while the proportion of Australian children is projected to decline from 18.9 per cent to 17.6 per cent during the same period. The proof of this trend already exists, with the proportion of children decreasing from 36 per cent of the total population in 1925 to 22 per cent in 1990 and 19 per cent in 2012, with further decline to 17.6 per cent projected by 2015 (ABS, 2013).

Figure 1.1 compares the age distribution of the Australian Aboriginal and Torres Strait Islander population with the non-Indigenous population of Australia. The Aboriginal and Torres Strait Islander population is characterised by higher fertility and mortality rates than the general Australian population. In the most recent analysis of population data in 2006, children and young people (defined as 0–24 years in this example) represented more than half (57 per cent) of the total 517 000 Aboriginal and Torres Strait Islander people in Australia. Children under 15 years of age comprised 38 per cent of this population, compared with only 19 per cent of the non-Indigenous population (ABS, 2011a). These powerful numbers place Aboriginal and Torres Strait Islander children and youth clearly at the core of their family, culture and community relationships. The median age of the Australian Indigenous population in 2006 was 21 years, compared to a median age of 37 years for non-Indigenous Australians.

Australian families

The demographic characteristics of 6.3 million Australian families reported in the 2009–10 Family Characteristics Survey reveal that 44 per cent were couple

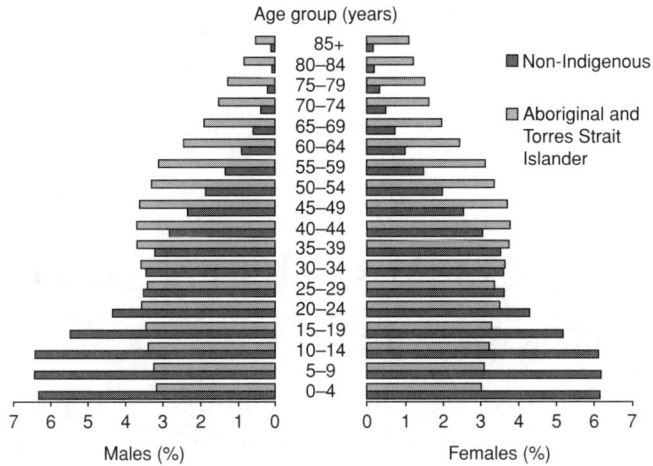

FIGURE 1.1 *Comparison of Aboriginal and Torres Strait Islander population with non-Indigenous population of Australia (2006)*

Source: ABS (2008b).

families with resident children. Just over 40 per cent of families had no resident children of any age and 14 per cent were sole-parent families with resident children. Of the 6.3 million families included in the 2009–10 report, 40 per cent (or 2.5 million) were migrant families demonstrating very similar characteristics (46 per cent couple families with resident children and 10 per cent sole parents). More migrant families live in multi-family (4.5 per cent) or group households (3.8 per cent) than Australian-born persons (2.3 per cent) (ABS, 2011c).

Reflection points 1.1

- Many Australian women are delaying having babies until later in life, and increasingly requiring assistance to become pregnant. Forty-seven percent of mothers over 40 years of age and 42.5 per cent of those choosing to deliver in a private hospital will have their baby delivered by caesarean section. What does this mean for nurses working in neonatal and paediatric care settings?
- The proportion of children and young people in the Australian population is declining while the proportion of adults over 65 years is increasing. What impact might this have on the health, wealth and wellbeing of Australians in the future?
- Children and young people (to the age of 24 years) constitute 57 per cent of the total Aboriginal and Torres Strait Islander population. What might this mean for Aboriginal and Torres Strait Islander people seeking to participate in the design and delivery of health-care services to their communities?

> • More than 25 per cent of those in the Australian population are born overseas. Working as a paediatric nurse in one of the most multicultural countries in the world may challenge you. What challenges have you encountered as a child growing up in Australia? How could you apply this knowledge to your work as a nurse?

The health of Australia's children and young people

An overview

Case Study 1.1 referred to Australia's international reputation as the 'lucky country', and generally Australian children are healthy and well. But there are large variations between health indicators for children living in remote or socially disadvantaged areas, between Indigenous and non-Indigenous children, and even between states and territories. Different health indicators are also important at different times across the lifespan. For example, infant mortality is an internationally recognised indicator of health and wellbeing in infancy. This is because a child's risk of death is greatest at the time of birth, and during the first year of life (AIHW, 2012). Similarly, weight at birth, breast-feeding and immunisation rates are indicators of a healthy early childhood (0–4 years) (AIHW, 2008). As children grow, injury and chronic diseases pose a more serious risk and, as they enter adolescence (13–18 years), indicators of mental and physical health include substance use, and overweight and obesity (AIHW, 2008).

The economic and social situation of the families and communities in which children and young people grow up is important to their health (teenage motherhood, employment, child care, parental health, disability and homelessness). Similarly, indicators of childhood safety and security (injury, child abuse and neglect, children as victims of violence, juvenile crime) sit alongside indicators of learning and development, which again vary across the lifespan. While early childhood education, literacy and numeracy rates, and youth participation in university education or work are equally important indicators of the wellbeing of children and young people, educational outcomes are not the focus of this text.

A number of major reports on child and youth health have been commissioned by the Australian government over the past five years, and no doubt others will have been completed by the time you read this text. This section draws on data from three major government reports to paint a picture of the current health and wellbeing of Australia's children and young people:

- Headline indicators for children's health, development and wellbeing 2011 (AIHW, 2011a)
- Aboriginal and Torres Strait Islander wellbeing: A focus on children and youth 2011 (ABS, 2011a)
- A picture of Australia's children 2012 (AIHW, 2012)

Mortality

Infant and child mortality rates are strongly associated with economic advantage and social determinants of health – access to clean water, nutritious food, a safe environment and health care. In Table 1.1, we outlined some of the common national indicators for measuring the general health status of children and young people in Australia. Mortality – especially infant mortality – is significant as one of few indicators that are routinely measured by OECD countries and which feature in most international comparisons of the health of children.

Infants

More than two-thirds of infant deaths in Australia occur in the first 28 days after birth (during the neonatal period) and almost half of these occur on the day the baby is born (AIHW, 2012). Despite this, a number of factors have contributed to Australia's progress in significantly reducing infant mortality over the past 30 years. These include improved effectiveness and participation in maternal antenatal care, better nutrition and the advantageous economic and environmental climate enjoyed by the majority of Australians (see Case Study 1.1).

Australia's infant mortality rate is currently 4.1 deaths per 1000 live births, a reduction from 8.8 deaths per 1000 live births recorded in 1986 (AIHW, 2012). Almost half of all infant deaths (46 per cent) are due to perinatal conditions (complications occurring during pregnancy or birth); a further 26 per cent are due to congenital anomalies and malformations. While hypospadias (a defect of male urethra) was the most common congenital anomaly reported in Australian infants in 2002–03 (Abeywardana & Sullivan, 2008), conditions of the heart and circulatory system were the most common malformations causing death. The remaining infant deaths are due to a range of mostly undefined abnormal signs and symptoms, including Sudden Infant Death Syndrome (SIDS).

Infant mortality rates vary across populations. In remote and very remote areas of Australia, the infant mortality rate is almost twice that of babies born in major cities at 6.8 per 1000 live births, and is similar for Aboriginal and Torres Strait Islander infants (7.2 deaths per 1000 live births) when based on combined data for New South Wales, South Australia and the Northern Territory (AIHW, 2012). A comparison of infant mortality in OECD countries in 2012 (OECD, 2013) revealed that infant mortality was highest in Mexico (14.1 deaths per 1000 live births) and lowest in Japan (1.1 deaths per 1000 live births), with Australian infant mortality rates equivalent to the OECD average.

Neonatal intensive-care units, with their associated specialised technology and staff, combined with the advent of emergency flight retrieval systems such as the Newborn and Paediatric Emergency Transport Service (NETS) in New South Wales, have contributed significantly to reducing neonatal deaths. Beyond birth, increasing awareness of national immunisation schedules and SIDS prevention through national health-promotion campaigns has contributed to reductions in vaccine-preventable diseases in infants, and to the rate of sudden and unexpected death in infants less than 1 year of age during sleep, previously known as 'cot death'. In 2010, the mortality rate from SIDS was 27 deaths per 100 000 live births, or 7 per cent of total infant deaths; almost three-quarters of these were male infants.

Children

The death rate for children 1–4 years of age (19 deaths per 100 000 children) is almost twice that of children aged 5–9 years or 10–14 years (both 10 per 100 000) (AIHW, 2012). This is attributed to higher rates of injury and **comorbidities** from congenital conditions affecting this age group. However, cancers and accidental drowning each accounted for three deaths per 100 000 in children aged less than 4 years in the *Making progress* report (AIHW, 2008). The mortality rate of Australian children under five years of age is equal to the OECD average.

Comorbidity The presence of one or more additional disorders (or diseases) co-occurring with a primary disease or disorder

Among Indigenous children, the mortality rate of 25 deaths per 100 000 is twice as high as the Australian average for children 0–14 years (13 per 100 000), but this rate is even higher for children living in remote or very remote regions (31 deaths per 100 000). Despite this, the rate of all childhood deaths (regardless of age group) has declined by an average of 52–60 per cent since 1986. This is largely due to reduced child mortality from traffic accidents, and coincides with the introduction of child safety seats in cars, as well as seatbelt and drink-driving legislation in Australia. While injury remains the leading cause of death (34 per cent) for Australian children, cancers (17 per cent) and diseases of the nervous system (11 per cent) also contribute significantly. It is of note that while death by suicide is relatively rare in children under 15 years of age (0.4 per 100 000 children), 17 of the 52 suicide deaths occurring between 2007 and 2011 in this age group were Aboriginal and Torres Strait Islander children (ABS, 2011b).

Young people

The independence of adolescence introduces a whole different set of risks to the health and wellbeing to young people aged between 15 and 18. Injuries from traffic or workplace accidents, the harmful effects of alcohol and other drug use and mental health problems are the leading causes of death in this age group.

In 2011 (ABS, 2011b), more than one-quarter (27.8 per cent) of all male deaths in the 15–24 years age group were due to suicide. In 2006, transport accidents and self-harm resulting in suicide accounted for 11 and five deaths per 100 000, respectively (AIHW, 2008). Unlike any other age group, mortality rates for male adolescents are twice as high as those for females of the same age. Between 2005 and 2009, the number of deaths among 15–24-year-old Aboriginal and Torres Strait Islander youth was almost three times higher than the non-Indigenous population. The mortality rate for young Indigenous people during this period was 115 deaths per 100 000, compared with 41 deaths per 100 000 for non-Indigenous people of the same age (AIHW, 2011a).

Chronic conditions

It may seem unusual to associate **chronic conditions** with children and young people but chronic diseases have the potential to interrupt normal growth and development, and to produce immediate and possible long-term effects on physical, emotional and social wellbeing. These impacts – especially on normal growth and development – are frequently overlooked as the unintended consequences of a chronic illness and its long-term treatment.

The Australian government nominates a range of health conditions (National Health Priorities) that are of specific relevance to the Australian population because of the burden these conditions place on the daily lives of families and communities, and their impact on the economic sustainability of the country. While reducing injury has been a National Health Priority since 1986, common chronic conditions affecting both adults and children in Australia (asthma, diabetes and cancer) collectively account for 20 per cent of

> **Chronic condition** Any ongoing physical or mental impairment that causes a functional limitation (or health burden), or necessitates the use of a service or care beyond that which is regarded as routine. The ABS defines a chronic condition as one that has lasted, or will last, for six months or more (ABS, 2009)

the burden of disease among children 0–14 years (AIHW, 2012). The impact of chronic conditions is often measured by hospitalisation rates (or **hospital separation rates**), as this provides an indication of the burden of illness experienced by the child or young person and their family.

> **Hospital separation rate**
> An episode of care in a hospital – usually the period from admission to discharge (transfer or death)
>
> **Young person (or youth)**
> A person 15–24 years of age

Importantly, the monitoring of hospitalisations also determines the need for health services in Australia, such as training for paediatric specialties, hospital, operating and intensive care beds, and community clinics and outreach care. Considering that in 2007–08, 37 per cent of Australia's children and **young people** had at least one long-term condition, and that this equates to more than 1.5 million children, you can start to see why chronic conditions of childhood are important (ABS, 2009).

The range of chronic conditions affecting children and young people is broad, and includes those resulting from neurological congenital anomalies such as spina bifida and neural tube defects, cardiac defects such as transposition of vessels, Tetralogy of Fallot and gastrointestinal, renal and limb deficits. Genetic conditions (Trisomy 13, 18 and 21, phenylketonuria, cystic fibrosis) also constitute an important burden for Australia's children and young people, and around 7 per cent of Australian children aged 0–14 years also have a disability of some kind. The most common types of disability are intellectual disabilities (affecting an estimated 161 000 children, or 3.9 per cent) and sensory or speech problems (affecting an estimated 119 000 children, or 2.9 per cent) (AIHW, 2012). All chronic conditions will impact on the way a child lives, grows and functions within their society.

We will briefly explore the three most common chronic conditions affecting Australia's children and young people – common not only because of their prevalence, but also because they collectively account for the highest number of hospitalisations. As a paediatric nurse, you will frequently care for children and young people who have one of these conditions.

Asthma

Asthma is by far the most common long-term condition affecting children and young people, with 10 per cent of Australia's children (0–14 years) reported to have asthma in 2007 and 2008 (ABS, 2009). While there are acknowledged gaps in the collection of population statistics for childhood asthma in Aboriginal and Torres Strait Islander communities, Indigenous children were estimated to have a 3 per cent higher **prevalence** of asthma (14 per cent) in 2004–05 and hospital separation rates were estimated at 589 per 100 000 compared with

506 per 100 000 for non-Indigenous children in this age group. Asthma is thought to be associated with environmental and lifestyle factors, although there is no difference in asthma prevalence between children growing up in remote areas or in a major city. At the same time, the prevalence of asthma is slightly higher among those children living in areas of low socio-economic advantage (AIHW, 2012).

> **Prevalence** The term used to describe the existence of a condition or problem in any defined sector of the population at any given point in time

While placing a considerable burden on the child and family, asthma can be managed with appropriate preventative treatment and medication, and fortunately deaths directly attributable to asthma are quite rare (26 deaths between 2008 and 10). The prevalence of asthma was highest in Australia during the 1980s and 1990s, but this trend has reversed, with age-standardised rates dropping from 13.5 per cent of all children aged 0–15 years during this decade to the current prevalence of 10 per cent (ABS, 2009). Asthma prevalence is highest among children aged 5–9 years (13 per cent), and is higher in boys (16 per cent) than girls (10 per cent).

Following this trend, hospitalisation rates for asthma decreased by one-third, to 331 per 100 000 children in the 5–12 years age group, between 1998–99 and 2006–07 (AIHW, 2011a). However, asthma separations still account for 4 per cent of all child hospital admissions, or more than 21 000 children per year.

Because indicators for the presence of asthma vary across the world, international comparisons can be difficult. For example, one study that showed prevalence rates in both Australia (20 per cent) and New Zealand (22 per cent) were above the global average of 11.5 per cent defined asthma as the presence of wheeze in 6–7-year-old children over the previous 12 months (ISAAC, 2011).

Diabetes

In contrast, there was a 54 per cent increase in hospital separations for diabetes (type 1 and type 2) between 2001–02 and 2007–08. Interestingly, the rate of hospitalisation was higher for girls, even though there is a higher incidence of type 1 diabetes in boys, especially in the 10–14 years age group (35 and 26 per 100 000 respectively). Type 1 diabetes accounts for the majority of childhood cases (more than 5700 children in Australia), and is estimated to account for 10 per cent of all diagnoses of diabetes in this country (AIHW, 2011b). However, there is early evidence to suggest that type 2 diabetes is increasing among children, thought to be due to increased levels of obesity and physical inactivity among Australian children and young people. In 2008, the prevalence of type 1 diabetes in those aged 0–14 years was 138 cases per 100 000 population, but this ranged from 62 per 100 000 children living in the Northern Territory to 188 per 100 000 living in Tasmania (AIHW, 2011b).

The key national indictor for diabetes is the number of new cases (or **incidence**) of type 1 diabetes among children aged 0–14 years (Table 1.1). According to the Australian National Diabetes Register, the incidence of new cases has increased from 19 per 100 000 in 2000 to 22 per 100 000 in 2009 (equivalent to 913 new cases) (AIHW, 2012). This increase occurred mainly before 2005, and rates have been relatively stable since. Incidence also increases with age: children in the 10–14 years age group are 2.6 times more likely to be diagnosed with diabetes than children in the 0–4 years age range (AIHW, 2012). Consequently, older children are 4.7 times more likely to be hospitalised than those under the age of 5 years (AIHW, 2012).

> **Incidence** The term used to describe the number of new cases of condition or problem in any defined sector of the population at a given point in time

As surprising as it may seem, there are no reliable estimates for the incidence of type 1 diabetes across geographic regions of Australia, by remoteness, family socioeconomic status or for Aboriginal and Torres Strait Islander children. Hospital data reveal that separations for type 1 diabetes were lower for Indigenous children aged 0–14 years than for all Australian children (52 and 74 per 100 000 respectively), and were slightly higher in major cities compared with remote and very remote regions (67 and 66 per 100 000 children), but were 34 per cent higher for children living in lower socioeconomic conditions than those living in higher socioeconomic areas (AIHW, 2012).

The International Diabetes Federation (IDF) is an alliance of more than 200 diabetes associations in more than 160 countries, which publishes an atlas of the latest global and regional diabetes statistics (IDF, 2013). According to the IDF, the incidence of type 1 diabetes in the 0–14 years age group in Australia is similar to that in the United States and United Kingdom; all of these countries rank above the OECD average incidence of 17 per 100 000 children. Korea has the lowest incidence of type 1 diabetes in the 0–14 years age group (1.1 per 100 000 children), while Finland has the highest (58 per 100 000).

Cancer

Cancers cause significant morbidity and mortality in children, and were collectively responsible for 17 per cent of deaths in those aged 1–14 years between 2008 and 2010 (AIHW, 2012). However, cancer is not just one disease, and in children the site of origin and course of illness can be very different from adult cancers. Acute Lymphoblastic Leukaemia (ALL) is the most common, accounting for 4.2 per cent of all cancers in children, with the next most common being cancers of the brain (1.9 per cent) and non-Hodgkin lymphomas (0.9 per cent) (AIHW, 2012).

Survival is used as a key indicator to measure the effectiveness of cancer treatment, specialised cancer services and early detection. Between 2004 and 2010, five-year survival for all cancers affecting Australian children aged 0–14 years was 81 per cent. While this represents a massive improvement from 68 per cent cancer survival during the mid-1980s, there are differences across cancer type and age group. Five-year survival from ALL, for example, had improved from 73 per cent in the mid-1980s to more than 90 per cent in 2012 (Hunger et al., 2012).

Another key national indictor for cancer is the number of new cases (or incidence) among children aged 0–14 years (Table 1.1). During the period 2004–08, an average 583 new cases of cancer were diagnosed in this age group. This equates to an incidence rate of 14 per 100 000 children, a rate that has remained relatively unchanged since the last major data collection in 1999–2003. There are also differences in cancer incidence across age groups. Children aged 0–4 years are almost twice as likely to be diagnosed with cancer (21 per 100 000) than older children (10–12 per 100 000). Between 2010 and 2011, cancer accounted for around 7000 hospital separations – mostly boys (57 per cent) aged 0–4 years – as indicated by incidence rates in this age group (AIHW, 2012).

Australia has similar rates of childhood cancer to those found in the United States and Canada, and ranks 25th among the cancer incidence rate of 33 OECD countries, and slightly above the OECD average of 13.4 new cases per 100 000 children. Germany has the highest incidence of childhood cancers (20.6 per 100 000) and Poland has the lowest incidence (5.6 per 100 000).

Again, there are no reliable national estimates for the incidence of cancer in Aboriginal and Torres Strait Islander children. However, hospital separation data reveal lower rates of hospitalisation for Indigenous children aged 0–14 years compared with all Australian children with cancer (114 and 164 separations per 100 000 respectively). Perhaps unsurprisingly, five-year survival rates for cancer were higher for children living in major cities (81 per cent) compared with those living in outer regional (78 per cent) and very remote areas (75 per cent) of Australia. Hospital separation rates were also higher for those living in major cities. There are no statistically significant differences between cancer survival rates for children of high or low socio-economic advantage (AIHW, 2012).

> **Reflection points 1.2**
> - Aboriginal and Torres Strait Islander children, as well as both Aboriginal and non-Aboriginal children living in remote and very remote regions of Australia, are, respectively, twice and three times more likely to die than the average Australian child. What factors do you think contribute to the higher child mortality rate of these populations?
> - How are measures of incidence and prevalence different?
> - What do you notice about the relative incidence and prevalence of asthma, diabetes and cancer? How does this relate to the actual number of Australian children with these chronic conditions?
> - Disability can be a result of a sensory, intellectual or mental impairment. Disability can also result from the treatment or chronicity of common childhood disorders such as the three discussed above. What disabilities do you think might arise from living with asthma, diabetes or cancer?

Emerging health priorities

Children's mental and physical growth and development are constantly challenged by transitions that occur both within their family and community, and through their increasingly broader engagement with the social world through school, sport and media. We have looked at some of the existing threats and now look at some of the areas emerging as priorities for the health and wellbeing of Australia's children and young people. The first (overweight and obesity) is somewhat obvious, as it is a frequent topic of media and public health research. The second (dental health) is perhaps less obviously related to health, but is important because of potential associations between gum disease and the development of chronic disease in later life. Social and emotional wellbeing is nominated as one of the national headline indicators for children's health, development and wellbeing (AIHW, 2011a), but no national data are currently available. As this indicator refers to the way children and young people feel about themselves and others (including their approach to stress), this third emerging health priority will be discussed under the topic of mental health (also see Chapter 7). Obesity and mental health are national health priority areas for Australia.

Overweight and obesity

While it is desirable that children's weight increases as they grow, excess weight gain will result from long-term imbalances between energy consumed and energy expended. We are all familiar with the social, cultural, environmental and economic drivers behind what is increasingly called the 'obesity epidemic'. This essentially results from increased consumption of high-energy foods and beverages and reduced physical activity. Parenting practices have a significant impact on establishing healthy eating patterns and promoting physical activity in early childhood. A survey of 880 000 Australian children (5–12 years) in 2008 showed that 42 per cent did not participate in any organised sport or dancing over the two-week data-collection period (AIHW, 2008). Being overweight or obese significantly increases the risk of developing serious and chronic health conditions such as asthma, cardiovascular disease, cancers and type 2 diabetes in both children and adults. In addition to increased stress on growing bones and joints, there can be significant associated self-esteem, behavioural and social impacts for children and young people who are overweight or obese. Obesity was named as a National Health Priority in 2008, and obesity prevention forms part of Australia's National Preventative Health Strategy (NPHT, 2009).

Body mass index (BMI) is the most common measure of overweight or obesity. While BMI is not a direct measure, like height or weight, international cut-off points based on age and sex are used to determine the number of children who are overweight or obese in any given population. In 2007–08, it was estimated that 23 per cent of Australian children aged 5–14 years had a BMI score above international reference points for being overweight (17 per cent) or obese (6 per cent) relative to their age and sex (AIHW, 2011a). This equates to a staggering 430 000 children in the 5–14 years age range, or 500 000 aged 5–17 years – approximately one in every four children and young people (ABS, 2009).

> **Body Mass Index (BMI)** Is calculated by:
> BMI = weight in kilograms/height in metres^2

There are no major differences in the numbers of overweight and obese children born in Australia or overseas, between boys and girls, or between children who live in couple or sole-parent families (AIHW, 2011a), but children living in the lowest socioeconomic areas are 1.7 times more likely to be overweight or obese (31 per cent) compared with same-aged peers in the highest socioeconomic areas (18 per cent) (AIHW, 2012). There appear to be slightly fewer overweight or obese children living in Tasmania compared with other states and territories of Australia, and in 2004–05, Indigenous teenagers (15–19 years) were 2.6 times more likely to be obese than non-Indigenous teenagers (AIHW, 2008). However, it is not possible to fully explore differences in overweight and obesity because of limited height, weight and socioeconomic indicator data available for children growing up in remote areas and the Northern Territory. Internationally comparable data for children and young people is also scarce.

A comparison of 15-year-old children living in 11 OECD countries between 2003 and 2007 ranks Australia as having the seventh highest rate of overweight and obesity (24 per cent of 15-year-olds) compared with the OECD average of 23 per cent (AIHW, 2011a).

There is considerable potential to reduce the adult health burden by preventing children from becoming overweight or obese, and the importance of establishing healthy eating and exercise behaviours in children should not be under-estimated. However, media reports suggesting that the childhood 'obesity epidemic' is out of control may be somewhat exaggerated. In a review of 41 studies reporting BMI in 2–18-year-old children and young people, Olds et al. (2010) concluded that trends in the prevalence of childhood obesity in Australia may have plateaued. Their meta-analysis shows almost no change in the prevalence rate of overweight (21–25 per cent) or obesity (5–6 per cent) over the past 10 years. There are specific trends emerging in different age groups, however. In 15–19-year-old youth, rates of overweight and obesity as measured by BMI are higher in males, but central obesity (measured by increased waist circumference) as a proportion of total adiposity appears to be increasing and is highest in girls (Garnett et al., 2011).

Dental health

The dental health of Australia's children and young people is measured by two main indicators. These are the proportion of children without tooth decay at ages 6 and 12 years (55 per cent and 61 per cent respectively in 2007) and the mean number of decayed, missing or filled teeth (DMFT) at 12 years of age (0.96 in 2007) (AIHW, 2012). There is a recognised pattern of increased tooth decay among girls, thought to result from the earlier eruption of permanent teeth compared with boys. There are also small variations in rates of dental decay between states, with South Australia having the lowest mean DMFT score of 0.8.

Most Australian children will attend their first oral examination on school entry (5 years of age) and 80 per cent of Australian children (0–14 years) will grow up in areas with fluoridated water – a public health introduced measure to prevent tooth decay. The latest Child Dental Health Survey conducted between 2003 and 2004 showed that the majority of Australia's 12-year-olds (58 per cent) had no evidence of tooth decay (AIHW, 2011a). This places the dental health of Australian 12-year-olds above the OECD average (DMFT score of 1.4), and ranks Australia eighth of 22 OECD countries using this measure for international comparison.

Pain from dental or gum problems can interrupt normal eating and sleeping, and may impact on nutrition (weight), school attendance and social interactions between peers. The prevalence of dental and gum disease in Australian children and young people has decreased over time, but risk factors related to diet (such as sugary food and drinks) and oral care (e.g. tooth and gum hygiene) remain. Potential associations between dental health and future cardiovascular problems, lung disease and diabetes is an area of current research, but for children and young people, it is ongoing disparities in dental health across age and population groups that remain of greatest concern.

Children living in regional and remote areas of Australia experience higher levels of tooth decay than those living in major cities (mean DMFT 1.2 and 0.9 respectively), a trend that may in part reflect differences in access to fluoridated water. The mean DMFT score of children living in the lowest socioeconomic regions in 2002–03 was almost 60 per cent higher (average of 1.1 teeth) than that of children from the highest socioeconomic areas (0.7), a trend that is evident across all states and territories of Australia. Indigenous children are at greatest risk of dental decay because of higher rates of socioeconomic disadvantage and remoteness. Nearly one-quarter of Aboriginal and Torres Strait Islander children (0–14 years) live in remote and very remote areas compared with only 2 per cent of non-Indigenous children of the same age (ABS, 2011a). Across a range of reports published between 2002 and 2004, Indigenous children were reported to have a mean DMFT score of 1.4 (for South Australia) and 1.8 (for Victoria, Queensland, South Australia and Northern Territory combined) compared with the mean DMFT of 1.0 for all Australian children. In 2008, some 30 per cent of Aboriginal and Torres Strait Islander children aged 0–14 years reported having teeth or gum problems (ABS, 2011a).

Social and emotional health

As we have already discussed, the teenage years mark a point of difference in morbidity and mortality patterns from those of childhood. Adolescents (13–18 years) are more likely to engage in risk-taking behaviours, but are also trying to adjust to individual physical and emotional change. Mental health disorders account for nearly 50 per cent of the burden of disease among 15–24-year-olds in Australia (AIHW, 2008). Anxiety and depression diagnoses account for 17 per cent of the mental health disease burden for young men and 32 per cent of the disease burden for young women in this age range.

Maintaining the mental health of Australia's children and young people is a national health priority, but the process of defining indicators and conceptualising the scope of such a multidimensional and complex area is largely incomplete. There is evidence to suggest that children who are socially and emotionally confident and well adjusted will cope more successfully with the daily stressors and challenges of growing up (AIHW, 2011a). Conversely, children with low levels of social and emotional wellbeing are more likely to be at risk of behavioural and mental health problems, to have poor resilience and coping skills, and to experience a reduced engagement and performance at school (AIHW, 2011a). The causes of mental and behavioural disorders are complex, but can be related to any combination of family, community, environmental, cultural, genetic or societal factors experienced by children and young people as they grow. Young people with mental health disorders such as depression, anxiety, bipolar disorder [BD] and schizophrenia, and behavioural disorders such as Attention Deficit Hyperactivity Disorder (ADHD), Obsessive Compulsive Disorder (OCD) and eating disorders, are more likely to experience poorer physical health, and reduced educational and employment attainment (AIHW, 2008).

In the absence of an agreed national indicator (and data) on the social and emotional wellbeing of Australia's children and young people, measures such as hospitalisation rates for mental illness offer a poor estimate of prevalence. The extent to which children and young people receive treatment in the primary health care or private sector is not well understood. The hospitalisation rate for mental and behavioural disorders among children aged 5–12 years has not changed significantly since the late 1990s, and we have previously noted that death by suicide is relatively rare in children under 15 years of age. In 2006–07, a total of 3900 children aged 5–12 years were hospitalised for mental and behavioural disorders, representing a rate of 178 children per 100 000 population (AIHW, 2011a).

The prevalence of mental and behavioural problems rises in the adolescent population, with mood disorders such as depression and bipolar disorder more common in girls aged 15–19 years, and psychological development disorders such as language, learning and autistic spectrum disorders more common in males of this age. In 2008, 10 per cent of all 13–19-year-olds were hospitalised for some type of mental or behavioural problem (AIHW, 2008). This equates to 19 400 young Australians, or a prevalence of 973 per 100 000 of the 13–19-year-old Australian population. The number of days in hospital for each episode of care is represented as a bed day rate. The bed day rate in 2008 was

5800 per 100 000 (AIHW, 2008). While the bed day rate for schizophrenic and substance use-related hospitalisations fell between1998–99 and 2006–07, there was a 20 per cent rise in hospitalisation for behavioural disorders and a 26 per cent rise in the mood disorder bed day rate among young women (AIHW, 2008). Mental health and behavioural disorders were 40 per cent more common in Aboriginal and Torres Strait Islander youth, and 33 per cent of suicide deaths between 2007 and 2011 were of young Indigenous Australians (ABS, 2011b).

Reflection points 1.3

- One-quarter of Australia's children and young people are overweight or obese. The potential to intervene and prevent overweight or obesity is greatest in early childhood. Do you think the current National Preventative Health Strategy adequately addresses this potential?
- The association between dental health and the development of future chronic disease is currently under investigation. What impact do you think ongoing disparities in dental health across Australia might have on the current and future health and wellbeing of children and young people?
- The National Mental Health Strategy and National Suicide Prevention Strategy recognise the importance of early intervention in preventing the development of mental health problems in children and young people. What do you know about these strategies, and how might they relate to your care of the mental health of children and young people?

Finally, it is important to acknowledge some other perhaps less obvious but equally important determinants of the mental health of Australia's children and young people. These include parental mental illness, teenage pregnancy and birth, poverty, crime and the misuse of drugs and alcohol, including a range of increasingly sophisticated and easily available psychedelic and hallucinogenic agents.

Applying new knowledge to practice

In this chapter, we have invited you to consider historical influences on the health and wellbeing of the children and young people of Australia. We have also asked you to think about the wider context of family, community, environmental, cultural and societal influences experienced by children and young people as they grow up in Australia. We hope you will read the following chapters with this broader vision in mind, and with a better understanding of the complex interactions that are possible between children, young people, their families and their environment.

Monitoring trends in health, estimating the effects of emerging infections or threats, and improving your knowledge of the many environmental or global factors that may impact on your care of families, children and young people provides a context for practice that will not come from your reading of any single research paper or systematic review. The Australian government provides a range of excellent resources to help you keep track of the health and wellbeing of children and young people living in Australia. These publications should become as much a part of your evidence base for practice as any emerging research (see Further reading). But, as with all evidence, it is important to develop a critical lens for your reading of these frequently published reports. You need to remain aware of differences in units of measurement and denominators used, and think carefully about the demographic characteristics of the groups you are aiming to compare. You have already seen the difference in age ranges used to report on various health indicators, and how the lack of quality data from some regions and sectors of the Australian population impacts upon the integrity and accuracy of reported statistics. You may also have identified that significant inequality within population groups can be masked or diluted by looking only at nationally aggregated population statistics and not at the specific sub-group.

As a paediatric nurse, you will find yourself in the privileged position of being invited to share the people, places and things that are most important to the children and young people for whom you care. Therefore, while it may seem odd to begin a paediatric text with a history lesson, throughout this book we will make reference to the context in which Australia's children and young people are growing up: their culture, home, family and friends. At times, this context will challenge you. The rosy social and economic picture Australia presents to the world will sometimes conflict with the impoverished or disturbing history of the young child for whom you are caring, or the presentation of an angry young person struggling to make sense of themselves and their place in the world. Looking at 'the bigger picture' is something a health professional invited into the life of a child or young person must be able to do. And, as in all nursing work, the person or patient in front of you – no matter how young or how old – is only ever one part of a much larger story.

Summary

- Australian government data collections are an extremely useful and important resource for recording and monitoring the demographic profile of children and young people living in Australia.

- Government data collections define a range of national indicators to describe the health and wellbeing of different age groups, focus on a particular condition of interest and capture trends over periods of time. National health indicators are developed to be consistent with international indicators in order to facilitate benchmarking or comparisons.
- The health of Australia's children and young people is good overall, but there are differences within and between socioeconomic, geographic and cultural sub-populations. It is sometimes difficult to navigate the breadth and complexity of sub-population data to get a clear picture of what is happening to a particular group of Australian children and young people, living in a particular place at any point in time.
- Overweight, obesity, dental health and social and emotional wellbeing (of which mental health is a component) are identified as possible emerging threats to the health and wellbeing of Australia's children and young people.
- Current and past influences on the health and wellbeing of children and young people in Australia constitute a broad contextual framework of family, community, environmental, cultural, genetic and societal factors. It is fundamental to the holistic and person-centred approach of the paediatric nurse to consider the complex interactions between these influences when caring for children, young people and their families.

Learning activities

1.1 Search the World Health Organization Statistical Information System (WHOSIS) website, <www.who.int/whosis/en> (data are also published in May each year in the World Health Statistics Report). Here you can search among more than 70 health indictors collected for WHO member countries. Answer the following questions:
- Choose two indicators measuring an aspect of health or wellbeing in children or youth. Describe three or more major differences between the results of these indicators in developed and developing countries.
- What have been some major successes or failures in terms of healthcare interventions for children and young people in these countries or regions? (*Hint:* for example, immunisation.)

1.2 Find a reference or report that details major health trends for children and young people within your state or region. You may wish to limit your

search to children or youth who have a particular disability or disease. Answer the following questions:
- How often is this report published?
- Who is the author(s)?
- What level of detail is reported (for example, death rates, specific diseases, age groups)?
- Does the report identify upward or downward trends in health statistics or health service delivery?

Further reading

The Australian government provides a range of excellent resources to help you keep track of the health and wellbeing of children and young people living in Australia. These are constantly updated and freely accessible through the following online resources:

- The Australian Bureau of Statistics Topics at Glance: <www.abs.gov.au/websitedbs/d3310114.nsf/home/topics+@+a+glance>
- The Australian Institute of Health and Welfare: <www.aihw.gov.au>
- The National Health and Medical Research Council (National Health Priorities): <www.nhmrc.gov.au/grants/research-funding-statistics-and-data/national-health-priority-areas-nhpas>
- The Productivity Commission: <www.pc.gov.au>.

In addition, there are a range of groups and organisations that regularly publish updates and reports about specific conditions or health priorities, including:

- The International Diabetes Federation: <www.idf.org/diabetesatlas>
- Asthma in Australian children: findings from Growing Up in Australia, the Longitudinal Study of Australian Children: <www.aihw.gov.au/publication-detail/?id=6442468289>
- The National Obesity Taskforce: <www.healthyactive.gov.au/internet/healthyactive/publishing.nsf/Content/healthy_weight08.pdf/$File/healthy_weight08.pdf>.

References

Abeywardana, S & Sullivan, EA 2008, *Congenital anomalies in Australia*, AIHW National Perinatal Statistics Unit, Sydney.

Australian Bureau of Statistics (ABS) 2008a, *Australian population pyramid*, ABS, Canberra, viewed 20 February 2014, http://www.abs.gov.au/websitedbs/ d3310114.nsf/home/Population%20Pyramid%20-%20Australia.

—— 2008b, *Experimental estimates of Aboriginal and Torres Strait Islander Australians, June 2006*, cat. no. 3238.0.55.001, ABS, Canberra.

—— 2009, *National Health Survey: Summary of results 2007–2008*, cat. no. 4430.0, ABS, Canberra.

—— 2011a, *Aboriginal and Torres Strait Islander wellbeing: A focus on children and youth, April 2011*, cat. no. 4725.0, ABS, Canberra, viewed 20 February 2014, http://www.abs.gov.au/ausstats/abs@.nsf/Lookup/4725.0Chapter100Apr%20 2011.

—— 2011b, *Causes of death Australia 2011*, cat. no. 3303.0, ABS, Canberra, viewed 20 February 2014, http://www.abs.gov.au/ausstats/abs@nsf/mf/3303.0.

—— 2011c, *The Family Characteristics Survey 2009–2010*, ABS, Canberra, viewed 20 February 2014, http://www.abs.gov.au/ausstats/abs@.nsf/Latestproducts/341 6.0Main±Features2Mar±2013#SURVEY.

—— 2013, *Australian population projections 2012 (base) to 2101*, cat. no. 3222.0, ABS, Canberra, viewed 20 February 2014, http://www.abs.gov.au/ausstats/abs@.nsf/ Lookup/3222.0main±features52012%20(base)%20to%202101.

Australian Council on Healthcare Standards (ACHS) 2012, *Australasian clinical indicator report 2004–2011*, Australasian Council on Healthcare Standards, Sydney.

Australian Institute of Health and Welfare (AIHW) 2008, *Making progress: The health, development and wellbeing of Australia's children and young people*, AIHW, Canberra.

—— 2011a, *Headline indicators for children's health, development and wellbeing*, AIHW, Canberra.

—— 2011b, *Prevalence of type 1 diabetes in Australian children 2008*, cat. no. CVD 54, AIHW, Canberra, viewed 20 February 2014, http://www.aihw.gov.au/ publication-detail/?id=10737419239.

—— 2012, *A picture of Australia's children 2012*, AIHW, Canberra.

Garnett, S, Baur, L & Cowell, C 2011, The prevalence of increased central adiposity in Australian school children 1985 to 2007, *Obesity Reviews*, 12(11), pp. 887–96.

Hunger, SP et al. 2012, Improved survival for children and adolescents with Acute Lymphoblastic Leukemia between 1990 and 2005: A report from the Children's Oncology Group, *Journal of Clinical Oncology*, 30(14), pp. 1663–9.

International Diabetes Federation (IDF) 2013, *International Diabetes Federation Atlas*, 6th edn, International Diabetes Federation, Brussels.

International Study of Asthma and Allergies in Childhood (ISAAC) 2011, *The global asthma report 2011*, ISAAC, Paris.

Li, Z, Zeki, R, Hilder, L & Sullivan, EA 2012, *Australia's mothers and babies 2010*, AIHW National Perinatal Epidemiology and Statistics Unit, Canberra.

National Preventative Health Taskforce (NPHT) 2009, *Australia: The healthiest country by 2020*, NPHT, Canberra, viewed 20 November 2013, http://www.preventativehealth.org.au/internet/preventativehealth/publishing.nsf/Content/nphs-overview/$File/nphs-overview.pdf.

Olds, TS, Tomkinson, GR, Ferrar, KE & Maher, CA 2010, Trends in the prevalence of childhood overweight and obesity in Australia between 1985 and 2008, *International Journal of Obesity*, 34(1), pp. 57–66.

Organization for Economic Cooperation and Development (OECD) 2013, *OECD health data 2013*, OECD, New York, viewed 2 November 2013, http://www.oecd.org/health/healthdata.

2 Child rights in Australia

Jennifer Fraser and Helen Stasa

Learning objectives

In this chapter you will:

- Be introduced to the concept of child rights, and in particular the rights of children and young people living in Australia
- Become familiar with the United Nations (UN) Declaration of the Rights of the Child
- Develop an understanding of how these rights translate into paediatric settings
- Develop an understanding of the purpose and intention of Australian policies that determine how, where and by whom children and young people will be cared for in the Australian health-care system
- Consider your professional priorities in relation to children's rights and child-protection legislation

Introduction

This chapter builds on the information about the context of paediatric nursing in Australia in Chapter 1. It is intended to provide a basis for understanding the ways in which children and young people's rights are upheld in Australia, and in particular within the health-care system. This extends to child protection, including nurses' legal responsibility to report child abuse and neglect.

As a nurse working with children, young people and their parents, you will be challenged to consider many important issues regarding your involvement with them as active participants in health. In your practice, you will decide which treatments or interventions are necessary, and whether the child or young person has the capacity to understand the importance and consequences of the choices that you make in collaboration with the family. Your assumptions about childhood and the role of parents will underpin the way in which you approach the child or young person and their family. These assumptions need to be critically evaluated and open to scrutiny and review, so that you can provide them with the best possible care within a variety of contexts. This can sometimes be challenging, as there is a disparity of power in the relationships between the child or young person, you and the family, and this disparity needs to be acknowledged and addressed.

The purpose of this chapter is to provide insight into the way in which human rights, and in particular child rights, inform paediatric nursing practice in Australia. The chapter explains how the current Australian legislation attempts to ensure that child rights are protected within the health-care system. It begins by looking at the international agreements and covenants regarding the protection of child rights that Australia has endorsed before moving on to examine the national legislation. The second part of the chapter looks at some of the ethical challenges regarding child and family rights that you will have to consider as a paediatric nurse in Australia. In particular, we look at issues surrounding access to family, advocacy and consent to treatment of specific diseases in some situations. Further, the chapter provides a basis for understanding the way in which children and young people's rights – including the right to be protected from all forms of violence and neglect – are upheld in Australia, particularly within the health and welfare systems.

International legislation

The United Nations Declaration of the Rights of the Child (UN, 1989a) and its guidelines provide a foundation for the way in which the dignity, wellbeing and human rights of children, young people and their families are respected globally. The Declaration sets out the standards of rights that are required to ensure that children and young people can live a minimally decent life.

As Professor Yanghee Lee, past chairperson of the UN Committee on the Rights of the Child, suggests, there has been a fundamental paradigm shift in how the relationship of children and young people with societal systems (such as the health system) is conceived (Lee, 2013). Whereas legislation previously served a protective function, ensuring the welfare status of the child, in recent times the paradigm has changed so that children are viewed as holders of rights, and actors in promoting and protecting their own rights, rather than mere passive agents. The Declaration is based around four general principles – non-discrimination; life, survival and development; the best interests of the child; and respect for the

TABLE 2.1 *The four principles of the convention of the rights of the child*

Non-discrimination	Best interests of the child
Article 2	Article 3
Life, survival and development	Respect for the child's view
Article 6	Article 12

child's preferences and viewpoints – and these underlie the Declaration's specific Articles (see Table 2.1).

Regarding health care, the Declaration explicitly states that the child 'shall be entitled to grow and develop in health … [and] shall have the right to adequate nutrition, housing, recreation and medical services' (UN, 1989b). The Convention was adopted by the United Nations in 1989 and has been ratified in all countries except Somalia and the United States. Australia ratified the Convention in 1991, followed by New Zealand in 1993 (UN, 1989b).

Other relevant international human rights laws applicable to the health of children and young people in the Australian context include Article 3 of the Universal Declaration of Human Rights, which states that 'everyone has a right to life' (and the treatment required to sustain life). Additionally, Article 12(1) of the UN International Covenant on Economic, Social and Cultural Rights recognises 'the right of everyone (of which children and young people are one group) to the enjoyment of the highest attainable standard of physical and mental health'. This Article is especially notable, as it makes specific reference to the fact that health encompasses both physical and mental aspects, rather than just focusing on the physical. Article 19 of the UN Convention on the Rights of the Child (UN, 1989a) expands upon this Covenant, and obligates state parties to take action and intervene to 'protect the child from all forms of physical and mental violence, injury or abuse, neglect or negligent treatment'.

The United Nations Convention on the Rights of the Child emphasises that children have their own rights and entitlements, and that, because of their youth, they need extra protection (UN, 1989a). These fall into four categories:

Non-discrimination. The Convention applies to all children, whatever their race, religion or abilities; whatever they think or say; whatever type of family they come from. No child should be treated unfairly on any basis.

Life, survival and development rights. These are rights to the resources, skills and contributions necessary for the survival and full development of the child.

The 'rights to survival' in the Convention not only include a guarantee to life, but also a guarantee of nutrition and health care at the highest level. Rights in this group include the right to survival, the right to have birth registration and nationality, the right to live with parents and the right to be taken care of. They include rights to adequate food, shelter, clean water, formal education, primary health care, leisure and recreation, cultural activities and information about their rights. These rights require not only the existence of the means to fulfil the rights but also access to them. Specific articles address the needs of child refugees, children with disabilities and children of minority or Indigenous groups.

Protection rights. The term 'child protection' is not limited to the prevention of physical and mental abuse; it includes the prevention and surmounting of disadvantageous conditions in children's lives. According to the Convention, these rights include, but are not limited to, the right to be protected from all kinds of abuse such as exploitation, violence, neglect and discrimination, and the right to be protected in circumstances of special difficulties, such as family separation, war and disasters. These rights include protection from abuse in the criminal justice system.

Participation rights. Children are entitled to the freedom to express opinions and to have a say in matters affecting their social, economic, religious, cultural and political life. Participation rights include the right to express opinions and be heard, the right to information and the right to freedom of association. Engaging these rights as they mature helps children bring about the realisation of all their rights and prepares them for an active role in society. The right of the child or young person to make their own decisions about treatment or non-treatment are enshrined in Article 13(1), which provides that:

> The child shall have the right to freedom of expression; this right shall include the freedom to seek, receive and impart information and ideas of all kinds, regardless of frontiers ... (UN, 1989a)

Clearly, at younger ages and in cases of cognitive impairment, a child may not have formed considered preferences regarding their medical care. In such situations, the health-care staff may need to rely on parents to provide information about the child's treatment. However, in some situations, the parents' preferences may conflict with what is thought to be in the best health-care interests of the child. In such circumstances, nursing staff have an important role to play in advocating to ensure that the child's rights are protected, while also acknowledging the rights of parents to have their views heard.

> ### Reflection points 2.1
>
> Moral and ethical nursing practice is based on an ethos of lawful scope of practice and ethical standards. We acknowledge Article 13 (1) of the UN Declaration of the Rights of the Child:
>
> The child shall have the right to freedom of expression; this right shall include the freedom to seek, receive and impart information and ideas of all kind: ... (UN, 1989a)
> - List specific groups of children and young people within Australian society that you believe need special safeguarding and care, as well as legal protection.
> - Identify ways in which Australian paediatric nurses can apply children's rights and health care, decision-making frameworks, ethical decision-making and informed consent for two of these highly vulnerable groups.

Australian legislation

Implementation of International Rights of the Child

The Australian legislation surrounding the protection of child rights is based on the international charters outlined above. Implementation of International Rights of the Child occurs through enacting child-specific treaties such as distinctive national policies, protocols and legislation. The Children in Hospital Protocol and the Australian Nursing Standards are two key documents that pertain specifically to the care of children and young people in the Australian health-care system. Both take a human rights-based approach to policy development.

Protecting children and their rights in the context of health care in Australian paediatric settings requires that the principle of family unity be recognised. This ensures that children and their families are not separated by hospital policy or discriminated against for any reason. Moreover, that they have access to appropriate services and service providers and where children's' agency is respected. Children must be allowed to have a say in the way in which they are cared for, and by whom.

First, the Royal Australasian College of Physicians publishes *Standards for the Care of Children and Adolescents in Health Services* (Royal Australasian College of Physicians, 2008). These articulate standards for high quality health care that is safe and appropriate for the child or adolescent. The standards emphasise that the medical and psychosocial needs of children and young people differ greatly from those of adults, and that it is important that health services are designed to accommodate these diverse needs. The standards aim to ensure that the rights of children and young people are respected, that the facilities in which they receive care are appropriate for their developmental age, and that specially qualified staff are responsible for care.

The second key Australian document related to the care of children and young people is a position statement entitled *Minimum Standard for Nurses Caring for Children and Young People,* published by the Australian College of Children and Young People's Nurses (2009). This statement emphasises the engagement of all relevant stakeholders (such as the child or young person, their family, nursing and medical staff, allied health professionals and others) in the planning and delivery of care. It details the knowledge expected of nurses working with children and young people, and elucidates the expectations surrounding communication, family involvement and advocacy. An extract from the position statement follows.

> The goal for nurses working with children and young people and their families is to achieve their optimal health and wellbeing. This will be achieved by engaging all relevant stakeholders in the planning and delivery of care.
>
> The following statements are related to minimum practice standards. The role descriptors are the same for all nurses working with children and young people; however the emphasis of the role will be influenced by the context in which the nurse practises. It states:
>
> Within their scope of nursing practice the nurse:
>
> - assesses children and young people's health, development and wellbeing, recognising deviations from the norm and acting appropriately on the findings
> - describes common health issues affecting children and young people, discusses the management and bases practice on the best available evidence
> - provides family centred care which recognises the impact of hospitalisation, home environment and community on children, young people and families
> - communicates effectively and works in partnership with children and young people and their families

- utilises contact with families to promote the health of children and young people using relevant health guidelines
- describes pharmacokinetics and pharmacodynamics; calculates and safely administers medications and other preparations to children and young people
- is competent in basic paediatric life support
- acts within relevant federal and state legislation and policies
- critically examines and utilises relevant evidence to inform and guide practice relating to the care and protection of children and young people
- practises in a culturally safe manner
- advocates for the health and safety of children and young people
- encourages developmentally appropriate self care/independence for children and young people within their family context
- liaises with others in the community in meeting children and young people's health needs
- works collaboratively with other agencies and disciplines to improve health outcomes for children, young people and their families.

(ACCYPN, 2009)

For nurses working in paediatric settings across Australia, these two documents are important references for the provision of high-quality care, which, taken together with the international documents (such as the UN Declarations) provide a mechanism for attempting to ensure that the rights of children, young people and their families are protected by the health-care system.

Reflection points 2.2

- List ways in which nurses can protect children's rights in hospital. Identify potential barriers to such protection and consider how these barriers may be addressed.
- Talk to a child or young person about a recent illness experience. How did they feel about the care they received? Did they feel in control of the treatment decisions and that they were listened to by their parents/caregivers and health agency staff?

Practice implications

Having briefly outlined the key international and national declarations regarding children, young people and families, and their applicability to the health-care setting, it is important to examine practical situations where, as a paediatric nurse, you may be required to make decisions that require a clear understanding of child rights and your associated responsibilities. In this section, we will examine some of the challenging situations that paediatric nurses may face regarding access to family, consent to treatment and advocacy for children at risk of abuse or neglect.

Access to family

Paediatric nursing care in Australia emphasises the importance of family-centred care. It is suggested that family-centred care emerged as best practice in children's health settings due to widespread interest in patient advocacy, with hospital visiting rights for parents one outcome of the advocacy movement. Within paediatric health-care settings, the term 'family-centred care' is used to describe an approach to nursing care that focuses on issues such the active involvement of parents in the care of the child; consideration of the child's perspectives and views; and increasing the children's involvement in their treatment and decision-making about their treatment (Kuo et al., 2012).

As a paediatric nurse, you may need to rely on the child's parents or guardians to make health-care decisions on the child's behalf, particularly if the child is very young or has a condition that prevents them from exercising their autonomous choice. It is assumed that the parents will make a decision based on the *child's* best interests. It is therefore fundamental to consider models of family-centred care that emphasise training of parents to assume responsibility for care and decision-making, and that move towards truly collaborative relationships between families and nurses.

The ways in which children's choices can best be acknowledged within the Australian paediatric health-care system are supported by a broad literature devoted to the topic. Much of this relies on well-executed qualitative research that provides key insights into the ways in which nurses negotiate and coordinate the views and decisions of children and their parents. Unfortunately, it seems that there is still a long way to go before we can be confident that children are not marginalised in the health-care system and therefore guarantee that their needs are not overlooked.

Using a critical ethnography to study children's in-patient hospital experiences, Livesley and Long (2013) concluded that children had little say in the way in which they were cared for. Children without an adult advocate, such as a parent, in attendance were least likely to be able to negotiate how they were treated in hospital. Children in the study were drawn from a cohort of patients in a nephro-urology ward in the north of England. They typically resorted to attention-seeking behaviours to try to get what they needed from nurses. Children who were less capable of asserting themselves were observed to receive minimal nursing care. What we can see is that some of the defiant and oppositional behaviour that we witness in paediatric settings may in fact be a way for children to demand better or more appropriate care according to their needs. Future research is needed to guide our understanding of how children communicate their need for care and attention, and how nurses can best interpret hospitalised children's behaviour. Nurses are placed in the situation of having to care for and control their patients at the same time (Gray & Smith, 2009). We will look at this aspect of caring for children in paediatric settings in more depth in Chapter 7.

In summary, using a developmental approach, children become increasingly involved in their own health-care decisions as health literacy develops. In line with a child rights perspective, children with the necessary capacity and capability should be involved despite their age. That is, rather than suggesting a particular age at which decision-making is encouraged, children capable of making their own decisions ought to be involved and consulted. Nevertheless, in Australia, children may assent (voluntarily agree) to treatment before legal autonomy; however, it is their parents who must give consent.

Australian age-of-majority legislation

For most Australian jurisdictions, 18 years is the age of legal autonomy, when the person can give consent for treatment without parental approval. This does vary, however. The age for making medical decisions in New South Wales is 14 (*Minors (Property and Contracts) Act 1970* (NSW), s 49) and in South Australia, under section 6 of the *Consent to Medical Treatment and Palliative Care Act 1995*, a person 16 years of age or older may make decisions about their own medical treatment (see Box 2.1).

BOX 2.1 *Age-of-majority legislation in Australia*

Consent to medical treatment

The age of consent for medical treatment differs across jurisdictions – for example, in Western Australia the age of consent remains at 18 years (the general age of majority in Australia); however, in New South Wales and South Australia, the age of consent for making decisions regarding medical treatment has been amended by legislation to 14 and 16 years respectively.

Generally, treatment provided to children below the age of 16 requires the consent of their parents or guardians. Parents may only consent to treatment that is in the best interests of the child.

In all jurisdictions, the consent of the child alone may be sufficient in circumstances where the child has 'sufficient understanding and intelligence to enable him or her to understand fully what is proposed' (*Gillick* test, from the case *Gillick v West Norfolk AHA* (1986) (see also Harrison, 1992). In South Australia, this test has been modified by statute to be: if the child consents, and (1) the medication practitioner is satisfied that the child is capable of understanding the nature, consequences, and risks of the treatment, and that the treatment is in the best interests of the child's health and wellbeing; and (2) that this opinion of the medical practitioner is supported by the written opinion of another medical practitioner who has also examined the child.

A parent may not consent to certain treatments of children. Where a treatment involves major, invasive and irreversible surgery that is not for the purpose of curing a malfunction or disease – for example, sterilisation or gender reassignment – neither a child nor a parent may consent, and it is necessary to obtain the consent of both the court exercising jurisdiction under the *Family Law Act 1975*, or authorised by legislation to consent, and the parents (*Gillick* test: see Harrison 1992).

Children generally may only participate in medical research with the consent of both the child and the parent in circumstances where the research is not contrary to the best interests of the child (Australian Government NHRC, 2001).

Sources: Law Library of Congress (2014); AIFS (2013).

As children make the transition towards adulthood, they develop the ability to be responsible for their actions. The parents' responsibility for the child gives way to autonomy. In the paediatric hospital setting, the adolescent may make a difficult transition into adult care – especially if they have had multiple hospital admissions and developed close relationships with their caregivers.

One particularly pertinent issue that arises with the transition to adult care concerns the competence of the adolescent to make informed, rational decisions about their care and treatment. Regarding consent to medical treatment, the term '*Gillick* competence' must be understood. A House of Lords ruling in *Gillick v West Norfolk Area Health Authority* (1986) states that if a child under the age of 16 can demonstrate sufficient understanding and intelligence (whether through words or actions) to understand fully the treatment proposed, they can give their consent to treatment in the absence of parental consent (Woolley, 2005: 717). This ruling only applies to medical treatment that has clear potential for direct benefit to the health of the child. It is also important to remember that the *Gillick* principle applies only to a decision to receive treatment: it does not apply in cases of refusing treatment. Indeed, as the NSW Law Reform Commission has stated, in some instances it may be possible for the courts to override a young person's decision to refuse treatment (for instance, if this decision is made on religious or spiritual grounds that prohibit receiving particular forms of health-care treatment) if it is believed that it is in the young person's best interests that they receive the care (NSWLRC, 2008).

In Australia, the law is clear that a child can give legally informed and effective consent to medical treatment using a *Gillick* assessment, although it is not obligatory. Australian law still has some way to go in upholding children's rights to medical treatment without parental consent.

The next section of this chapter looks more closely at the relationship between children and their parents, and presents the responsibilities of health-care professionals, including registered nurses, in protecting children from harm.

Priorities in relation to children's rights and child-protection legislation

Child abuse and neglect refer to a wide range of behaviours. These include acts of commission related to physical, sexual, emotional or psychological harm to children, as well as acts of omission related to physical and emotional neglect. The categories of neglect, physical injury, sexual abuse and emotional abuse are widely used for the purposes of child abuse notification, substantiation of child abuse cases and prosecution. Notwithstanding, there are variations between Australian states and territories regarding what constitutes child abuse and neglect. Not only do the definitions vary; there are also some differences in what nurses are mandated to report to the child-protection authorities. This is because each state and territory of Australia has separate legislation aimed at protecting children from abuse and neglect.

Child abuse and neglect notifications are substantiated when, 'in the professional opinion of the officers concerned, there is reasonable cause to believe that the child has been, is being or is likely to be abused or neglected' (AIHW, 2013). Australia has an estimated child abuse and neglect incidence rate of 7.4 per 1000 children in age group from birth to 16 years (AIHW, 2013).

Being able to recognise abuse and neglect of children is the most important first step to being able to provide early intervention to reduce the harm they cause. Prevention is even better, so once a child and family are recognised as needing extra support, there is a chance that risk factors for child abuse and neglect can be reduced. At the same time, it must be recognised that the parent, child and environment transact over time. The scope of child abuse and neglect becomes even more extensive as research reveals the impact of maltreatment on children's development. These issues then further impact on other parts of the child's personality and behaviour in a dangerous spiral.

The role of Australian health professionals – in particular medical and nursing personnel – in reporting child abuse and neglect has increased substantially over the past two decades. The responsibilities of not only recognising but reporting all forms of child maltreatment by doctors and nurses are articulated through policy and legislation to report their knowledge or suspicion of child maltreatment. As well, health services impose policies in line with legislation specific to their jurisdiction to assist clinical staff in responding when they know of, or have a reasonable suspicion of, harm being caused to a child. In most Australian states and territories, if doctors and nurses know or suspect that a child is suffering, has suffered or is likely to suffer significant harm, then they have a legal obligation to report this to child-protection authorities.

Mandatory reporting of known and suspected child abuse and neglect is now well established in all states and territories of Australia. Health professionals, including registered nurses, need to be able to identify, evaluate and document injuries and manage the protection of children in their care to intervene early and prevent further harm. Collaboration with law enforcement bodies, social service agencies, advocacy organisations where they exist and the criminal justice system is essential to provide a network of support. The intent of legislation that mandates reporting to child-protection authorities is to promote early intervention and prevent further violence and abuse.

The responsibility to report child maltreatment

It must be understood that, in Australia, registered nurses are mandated by state and territory laws to report knowledge or suspicion of a child who is experiencing, has experienced or is likely to experience significant harm to a designated authority. Legislation in some jurisdictions is limited to type of abuse and significant harm. Nevertheless, where this is the case – that is, where there is not a legislative duty to report certain forms of abuse – occupational and health service policy requirements exist. Yet, despite these legal and policy obligations, only 13.5 per cent of all reports to statutory child-protection authorities came from health professionals compared with 24.6 per cent from police and 15.1 per cent from schools in the latest reports (AIHW, 2013). This also occurs in Canada, where school personnel, police and social workers report more child abuse and neglect than health-care professionals do (Tonmyr et al., 2009). There is growing research interest in determining the underlying reasons for this, given nurses' exposure to children and families across a range of settings. It is important to tease out whether these factors are related to nurses' skills, knowledge and attitudes, or there are more systematic workplace issues creating barriers to reporting. Do nurses in Australia view child protection as part of their role to the same extent as doctors, police, social workers and others? Are nurses conflicted about their role as advocates for families and children, versus that as advocates for their profession or the health-care agency? These and other questions have been studied in recent Australian research.

In a study of Queensland nurses, 21.1 per cent of nurses surveyed had never reported maltreatment and 26.6 per cent who had made notifications had failed to report on at least one occasion (Fraser et al., 2010), despite being aware of the legal responsibility to do so. Nurses are not alone in their reluctance to report. Even though 97 per cent of general practitioners surveyed in Queensland were aware of the responsibility to report child abuse and neglect, 26 per cent had decided at least once not to do so (Schweitzer et al., 2006). Alarmingly, one of the reasons they gave for not reporting was that they considered the abuse to be a one-off event and viewed further harm to the child as very unlikely.

Compliance with legislation to report child abuse and neglect is compromised by a number of individual and contextual factors. These have also been studied in Australia with nurses and other professional groups (Nayda, 2004; Land & Barclay, 2008), and overseas (Feng & Levine, 2005; Lee et al., 2007).

At the level of the individual – let's call this a proximal factor – is the ability to recognise past, current and future abuse and neglect. Knowledge of child abuse and neglect recognition is variable, and depends on whether the topic is covered in professional development courses or staff training. There is sufficient evidence to indicate the relationship of injury presentations and physical and sexual abuse for example, but staff need to have this knowledge. Certain physical injury presentations are more likely to have resulted from maltreatment. All fractures in a pre-ambulatory child should be treated as suspicious. The child-protection registrar, where available, or a senior medical officer must be notified immediately of any such presentation. Fractures of the femur (Leventhal et al., 2011), rib fractures and those caused by twisting forces, skull fractures or a combination of a skull and long bone fracture are associated with abuse (Bandyopadhyay & Yen, 2002). Head injury is the most common cause of fatal inflicted injury in children (King et al., 2006). Unfortunately it is seen in those under 2 years of age due to the vulnerability of infants (Berkowitz, 1995; DiScala et al., 2000).

Acceleration–deceleration injuries indicate that the infant has been shaken, and a diagnosis of Shaken baby syndrome will be investigated. When considering the causes of injury, it is not enough to undertake a physical assessment of injury and risk alone. Shaken baby syndrome often presents with subdural or subarachnoid bleeding, cerebral oedema, long bone and/or rib fractures, retinal bleeding and little or no cranio-facial trauma (Cadzow & Armstrong, 2000; Kairys et al., 2001; Reece & Sege, 2000). Careful documentation is necessary, as the case may not be clear and symptoms can be diverse, such as abdominal pain and loss of consciousness (Jenny et al., 1999; Kairys et al., 2001; Keenan et al., 2004). Detailed recording of the history – that is, the parents' story – is necessary every time it is told. Inconsistencies across time and between the parents' recall are suspicious (Scott, 2013; Scott et al., 2012).

Cases of neglect and emotional abuse have emerged as the most problematic forms of child maltreatment in Australia (AIHW, 2013). While progress has been made in identifying and reducing both child physical and sexual abuse, substantiated notifications of neglect and emotional abuse are increasing. It is crucial to be able to recognise the risks of abuse and neglect, and make a report of suspicion. In all cases of reporting, it is not the nurse's individual responsibility to substantiate the suspicion, but rather to detail the seriousness of the harm or potential harm to the child.

A nurse's dilemma

Case study 2.1

Chung is an 8-year-old boy born to Chinese parents in Australia. He is often struck by his father with a rod, sometimes for only minor discretions such as being late home from school. Over a period of time, Chung starts to feel sad a lot and loses confidence in himself. He subsequently suffers a loss of faith in humanity, and lacks trust in his relationships with friends, which leads him to distance himself from them. His friends do not understand why this is happening, and start to tease him. Chung responds to this with physical violence, which gets him in trouble with the teacher at his school, and consequently into more trouble with his father.

Wang Li (Lianne) is a registered nurse working in the emergency department of a busy children's hospital in metropolitan Sydney. Wang Li has a legal obligation to report child abuse and neglect to the child-protection authorities, depending on the severity of harm to the child. If the abuse or neglect is deemed to be serious, then she is compelled by legislation and of course hospital policy to make a report. Chung has presented to the hospital where she is working. He is anxious and struggling to breathe. He presents regularly at the hospital, always accompanied by his mother. He has asthma and also a strong history of eczema. His mother says both conditions are really playing up at the moment and that Chung is very anxious. He has been doing net-testing at school and is worried he has not done well.

Using their shared Mandarin language, Wang Li asks Chung's mother whether she knows what might be upsetting him. In Mandarin, Chung's mother discloses the extent to which her husband beats young Chung and makes him spend hours doing homework, even when he is too tired to concentrate. She wants him to stop but is afraid of his reaction if she says anything. She appeals to Wang Li not to mention it to anyone, as she is so ashamed and believes that no other Chinese parent living in Australia would treat their child in this way.

Wang Li is aware of her legal obligation to report the abuse, which she understands to be causing serious harm to Chung's wellbeing. However, she is uncertain whether reporting the concern would be in the best interests of this family. She too was brought up to believe that if you spare the rod you spoil the child – that is, that harsh punishment of children is necessary for their growth and development. Her father was very stern but loving towards her. She has developed a trusting relationship with Chung's mother and feels that she would betray her trust by making a report. Wang Li is not certain whether she can discuss the report with colleagues and whether her identity would be protected.

The multidisciplinary response to child protection

Concerns expressed by Wang Li, in this scenario, are known to be barriers to reporting. Approximately one-fifth of the population of nurses surveyed in Australia and overseas (Feng & Levine, 2005; Fraser et al., 2006; Lee et al., 2011) admit to having not reported their suspicion of abuse or neglect, even when mandated to do so.

Case study resolution

The registered nurse is mandated to report the abuse to the appropriate child-protection agency. In most jurisdictions in Australia, this is enabled by the fact that the nurse can confer with other health professionals and follow a protocol. The registered nurse in this case is mandated to report child abuse and neglect she identifies or suspects in the course of her professional work. Some jurisdictions may have legislation that compels the nurse to report even if it is not part of the professional role. Details of the current legislation for the jurisdiction within which you are working should be well understood and opportunities for training taken.

Wang Li's identity in this case would be protected by Australian law, and she would not be liable for making a report that could not be substantiated if she makes the report in good faith. Depending on the jurisdiction, if she fails to report, a penalty may be incurred. It is important to note that to make a report in Australia, the registered nurse does not have to be able to substantiate the abuse or neglect. She makes a report so that an investigation can be commenced. A Chinese family was presented in the case study to highlight some of the cultural considerations nurses may need to make when reporting. The case study highlights that child abuse and neglect occurs across cultures and religion.

Apart from the legal responsibility, the ethical and moral obligation to report abuse to the appropriate child-protection authority should actually enhance the nurse–family relationship because it should allow for the provision of much-needed assistance to families struggling to provide good parenting for their children. Unfortunately, we know that a number of health professionals, doctors and nurses do not share this optimism, and there remains a critical debate about further expansion of mandatory reporting laws for child abuse and neglect (Mathews, 2012).

Summary

- This chapter introduced the concept of child rights within the scope of paediatric nursing, and in particular the rights of children and young people experiencing paediatric nursing care in Australia.
- The relationship between the UN Declaration of the Rights of the Child, to which Australia is a signatory, and policies on the quality of health care received by children and young people in Australia, were explored.
- The chapter explained the way in which child rights are integrated into Australian policies that determine how children and young people will be cared for in Australian paediatric health-care settings and outlined the mandatory reporting legislation that promotes nurses as advocates for children.
- It is anticipated that you will consider your professional priorities in relation to children's rights and child-protection legislation.
    - This chapter introduced the way in which child rights are upheld in the Australian health-care system.

> The way in which nurses working in Australian paediatric settings align working with children and young people, Australian legislation and policy and the key elements of the UN Declaration of the Rights of the Child were explained.
> Professional priorities, in particular the legal responsibility to report child abuse and neglect to appropriate authorities, were considered.

Learning activities

2.1 Describe standards of nursing practice that relate to the care of children in Australia.
2.2 Describe standards of nursing practice related to the care of young people in Australia.
2.3 Discuss professional boundaries in the therapeutic relationship when providing nursing care for children and families.
2.4 Analyse nursing roles and responsibilities in protecting children from harm.
2.5 Do you think it should be the responsibility of nurses to report child abuse and neglect? Discuss.

Further reading

- For more detailed information about child maltreatment and the obligation you have as a health professional to recognise and respond to known or suspected cases, access the excellent training materials provided by the International Society for the Prevention of Child Abuse and Neglect at <www.ispcan.org/?page=Training_Materials>.
- For further information about Human Rights and Child Rights go to <www.unicef.org/crc/index_30160.html>.
- The International Council of Nurses (2012) publishes position statements relating to nursing practice. The following links take you to the key international statements on nursing ethics and position statements relating to child rights:

    <www.icn.ch/images/stories/documents/about/icncode_english.pdf>
    <www.icn.ch/images/stories/documents/publications/position_statements/E12_Rights_Children.pdf>

<www.icn.ch/images/stories/documents/publications/position_statements/E10_Nurses_Human_Rights.pdf>
<www.icn.ch/images/stories/documents/publications/position_statements/A16_Prevention_Disability_Care.pdf>.

References

Australian College of Children and Young People's Nurses (ACCYPN) 2009, *Minimum standard for nurses caring for children and young people*, position statement, ACCYPN, Brisbane.

Australian Government National Health and Research Council (NHRC) 2001, *Human research ethics handbook*, Commonwealth Government, Canberra, viewed 1 June 2014, http://www.nhmrc.gov.au/publications/hrecbook/misc/contents.htm.

Australian Institute of Family Studies (AIFS) 2013, Age of consent laws, viewed 1 June 2014, http://www.aifs.gov.au/cfca/pubs/factsheets/a142090/#table-1.

Australian Institute of Health and Welfare (AIHW) 2013, *Child protection Australia: 2011–2012*, AIHW, Canberra.

Bandyopadhyay, S & Yen, K 2002, Non-accidental fractures in child maltreatment syndrome, *Clinical Pediatric Emergency Medicine*, 3(2), pp. 145–52.

Berkowitz, C 1995, Pediatric abuse, *Emergency Medical Clinics of North America*, 13, pp. 321–42.

Cadzow, SP & Armstrong, KL 2000, Rib fractures in infants: Red alert! The clinical features, investigations and child protection outcomes, *Journal of Paediatrics and Child Health*, 36(4), pp. 322–6.

DiScala, C, Sege, R, Li, G & Reece, RM 2000, Child abuse and unintentional injuries: A 10-year retrospective, *Archives of Pediatric and Adolescent Medicine*, 154(1), pp. 16–22.

Feng, JY & Levine, M 2005, Factors associated with nurses' intention to report child abuse: A national survey of Taiwanese nurses, *Child Abuse and Neglect*, 29(7), pp. 783–95.

Fraser, JA, Mathews, B, Walsh, K, Chen, L & Dunne, M 2010, Factors influencing child abuse and neglect recognition and reporting by nurses: A multivariate analysis, *International Journal of Nursing Studies*, 47(2), pp. 146–53.

Gillick v West Norfolk and Wisbech Area Health Authority [1985] 3 All ER 402 (HL).

Gray, B & Smith, P 2009, Emotional labour and the clinical settings of nursing care: The perspectives of nurses in East London, *Nurse Education in Practice*, 9(4), pp. 253–61.

Harrison, M 1992, What's new in family law? Parental authority and its constraints – the case of *Marion*, *Family Matters*, 32, pp. 10–12, viewed 3 August 2007, http://www.aifs.gov.au/institute/pubs/fm1/fm32mh.html.

International Council of Nurses (ICN) 2012, *The ICN Code of Ethics for Nurses*, ICN, Geneva.

Jenny, C, Hymel, KP, Ritzen, A, Reinert, SE & Hay, TC 1999, Analysis of missed cases of abusive head trauma, *JAMA: The Journal of the American Medical Association*, 281(7), pp. 621–6.

Kairys, S.Alexander, R, Block, R, Everett, D, Hymel, K & Jenny, C 2001, Shaken baby syndrome: Rotational cranial injuries – technical report, *Paediatrics*, 108(1), pp. 206–10.

Keenan, H, Runyan, D, Marshall, S, Nocera, M & Merten, D 2004, A population-based comparison of clinical and outcome characteristics of young children with serous inflicted and non-inflicted traumatic brain injury, *Pediatrics*, 114(3), pp. 633–9.

King, W, Kiesel, E & Simon, H 2006, Child abuse fatalities: Are we missing opportunities for intervention? *Pediatric Emergency Care*, 22(4), pp. 211–14.

Kuo, DZ, Houtrow, AJ, Arango, P, Kuhlthau, KA, Simmons, JM & Neff, JM 2012, Family-centered care: Current applications and future directions in pediatric health care, *Maternal and Child Health Journal* 16(2), pp. 297–305.

Land, M & Barclay, L 2008, Nurses' contribution to child protection, *Neonatal, Paediatric and Child Health Nursing*, 11(1), pp. 18–24.

Law Library of Congress 2014, Children's rights: Australia, viewed 12 March 2014, http://www.loc.gov/law/help/child-rights/australia.php#f9.

Lee, PY, Fraser, JA & Chou, FH 2007, Nurse reporting of known and suspected child abuse and neglect cases in Taiwan, *Kaohsiung Journal of Medical Sciences*, 23(3), pp. 128–37.

Lee, Y 2013, Keynote presentation: Child indicators in a globalized world: Implications for research, practice and policy, UN Committee on the Rights of the Child 2007–2011, presented at the 4th ISCI Conference, Seoul National University, Seoul.

Leventhal, JM et al. 2011, Are abusive fractures in young children becoming less common? Changes over 24 years, *Child Abuse & Neglect*, 35(11), pp. 905–14.

Livesley, J & Long, T 2013, Children's experiences as hospital in-patients: Voice, competence and work. Messages for nursing from a critical ethnographic study, *International Journal of Nursing Studies*, 50, pp. 1292–303.

Mathews, BP 2012, Exploring the contested role of mandatory reporting laws in the identification of severe child abuse and neglect. In M. Freeman (ed.), *Law and childhood studies*, Oxford University Press, Oxford, pp. 302–38.

Miller, AJ & Kaufhold, M 2013, *Child maltreatment medical curriculum*, ISPCAN, viewed 1 April 2013, http://www.ispcan.org/Medical_Curriculum.

Nayda, R 2002, Influences on registered nurses' decision-making in cases of suspected child abuse, *Child Abuse Review*, 11, pp. 168–78.

—— 2004, Registered nurses' communication about abused children: Rules, responsibilities and resistance, *Child Abuse Review*, 13(3), pp. 188–99.

NSW Law Reform Commission (NSWLRC) 2008, *Young people and consent to health care*, report no. 119, NSWLRC, Sydney.

Reece, RM & Sege, R 2000, Childhood head injuries: Accidental or inflicted? *Archives of Pediatric and Adolescent Medicine*, 154(1), pp. 11–15.

Royal Australasian College of Physicians 2008, *Standards for the care of children and adolescents in health services*, viewed 1 June 2014, http://www.racp.edu.au/index.cfm?objectid=393E4ADA-CDAA-D1AF-0D543B5DC13C7B46.

Schweitzer, R, Buckley, L, Harnett, P & Loxton, N 2006, Predictors of failure by medical practitioners to report suspected child abuse in Queensland, *Australian Health Review*, 30(3), pp. 298–304.

Scott, D 2013, Meeting children's needs when the family environment isn't always 'good enough': A systems approach, viewed 20 December 2013, http://www.aifs.gov.au/cfca/pubs/papers/a144433/cfca14.pdf.

Scott, D, Higgins, D & Franklin, R 2012, The role of supervisory neglect in childhood injury, viewed 20 December 2013, http://www.aifs.gov.au/cfca/pubs/papers/a142582.

Tonmyr, L, Li, A, Williams, G, Scott, D & Jack, S 2009, Patterns of reporting to child protection services in Canada by healthcare and non-healthcare professionals, *Paediatrics & Child Health*, 15(8), pp. 25–32.

United Nations (UN) 1989a, *Convention on the Rights of the Child*, United Nations, New York.

—— 1989b, *Treaty Collection*, viewed 1 June 2014, https://treaties.un.org.

Woolley S 2005, Children of Jehovah's Witnesses and adolescent Jehovah's Witnesses: What are their rights? *Archives of Disease in Childhood*, 90, pp. 715–19.

3 Psychosocial development and response to illness

Jennifer Fraser and Robyn Rosina

Learning objectives

In this chapter you will:

- Be introduced to the way in which children, young people and their families respond to disruptions in health

- Explore the relationship between responsive nursing practice and psychosocial development of children and young people

- Examine cultural factors that influence the way in which children, young people and their families respond to disruptions in health

- Consider child behaviour and child development, and the impact of nursing practice on responses to experiences of illness

- Identify health-promotion and health-education strategies that aim to improve the health and wellbeing of Australian children and young people

Introduction

This chapter pays special attention to the responses of children, young people and their families to disruptions to the child's health. When a child experiences an acute or chronic illness, we can expect a number of **emotional** and **behavioural responses**. The paediatric nurse's knowledge of child behaviour and child development can be of great benefit in assisting parents and caregivers to promote resilience in the child or young person.

This chapter presents a series of case studies and case study resolutions to provide guidelines and recommendations for managing emotional and behavioural disorders related to children's experiences of illness. The case studies are presented within a framework of psychosocial development to best illustrate the relationship between child development and response to illness. The relationship is bidirectional – that is, responses are shaped according to the developmental stage

Emotional response A reaction to an internal feeling, accompanied by physiological changes that may or may not be outwardly manifested

Behavioural response A person's actions or reactions in response to external or internal stimuli

of the child or young person, and development is impacted by the experiences of both acute and chronic illness. Consideration is given to cultural and social factors that influence the child's response to the experience of illness. This includes Aboriginal and Torres Strait Islander health practices and their potential implications for care provided to children, young people and their families.

The psychosocial development of children and young people experiencing disruptions to health

Opportunities for developmental experiences that promote healthy psychosocial development may be limited or compromised by childhood illness, and possibly also by nursing practice. The presence of chronic illness may disrupt the pace and timing of – and may cause regression in – developmental milestone achievements. Long absences from school and limited opportunities for self-responsibility or the experience of achievement can compromise psychosocial developmental mastery. For some younger children, the inability to play and the absence of a playgroup can reduce opportunities for developmental progress. The feelings of difference from peers and the experience of an inconsistent peer group make it even more difficult for some young people to achieve developmental milestones.

The sequencing and progression of psychosocial development is shaped by day-to-day life experiences and interactions, both within families and with other people in the community (Erikson, 1968). Children and young people with **chronic illness** often have long hospital admissions, which means they are isolated from family members and peer groups. Periods of life-threatening crises, persisting anxiety and distress, endurance of pain and long **hospitalisations** can limit developmental experiences for psychosocial task experimentation and mastery.

Further challenges emerge when the physical effects of the disease and treatments – such as short stature, weight gain or loss, disabilities, jaundiced skin colour and (for some) hair loss – can increase the sense of difference from well peers (Gurney et al., 2003). There are numerous environmental mediators that can act as, or become, protective factors when an individual is faced with developmental compromise. These environmental factors can also be risk factors (Turkel & Pao, 2007). Other factors,

> **Chronic illness**
> Any illness that persists over a long period and affects physical, emotional, intellectual and social functioning
>
> **Hospitalisation**
> A period of medical care in a hospital

such as the severity and visibility of the illness, current health state, duration of the illness and time since diagnosis, can also impact on the developmental environment to predispose or protect the young person from the adverse effects of illness on **psychosocial development** (Falvo, 2013). However, the relationship between these factors and moderation of the environment is complex.

> **Pscyhosocial development**
> The acquisition of social attitudes and skills, and the development of the personality from infancy through maturity

Following the stages proposed by Erikson's (1968) theory of psychosocial development from infancy through to young adulthood, the chapter will now examine the impact of pain, illness and disability, and the responsiveness of nursing practice. The six psychosocial developmental stages are:

1 trust versus mistrust: infancy (first year of life)
2 autonomy versus shame and doubt: infancy (second year of life)
3 initiative versus guilt: early childhood – the preschool years (3–5 years)
4 industry versus inferiority: middle and late childhood (infants and primary school – 6 years to puberty)
5 identity versus identity confusion: adolescence (10–20 years)
6 intimacy versus isolation: early adulthood (twenties and thirties).

Trust versus mistrust: Infancy (first year of life) and the sick infant

Erikson's first psychosocial developmental stage, from birth to 1 year of age, begins with the conflict of basic trust versus mistrust. This conflict is resolved if the infant experiences a sense of trust about having their needs met without high levels of anxiety or distress. For example, the situation of distress may arise for infants while waiting for care in busy hospital wards or with inconsistent caregiving or in the absence of parental care. Delays in the gratification of the infant's needs and persisting anxiety can induce a poor or negative resolution of the conflict of trust versus mistrust. A negative resolution of this stage can result in feelings of mistrust and anxiety about the responsiveness of the environment to meet the infant's needs in the future (Erikson, 1968).

The resolution of this first developmental stage is also important to the process of attachment to a caregiver in infancy. Bowlby (1969), a major attachment theorist, proposed that it is in fact the infant who elicits care by a series of built-in behaviours such as crying, sucking, clinging, gazing and smiling. These behaviours trigger a caregiving response – that is, rather than the parent initiating caregiving, it is the infant who initiates this responsivity to cues. The caregiver, however, needs to be sensitive to these cues in order to respond appropriately to their needs. In the case of a sick infant, distance from the primary caregiver can result in separation anxiety and an anxious attachment (Bowlby, 1969). This situation may compromise the development of trust inherent in Erikson's stage of trust versus mistrust. The post-natal stage of development is a 'sensitive period', when bonding can occur and attachment to a consistent caregiver – ideally a parent – can begin (Newman & Newman, 2011). Clearly, illness and hospitalisation during early infancy can put at risk the quality of attachment and the development task to accommodate a sense of trust in the environment for sick infants.

Child development throughout infancy and toddlerhood is grounded in the security of parent–infant attachment (Ainsworth et al., 1978; Bowlby, 1951, 1969, 1988). Research on the developmental effects of chronic illness, disability and hospitalisation typically integrates the theories of human attachment (Ainsworth et al., 1978; Bowlby, 1969, 1988) and social learning (Bandura, 1977) into an ecological framework of child development. Developmental problems among hospitalised infants and toddlers appear to relate to limited opportunities for nurturance by caregivers, as well as to the way in which the child adapts to the environment over time. These two themes of parent–infant attachment and adaptation to the environment dominate the literature on effects of frequent hospitalisation on children's development.

Luka

Case study 3.1

Luka was born with a congenital cleft lip and palate. He is admitted to the paediatric surgical unit for the first of a series of operations to repair the anomaly at 10 weeks of age. On admission, you notice that his mother always faces him away from her own face, towards you. She doesn't kiss him or speak to him warmly. She hardly speaks to you or the other nurses about him or his care unless encouraged to do so. In fact, she is noticeably avoidant of her young son. When he tries to engage her with a little smile or with his eyes, she turns away and looks at her mobile phone. She doesn't respond to any of his desperate cues to gain her attention.

As a paediatric nurse, you will recognise subtle cues and understand the developing capabilities of children in different stages. An infant with a mild temperament, engaging communication style (e.g. smiles often and maintains eye contact) and an attractive physical appearance will elicit more positive interactions with caregivers and staff compared with infants who do not engage well, who cry often or whose medical condition requires minimal handling. Optimise opportunities to promote the growth and psychosocial development of hospitalised infants through careful observation and timing of nursing interventions. With access to the hospitalised child around the clock, your actions can ameliorate the psychological impact of hospitalisation and potentially reduce the stress of the child's suffering.

Recognition of a child's stress response is the trigger to identify measures that can modify stressors and help decrease the impact of experiences such as pain and emotional distress. Accurate assessment data are needed. These are usually gathered from parents or caregivers, and include details of familiar routines that are usual or normal for the child, as well as developmental milestones. Communication and cognition skills are not fully developed in the young child, leaving the nurse to rely on parents or other significant caregivers for information. Even children with verbal skills and the ability to communicate easily may not be capable of explaining their symptoms and the impact of hospitalisation or the experience of illness. This ability relies on a range of developmental factors.

Reflection points 3.1

- Family-centred care is based on the tenets of **attachment theory**, in recognition of the importance of maintaining a secure attachment relationship in infancy and childhood.
- Sick infants and toddlers need ongoing opportunities for nurturance by caregivers to prevent developmental problems associated with hospitalisation.

Attachment theory The theory of the relationships between humans. Ainsworth et al. (1978) suggested a number of attachment patterns in infants that impacted their future development

Case study 3.2

11-month-old Evie was admitted to hospital at 4.00 am with respiratory distress and diagnosed with bronchiolitis. Her oxygen saturations go down when she gets upset. Her mother has had to go home to care for her other three young children. Evie's parents both work shifts. Her father will be able to arrange to take some time off from his job to assist with child care, but for now Evie's mother needs to be at home to take care of Evie's siblings. Evie eats a normal family diet supplemented with bottles of formula four times a day. She has been screaming and crying out for her mother ever since she left 20 minutes ago. The nurse must decide how best to care for Evie until her mother can return in the evening.

Reactions to hospitalisation depend not only on the developmental maturity of the child but also on:

- their previous experience of hospitals and illness
- separation and their resilience to being separated from the primary caregiver
- their innate and acquired coping skills
- the seriousness of the illness or disability, and
- the quality of support networks the family can access.

As mentioned previously, separation from the primary caregiver creates the greatest stress for young children in the first year of life and in the preschool age group. Separation anxiety manifests as initial protesting and crying when the caregiver leaves the infant. This is especially characteristic between 9 and 11 months of age, but can be experienced throughout childhood. This is followed by a period of despair and withdrawal, when the child will appear depressed. They may be less communicative and regress developmentally. If separated further – that is, if the parent fails to reappear – the child will become detached from the external environment and develop superficial relationships with others as they adjust to separation.

Factors that can exacerbate these reactions to hospitalisation, injury and pain include inconsistent caregivers, inconsistent care and not following routine daily activities. These are just some of the considerations a paediatric nurse needs to give to the care of a child in hospital. Strategies to reduce the impact are based on a detailed assessment of the seriousness of the child's condition, the family's previous experience of childhood illness and hospitalisation, and the medical procedures that will be necessary for an optimal recovery. It has been recognised for some time that affectional ties with parent substitutes such as grandparents and older siblings, which encourage trust, autonomy and initiative, aid in the healthy and optimal development of young children (Werner & Smith, 1992: 192).

Nursing assessment and interventions

Where the parent is unavailable during the child's hospitalisation, there are a number of nursing interventions that can be implemented to assist with caring for the child. Importantly, the child's routines – and especially their dietary requirements – must be documented carefully. Planning care around usual activities and familiar routines may be challenging, but the benefits of having a relaxed child will outweigh the inconvenience. Check with her mother before she leaves the hospital that you have all the information you will need to care for Evie. Make sure that you can contact her at any time if necessary and reassure her that she can keep in touch with the hospital as frequently as she wishes. A favourite toy and some familiar books might assist in soothing Evie while her mother is absent. If possible, assist the mother to problem-solve so that she can make staying with Evie in hospital a priority. For example, prompt her to think of responsible friends or relatives whom she could trust to care for her other children. Seek advice about any other relatives familiar to Evie who might be able to stay in hospital at times when she cannot. Parents, as well as their children, are stressed at times of illness and hospitalisation, and assisting with problem-solving can be very helpful and comforting.

Autonomy versus shame and doubt: Infancy (second year of life) and the sick toddler

Erikson's second stage of psychosocial development, from the age of 1 to 3 years, involves resolving the conflict of autonomy versus shame and doubt (Erikson, 1968). The child's discovery of a will of their own marks this stage. The child begins to walk and climb, and develop the mental powers to make decisions. Autonomy begins to form during this stage when parents or caregivers offer guided choices and do not overly restrict, force or shame the child (Erikson, 1968). Children who are restrained too much or punished too harshly may be at risk of developing of a sense of shame and self-doubt (Erikson, 1968). For young children with chronic illness, the achievement of milestones such as walking and climbing may be impossible or delayed by the impact of the disease process. Incapacity and physical limitations may also compromise the attainment of a sense of competence for children with chronic illness.

The diagnosis and treatment of chronic conditions often involves multiple painful and traumatic procedures that may embarrass and shame young children. The hospital experience can become an extremely stressful period for both the child and the family. The anxiety that a child may experience during invasive and traumatic procedures can have psychological effects that linger for months after discharge from the hospital (Turkel, 2007). It is important to consider the developmental impact of stressful and traumatic experiences for young children in hospital. However, for young children this cannot be considered in isolation from family considerations with regard to the developmental impact of health care.

A common reaction to stress in children is regression of developmental gains. The young child who was toilet trained may need to wear nappies again until they become more resilient in the stressful situation, and the toddler who was beginning to dress independently may need some assistance while in hospital. The extra attention paid to the child will assist with the adjustment to hospitalisation. Parents can become quite distressed to see their children regress in this way, and need to be reassured that this should be a temporary and expected response to the stress of illness and hospitalisation. Patience and understanding are needed, and the nurse may use strategies such as modelling the behaviours and providing anticipatory guidance – thus preparing the parents for the extra care and attention the child will need to overcome stress (see Box 3.1).

BOX 3.1 *Nursing assessment and interventions*

- If possible, prepare the child for hospitalisation.
- Prevent or minimise separation from caregivers.
- Prevent or minimise loss of control.
- Provide excellent pain management.
- Provide age-appropriate play equipment.
- Provide opportunities for the child to play.
- Allow regression and assist parents to accept immature behaviours.

Initiative versus guilt: Early childhood – the preschool years (3–5 years)

According to Erikson's theory of psychosocial development, the third stage, from around the ages of 3 to 5 years, is marked by courage and independence (Erikson, 1968). The child gains initiative and is capable of planning and problem-solving. With this stage also comes a new emotion: guilt. Children at this stage of development may experience a feeling of guilt when their initiatives are unsuccessful.

Case Study 3.3 involves David, an 11-year-old boy with an intellectual disability, Down syndrome. Erikson's conflict of industry versus inferiority is a particularly important and critical stage and milestone for many children with disabilities. David's story highlights the importance of recognising developmental mastery among children with disabilities, and the key role played by nursing practice in influencing the hospital experiences for this group. The case example of David highlights not only the importance of identifying anxiety but also how difficult it is to recognise behavioural developmental cues and to ensure responsive nursing care.

Case study 3.3: David

David was admitted to hospital for further medical management of congenital heart defects that were now impairing his cardiac function. Prior to admission to hospital, David was able to assist with dressing and, after prompting by his mother, Kath, could almost use the toilet by himself. Early in the admission, the insertion of a cannula was required to administer antibiotics. David thrashed about violently and needed to be restrained for the procedure. After the procedure, David remained aggressive and incontinent, spitting and refusing to swallow medication. He eventually pulled out the cannula. Kath became visibly distressed and later disclosed feelings of helplessness, powerlessness and an inability to control or even influence her son's experience in the hospital. When at home, even when David was sick, she was able to control or at least soothe and make things easier for her son. Kath also felt her son was aware of her distress and her inability to protect him, which always made his behaviour worse.

The anxiety levels of mothers are reported to be a powerful predictor of anxiety among children in this age group (Smith & Kaye, 2012). Insight into maternal anxiety can also provide a window to assist the nurse to understand, predict, identify, and perhaps intervene with distressed children (Luyckx et al., 2008). Understanding and ameliorating maternal anxiety may potentially be another environmental mediator that could help reduce the anxiety of hospitalised children and facilitate resolution of the conflict of industry versus inferiority. At the very least, it may prevent developmental regression and the loss of previously acquired or current achievements. In the case of David, it may have been a loss of previously attained skills and current developmental mastery, such as toileting, feeding himself, feeling safe and being able to control his behaviour.

The perspectives and knowledge of parents and carers of the child's mood and behaviour, and particularly information about premorbid function, are extremely valuable in understanding the child's psychosocial functioning and current state. In particular, with children such as David, it could be useful to explore previous developmental achievements – specifically emotion regulation, feeding, bathing or the level of support required for these activities. Young children often find it more difficult to articulate their distress in a meaningful way; this is particularly apparent for children with developmental delays. A mild sedation for David and appropriate preparation for the traumatic procedures, both for David and his mother, may have reduced the need for restraint and the level of anxiety that ensued. Routine monitoring of mood, emotions, behaviour and functioning before and after traumatic procedures can identify rising anxiety for both parents and their children. Identifying anxiety can create opportunities to ameliorate distress and avoid losses in developmental mastery during hospitalisation and at home after discharge.

Nursing interventions that target maternal anxiety are important in moderating the anxiety of children undergoing traumatic procedures. Small (2002), in a literature review, identified that anxious and depressed parents influenced poor coping outcomes for their children during and/or following medical procedures and hospitalisations. A randomised control trial was conducted to explore the effect of interventions targeting maternal anxiety and depression among 163 mothers of hospitalised children in two paediatric hospitals. The level of anxiety and depression among the group was measured at intervals of one, three, six and 12 months after hospitalisation (Melnyk et al., 2004). The study showed that the use of specific interventions to reduce maternal anxiety strongly reduced child anxiety and resulted in fewer negative behaviours after discharge. The researchers concluded that with routine provision of interventions that reduce maternal anxiety, negative outcomes such as developmental regression following discharge could be reduced substantially (Melnyk et al., 2004). Nursing interventions that empower the child and/or normalise the hospital experience as much as possible – particularly for children with developmental delays – may promote developmental opportunities. Interventions that consider the challenges to development progression can also promote the retention of previous levels of developmental mastery. Developmental regression can weaken opportunities to resolve and master later developmental conflicts and milestones, such as moving from childhood to adolescence, so this stage is clearly critical in optimising children's self-care and independence as adults.

> **Reflection points 3.2**
> - The nurse cares for both the parents and the child in paediatric nursing settings in an effort to optimise the child's health.
> - Acknowledging maternal anxiety can reduce the anxiety of hospitalised children.
> - Children's development can regress due to pain, illness and isolation. Parents need to understand that some of the gains of development may be temporarily lost while the child is in hospital.

Parents and caregivers are the cornerstone of their children's health decisions and behaviours. Working with parents to achieve optimal health, growth and development requires an understanding of the impact on parent functioning of caring for a child with a chronic condition or disability. Not only are the parents responsible for the child's treatment regimen, emergency care responses and daily care routines, but also for the day-to-day management of the child's condition. An important consideration for nurses caring for David is the fact that children with chronic illness and disability are at higher risk for child physical abuse (Svensson et al., 2010). As discussed in Chapter 2, the paediatric nurse has a responsibility to detect and respond to the recognition of child abuse and neglect. Children are vulnerable due to their dependence on adults for care, to have their developmental needs met and to live in harmony.

There is ongoing concern for the increased vulnerability of children with chronic illness and those with longer-term disabilities. Svensson and colleagues' (2011) Swedish survey of 2510 children with a chronic illness and/or disability aged from 10 to 15 years found that the risk for physical abuse was high compared with unaffected peers. Likewise, a retrospective study of all children reported as abused or neglected between 1977 and 1984 revealed that chronic illness placed children at higher risk for neglect during the same period. Taken together, the evidence for children with chronic illness and disability being at risk for emotional, behavioural and social delay, and their increased likelihood for suffering child abuse and neglect, demonstrates their overwhelming risk. It also points to the importance of paying attention to the family environment and family functioning.

A review of related literature (Morawska et al., 2014) highlights that the characteristics of the family environment and the severity and chronicity of the illness, and not the specific childhood illness, are the best predictors of adjustment to chronic illness in childhood (Svavarsdottir & Orlygsdottir, 2006). These are important findings, guiding our understanding of the poor emotional or behavioural adjustment compared to children without a chronic illness across a variety of settings (Blackman et al., 2011; Hysing et al., 2007, 2009). That is, whether the child is cared for in the respiratory, endocrine, oncology or medical ward, we can expect to have to manage children and families struggling with adjustment disorders. Internalising conditions, such as depression and anxiety, and externalising disorders that feature behaviour problems and aggression (Pinquart & Shen, 2011), social difficulties (Meijer et al., 2000) and using the illness to avoid school and other responsibilities (Eksi et al., 1995), will need to be acknowledged and managed. Of particular importance during hospitalisation is the risk for poor social development. Children who present with poor social skills will find hospitalisation extremely stressful and should receive extra attention (Lambert et al., 2013; Meijer et al., 2000). Externalising behaviours may also be experienced. Reactions to injury and illness include crying, resistance and oppositional behaviour, and aggressive outbursts. As the child develops, the concerns become more sophisticated. The young child may fear disability and lack of privacy, and use words more effectively to describe fear and pain. School-aged children are especially vulnerable to stress as they struggle for independence and seek peer acceptance.

Industry versus inferiority: Middle and late childhood (infants and primary school – 6 years to puberty)

For children in the fourth stage of psychosocial development, social and cultural factors also play a key role in the way they respond. According to Erikson (1968), this is an important stage in the development of self-confidence. The child is now able to form moral values, and works hard to get things right. They are capable of recognising cultural and individual differences and express their individuality and independence.

Fine motor coordination increases during this stage, and children in this age group are capable of completing complex motor tasks. This improves their ability to play games that require hand–eye coordination, such as soccer and handball, and extends to having the physical skills to become involved in complex health procedures, such as applying creams and independently managing bandaging.

Perceptual thinking moves towards conceptual thinking – that is, the child moves from a way of thinking based on what they see (perceptual) to judging a situation based on their own reasoning (conceptual). Towards adolescence, concrete thinking matures. Abstract thought and a greater understanding of their health condition mean that children of this age have more agency in determining their own health behaviours. They are able to contribute more to discussion and decision-making. Children of this age often have a strong sense of industry, and enjoy accomplishment that can be harnessed into positive health behaviours and greater responsibility. Treatment adherence problems often begin to emerge at the end of this stage as young children attempt to participate in, or are strongly encouraged to take some responsibility for, their treatment and general health care. Behaviour problems are common as children strive to test their skills in their own way.

Interestingly, in relation to parenting style, authoritative parenting styles are associated with better management of childhood illness, and indeed with superior child adjustment (Botello-Harbaum et al., 2008; Park & Walton-Moss, 2012). Higher rates of emotional and behavioural problems among children with chronic illness may be explained by their parents' expectations of behaviour and reluctance to discipline a sick child (Ievers et al., 1994). Understandably, parents may set different expectations for their child's behaviour, especially during hospitalisation. High parenting stress and low parenting self-efficacy are known to reduce parents' ability to manage their children's behaviour, and to manage treatment regimens crucial to the management of childhood illness (Helgeson et al., 2011; Streisand et al., 2005).

Australian Aboriginal families

The determinants of health for Aboriginal families in Australia are tied to cultural, historical, social and economic conditions. The social determinants of health include:

- employment
- a sense of feeling safe in their community without discrimination
- participating in or already having a good education
- having enough money for their needs
- feeling connected to friends and family
- a connection to their land and the historical past that took people from their traditional lands away from their families. (Carson et al., 2007)

The national strategic plan for health and health services in Australia, the National Aboriginal and Torres Strait Islander Health Plan 2013–2023 (Australian Government, 2013) has set out an agenda for responsive health care. Aboriginal and Torres Strait Islander children and families are over-represented in health and welfare services, as detailed in Chapter 1. Nurses working in paediatric settings throughout Australia are encouraged to familiarise themselves with this plan. Aboriginal people continue to have lower life expectancies and poorer health than other Australians. The social determinants of Aboriginal health include historical factors, education, employment, housing, environment, social and cultural capital, and discrimination (Australian Government, 2013). The consequences of Aboriginal people being taken away from their traditional lands have been devastating, not only in terms of social and economic conditions, but also for subsequent health status. This situation has led to fewer life opportunities for this group, and has directly contributed to health disparities for Indigenous children in many communities across Australia:

> Aboriginal health means not just the physical wellbeing of an individual but refers to the social, emotional and cultural wellbeing of the whole community in which each individual is able to achieve their full potential as a human being, thereby bringing about the total well- being of their community. It is a whole-of-life view and includes the cyclical concept ... (Department of Health, 1989)

As a result of inequities in the social determinants of health experienced by Aboriginal people in Australia, they not only experience health problems but also face greater barriers to accessing services that could assist them to improve the health of their children and families. The following case study of Lana illustrates the struggles Aboriginal families faced living in rural and remote New South Wales.

Lana

Case study 3.4

Nine-year-old Lana, a member of the Wiradjuri group of Aboriginal Australians in north-west New South Wales, has chronic eczema. She is now experiencing her third admission to a city paediatric hospital with infected eczema. Lana lives with her parents and five siblings on a mission on the outskirts of a small rural town. A number of issues were identified that prevent treatment adherence for Lana's eczema and result in recurrent skin infections:

Psychosocial and family issues

> Lana's mother has difficulty accessing and paying for sufficient creams and bandages to comply with the eczema treatment regimen.

> Lana's father is out of work and without transport to seek work.

> A couple of Lana's siblings have recurrent ear infections.

> The mission has difficulty obtaining regular garbage collection, and as a consequence the garbage is stacked up at the entry to the mission. The children are attracted to the garbage to explore and play.

> A number of dogs wander through the mission and are also attracted by the garbage. The children love patting the dogs.

Lana's parents, and indeed the whole community, have numerous pressures placed on them. The ability to provide complex care is compromised by poverty and poor housing. Paediatric nursing care involves the child or young person and their family, because it is the family environment that shapes child health outcomes and emotional and behavioural adjustment. The child's response to illness experience is shaped by the influence of parenting capacity as well as family stress (Morawska et al., 2014).

Lana requires a family and community response that engages with a range of agencies to improve the resources available to her family if they are to effectively care for Lana's chronically infected eczema. Lana's treating doctor provided a plan for the treatment of her eczema; however, this time an inter-agency response was developed to assist her family to comply with the plan. Below are the people and agencies that came together for the case conference (or relayed input by phone) at the Aboriginal health centre in the nearest town.

Interprofessional connections

These included:

- Lana and Lana's parents
- paediatric outreach clinical nurse consultant via teleconference from the paediatric hospital and then handed over the Aboriginal health worker
- Aboriginal health worker
- Aboriginal welfare officer
- local hospital pharmacist
- Local pharmacist
- NGO employment agency
- Aboriginal elders (Lana's aunties on the mission)
- mission worker with local council
- general practitioner (GP) (for Lana and her siblings).

Following discussion, a community plan was put in place for Lana and her family. The plan enabled her father to regain employment; the council to manage the rubbish and the roaming dogs on the mission; Lana's aunties (also living on the mission) to assist Lana's mother with the care of the children; transport for Lana and her siblings to reconnect with their GP; and the mission workers to negotiate with the local council to ensure regular garbage collection for the mission.

Lana's situation – or rather, her family's determinants for health – improved immensely. Resources were made available for the family to determine their own health. The role of the paediatric CNC was reduced to periodic reviews and assistance with supply issues obtaining the necessary creams and bandages. Lana was seen at the paediatric hospital two years later for a hearing problem. Her eczema had almost resolved, and she had not had any further infections.

Note: Throughout the case study, we have used terms for Aboriginal and Torres Strait Islander people as advised and with respect. Because some people feel the term 'Indigenous Australian' diminishes their Aboriginality, we have used it only as necessary – such as within referencing. Because Aboriginal people are the original inhabitants of New South Wales, we use the term 'Aboriginal' to describe the New South Wales-based case family. We hope this does not offend Torres Strait Islander or Aboriginal and Torres Strait Islander people.

Sources: Northern Sydney Local Health District Aboriginal Health Services (2013: 6) and personal communication with the author, 5 May 2014.

Cultural considerations

Cultural considerations – cultural influences and family factors – play a large part in the way children experience health and illness. Cultures are not homogeneous, but those of the same culture often experience similar health and social issues. The family unit itself is culture at a foundational level, and health beliefs and parents' health practices for their children vary within and between cultures. Recognising and accepting heterogeneity within and between families enables the paediatric nurse to provide care that the family is more likely to accept. There are direct and indirect aspects of culture that impact on the individual's actions and beliefs. These include race, family values, customs, health beliefs and practices, child-rearing and susceptibility to certain health problems.

> **Cultural considerations**
> The cultural factors that affect our experiences of the society in which we live and the events we experience

Around the world, many people are moving from country to country to seek better living conditions and opportunities to improve the health and social status of themselves and or their families. A number of these people settle in Australia, bringing with them health and social issues from their country of origin and the countries en route to seeking asylum in Australia, as well as the additional concerns of settling in new country and culture. As nurses, we can expect to be confronted with complex issues requiring responsive clinical assessment and practice.

Aarfah

Case study 3.5

Aarfah is a 9-year-old girl who came to Australia by boat from Iraq via Indonesia and lives in a detention centre. She is brought to the hospital with her mother after three days of abdominal pain and vomiting. The detention centre nurse had decided the dehydration could not be managed at the centre and required hospitalisation. Aarfah's family had experienced significant trauma as a result of war in their home country and fear of discovery while waiting in Indonesia for a boat to Australia. Aarfah's living conditions had become quite poor and she and the other children had suffered from many infections. Aarfah's mother explains through an interpreter that her daughter has suffered night terrors since leaving the family home in Iraq and her much-loved school friends.

Aarfah's struggles with health had preceded her current abdominal pain and vomiting. Her viral illness was soon diagnosed and resolved quickly with the appropriate treatment. Her abdominal pain became more general 'pains', which continued despite her recovery from the virus. It was clear that Aarfah was not re covering as expected for a 9-year-old. She was disinterested in playing with her peers, teary and at times was seen hitting her mother. Aarfah's 'pains' and night terrors persisted.

A referral was made to a child psychiatrist in consultation with Aarfah's mother, using an interpreter. Following extensive family and child assessments, a diagnosis of Post Traumatic Stress Disorder (PTSD) was made and appropriate treatment commenced. Aarfah was discharged back to the detention centre with a care plan that included ongoing counselling and child and family psychological interventions. Some three months later, Aarfah attended a clinic appointment for immunisation and was seen by the Consultation Liaison Child Psychiatry CNC and Registrar (CL Team). Aarfah's physical health and mental state had improved and she was interacting normally with her mother, clinic staff and in play. Her mother reported that her daughter no longer experienced night terrors; she was playing with her siblings and was now participating in school activities at the centre.

The determination process for asylum seekers to achieve refugee status is lengthy in many countries like Australia. Asylum seekers and refugees have a higher risk of physical disease and mental illness as a result of poor living conditions, poor nutrition and an inability to access appropriate health care and economic resources to effectively care for themselves and their families (Hadgkiss et al., 2012). They often suffer from enduring stress as a result of their experiences in their war-torn homelands, on their journeys to Australia and while in detention. Children are especially vulnerable to PTSD and other mental disturbance and behaviour problems (Hadgkiss et al., 2012).

Reflection points 3.3

- Paediatric nurses require a comprehensive understanding of the lives of asylum seekers and refugees alongside information about their health and social needs.
- The domains of physical, mental and psychosocial health and disruptions to health are intricately linked, particularly during childhood.
- Consequently, each domain requires careful assessment and interventions to ensure good physical and mental health, and to ensure optimal psychosocial development.

Identity versus identity confusion: Adolescence (10–20 years)

As children move from childhood into the adolescent years, different developmental issues arise. Assuming the management of their own health and treatment regimens becomes increasingly important. The impact of their illness on their physical and psychosocial development becomes more tangible and personally real to the young person. For some young people and their families, this can be quite overwhelming.

Erikson (1968) marks the period of adolescence, from ages 10 to 20 years, as the fifth stage of human psychosocial development. This stage presents the conflict of identity versus identity confusion, and the transition from childhood to adulthood. The achievement of the earlier developmental tasks, regardless of the quality of mastery, becomes integrated into a lasting sense of identity and an emerging recognition of one's place in the society. A more negative outcome is recognised by identity confusion, sexual identity and future occupational potential.

The achievement of a sense of identity is a particularly critical stage for optimal independent functioning and mental health for young people with chronic illness. Young people with chronic illness may spend long periods in hospital or be confined largely to their homes. This situation limits the experience of a social context of peers and the community to work on the developmental conflict of identity versus identify confusion. Other vital experimentation with roles, normal levels of risk-taking behaviours and the development of cognitive abilities has the potential to be limited. The cumulative effect of experiencing fewer developmental experiences and poorer psychosocial development becomes apparent during adolescence. Given that some children and young people spend so much time in hospital during infancy, childhood and adolescence, nursing practice has the capacity to create opportunities for psychosocial growth and development through day-to-day hospital experiences.

Erikson believes that it is not the rapid growth and sexual impulses *per se* that disturb adolescents, but an acute fear of being different or of not conforming to a peer group. Clearly, for the chronically ill young person, this situation can cause increased anxiety. Young people also worry about the future and how they will be able to lead an independent life (Erikson, 1968). The visibility of a disease, in terms of physical difference from peers and forced dependence on others for care, presents major developmental challenges to the conflict of achieving a sense of identity. More often, the developmental trajectory does not conform to the timing and tempo of peers' development. Clearly, an openmind and astute developmental mastery skills are essential to adolescent health nursing practice.

In Case Study 3.6, Ellen, her family and the nurses, within an interprofessional team, work through a number of challenges. For Ellen, these include psychosocial developmental; for her family, anxiety and grieving issues;

Ellen – a young person

Case study 3.6

Ellen is a 16-year-old young woman with cystic fibrosis (CF). The treatment of CF for Ellen includes physiotherapy three times a day, nine enzyme replacement tablets with each meal as well as nebulised medicines twice daily and an average of four hospital admissions each year. Ellen prefers to keep her illness a secret from her peers. She had an earlier experience with a young man who, when he learned Ellen had a terminal inherited disease, did not want to continue seeing her. The young man believed Ellen might die during sexual intercourse, or worse, that she might become pregnant and the disease would affect the child. Ellen has dreamt of having a husband and children before she dies. Ellen's illness has prevented long-term friendships with peers. The experience of being called a 'freak' following a prolonged period of coughing has forced Ellen to fabricate stories to prevent disclosure of the illness to her peers. Ellen's family is quite over-protective, and has provided most of Ellen's health care at home and during admissions to a paediatric hospital.

At the age of 16, Ellen was told her next admission would need to be at the local adult hospital; she had progressed through the hospital's transitional care program to the adult health-care service, but she held reservations about an adult hospital admission.

Ellen was admitted to an adult hospital with a chest infection, her first to an adult hospital. She was very anxious about the admission, resisting until she was very ill.

The adult hospital encouraged independence, and a high level of self-management was expected. Some two weeks into the admission, Ellen became aggressive and refused or delayed her medications, and became almost childlike in her dependency needs. The nurses were surprised and somewhat annoyed to see Ellen's parents bathing and dressing her after they had insisted she practise self-care. Comments from nursing and medical staff included that Ellen was manipulative, immature and lazy, and that she cared little about her health, and that her parents perpetuated the situation. Later psychosocial assessment revealed that in fact Ellen was preoccupied with thoughts of her death as an adult and associated the adult hospital with the end of her life. Ellen preferred to have her parents provide total care, particularly when she was unwell, feared close relationships with adults – especially her peers – and had had thoughts of suicide using her own medication. Ellen felt more protected by assuming the behaviours of a younger developmental stage.

Many unresolved developmental conflicts are clearly evident in Ellen's story: struggles with dependence and independence, identity issues, fears about intimacy and overprotection by understandably very anxious parents with significant enmeshment. Ellen's parents preferred to maintain her dependence to protect her from growing up and having to take care of herself, knowing that she would only get sicker as she got older. Ellen's father commented on the difficulties of caring for Ellen: 'At least we have got her this far and there is no point building her up for a life that is not possible, she was fine until we brought her here.' Ellen confided that adult hospitals expected people to look after themselves, even when they didn't look after themselves at home. She felt self-care was too difficult, and by remaining a child, she kept the family happy. Clearly, these views are understandable responses to an increasingly difficult situation for Ellen and her family, who refused to see a psychiatrist.

The regularity of the hospital admissions and outpatient clinic visits for Ellen and her family provided an opportunity for support, including the final acceptance of a referral to the adolescent consultancy team at the hospital. Subsequent psychosocial and mental state assessments identified high levels of anxiety, long-standing depression and suicidal ideation. Collaboration between the adolescent team clinical nurse consultant, the respiratory physician and the respiratory clinical nurse consultant, and a community youth counsellor enabled treatment for depression and ongoing counselling. Ellen agreed to attend the hospital adolescent group room to mix with other young people with chronic illness, and to continue her schoolwork. Debriefing and group clinical supervision were also extremely valuable for the nurses caring for Ellen.

Ellen's family members were her closest and strongest supports, and eventually, as the nurses came to understand the complexity of the parent–child relationship, they became supportive of both Ellen and her parents. Even more importantly, the nurses understood how to support the family as a unit, in what became a nurse–interdisciplinary team–family relationship. The role of the family working in collaboration with the nurses was invaluable to the psychosocial aspects of her care. Completion of the tasks of adolescent development and the resolution of earlier developmental conflicts for Ellen may not occur until she is well into her twenties or thirties, with total independent functioning most likely impossible. A family therapist was eventually accepted to explore feelings of guilt, grief and loss that had persisted for many years, preventing any sense of hope or normalising of family life.

Cases such as Ellen's are complex, with the effects of the illness and treatment in conflict with the normal trajectory of psychosocial development and, clearly, the expectations of others. In such cases, health services may not have a right to decide what is right or wrong, given the terminal and severe disabling nature of many chronic illnesses, such as cystic fibrosis and cancer. Perhaps what families need from health staff is respect and acceptance for their predicament and the offer of supportive opportunities to meet current developmental needs rather than an assumption of what the young person should be able to achieve and an expectation of the role of parents.

Translation to practice

The developmental environment for many young people with chronic illness is dominated by hospital experiences. These experiences have the opportunity to inhibit or facilitate developmental task mastery. Through their ongoing contact with chronically ill young people and their families, nurses are influential in the health-care context of the young person's developmental world, and they need a thorough understanding of adolescent psychosocial development and risk assessment. Moreover, nurses are perfectly placed to identify young people struggling with psychosocial development, whether represented by treatment adherence or difficult and/or at-risk behaviours. However, given Ellen's story, it is sometimes difficult for nurses to accept that, at times, psychosocial nursing interventions are most appropriately aimed at adding dignity and respect to a clinical situation, rather than promoting developmental mastery.

Intimacy versus isolation: Early adulthood (twenties and thirties) and the sick young adult

Erikson's sixth stage of psychosocial development, spanning the years of the twenties and thirties – the final stage for the focus of this discussion – involves the conflict of intimacy versus isolation (Erikson, 1968). The resolution of this stage is achieved with the establishment of a meaningful life, with a sense of connectedness to other people. Erikson describes this stage as finding oneself, yet also losing oneself in another person (Erikson, 1968). Young adults unable to resolve this conflict are less able to establish close relationships, often fearing rejection and isolating themselves from other people.

During this developmental period, young adults predominately focus on seeking a career and developing intimate relationships with other people. The major developmental task at this stage is a psychological readiness and a commitment to mutual intimacy. This level of intimacy prepares the young adult for marriage or its alternatives to attain and retain individual identity within joint intimacy. If the young adult finds satisfying friendships, but is also able to achieve intimacy with another, the negative resolution of social isolation will be avoided. A negative resolution results in the young person being unable to establish close relationships, increasing the risk of social problems and relationship difficulties (Erikson, 1968).

For some young people with chronic illness, the ability to have an intimate relationship while remaining largely physically dependent on parents or carers is extremely difficult – for some, most likely impossible. This situation may be a result of delayed emergence of adulthood identity as a consequence of prolonged poor self-esteem. Long-term poor self-esteem has been linked to the intractable challenge for some young adults experiencing poor health to find a comfortable identity and a place in society for themselves to emerge into adulthood (Luyckx et al., 2008). Luyckx and colleagues' study – despite some limitations – identified this link and its precursor to adult depression and potentially other psychopathology.

Case Study 3.7 illustrates these challenges for Maria, and the challenge of response and/or helpful nursing care as she is admitted and re-admitted to hospital several times in paediatric and then adult care.

Maria – a young adult

Case study 3.7

Maria was diagnosed with liver failure and subsequently underwent a liver transplant during her late teens. After a period of physical wellness, Maria is diagnosed with severe rejection of the new liver.

At the age of 22, Maria's struggles with life highlight her experience of losing or delaying psychosocial developmental mastery. Maria found herself seeking the safety of more childlike ways of coping with the threat of illness and death. During each hospitalisation, Maria would behave almost like a child, rejecting any efforts by nurses to involve her in self-care; instead, she would cry and ask for mother to care for her. Her mother, clearly distressed, longed to feel needed again and provide all care, including showers and feeding, as the only way she knew to support Maria.

This situation, or identity of being sick, suited Maria and her mother, who were now quite enmeshed. However, in hospital this became a problem as the health goals were for independent functioning and discharge as soon as Maria was medically stable. Nursing staff experienced the brunt of Maria's and her mother's emotions. Despite nursing efforts, Maria's mental state become fragile, increasing her mother's anxiety and bid to reject nursing assistance. This caused great distress among the nursing staff and frustrated bewilderment among the rest of the treating team.

During the final admission, Maria self-harmed, and deliberate attempts to sabotage her treatment while at home became clear. A youth health clinical nurse consultant was called to review care. Subsequent assessments of Maria's psychosocial and mental state revealed her long-standing depression and suicidal ideation rather than a long-standing diagnosis of adjustment disorder without treatment. The consultation liaison psychiatrist and the youth health clinical nurse consultant began to meet regularly with Maria and her mother, some antidepressant medication was commenced and counselling began, which was later continued in the community. A 'care contract' with Maria and her mother was agreed upon, which took Maria's dependence levels into account and moved forward with short- and long-term goals leading to independent functioning and more confidence in self-care with the treatment regimens. It was a lengthy admission, but it was the last one for a long time.

Maria's story highlights the risks and vulnerabilities of cumulative poor developmental task mastery or a regression in developmental mastery. Maria's story begins during her recovery, with intermittent periods of organ rejection. During this recovery, Maria described how being better was the 'greatest challenge of all'. She believed her difficulties had begun not when she was given her diagnosis or during treatment, but when she was considered medically well enough to return to her normal life. Maria felt her problems centred on a loss of who she was and on her inability to see a future of how to be in the world. She was not the person she had been before her health problems emerged, not the heroic person who had survived a transplant, but another person who had to get back to normal – whatever 'normal' had now become.

When the severe rejection emerged, Maria felt more confident and was relieved to return to the identity of the sick person, receiving great support and respect from all around her. Once reluctantly 'cured' again – or rather, the rejection brought under control – Maria began to experience outbursts of temper. She punished herself with work, began to self-harm and refused to eat or to comply with the treatment regimen (medications, routine blood tests, and so on). She was unable to share her feelings with anyone, as she thought they would see her as ungrateful for having receiving a liver from someone who had died and given her this gift of life. Over time, Maria began to develop a new identity and to move on from a state of profound sadness to a desire for the 'sick person identity' to return. She asked, 'Why does the system build you up to be a hero and survivor forever grateful to your donor while you are sick, without preparing you for the fall, when you get better?'

Little and colleagues (2002) define this time of identity confusion and relative safety with the illness as a state of liminality. 'Liminality' is a term that comes from cultural anthropology, and refers to a state of feeling 'betwixt and between' – rather like a social initiation to a new life. The state of liminality occurs when the individual feels they cannot identify with the person they were before the cancer, but feels a sense of fragile security in the identity of a sufferer (Little et al., 2002).

Persistent anxiety and depression – either because of unresolved developmental crises or associated with the loss of previously achieved developmental milestones – may well be the antecedents of adult psychopathology. A lifetime of chronic illness or a new diagnosis during the developmental period of adolescence or young adulthood can bring some similar and other unique challenges. Clearly, a thorough understanding of psychosocial developmental process and mastery, as well as the antecedents and recognition of mental illness in non-mental health settings, is critical to ensure positive psychosocial and medical outcomes.

Reflection points 3.4

- How does psychosocial development influence the way in which children and young people respond to disruptions in health?
- What is the relationship between responsive nursing practice and the psychosocial development of children and young people?
- What role does culture play in influencing the way in which children, young people and their families respond to disruptions in health?

Summary

- At the beginning of this book, we emphasised the growing concerns that exist about the growth in the number of Australian children suffering the burden of chronic illness. Three of the most common chronic conditions impacting Australian children and young people and the health care services supporting them are asthma, diabetes and cancer.
- Developmental disabilities, mental health disorders and eczema are other well-known chronic illnesses of childhood known to affect children's broader health and social wellbeing, daily routines, behaviour and emotional adjustment (Morawska et al., 2014).
- Like adults, children in hospital must adapt to stressful events related to illness, pain and contact with health professionals who are, in the main, strangers to them.
- Major stressors for children are separation, loss of control, injury and pain.
- The way in which the child expresses anxiety and reacts to stress will depend on their growth, stage of development, maturity and repertoire of previous similar experiences.

- In this chapter, we have used a framework of psychosocial development to present responses to illness experiences for children and young people. Respectful and therapeutic responses to these by nurses have been discussed:
    > The welfare of the child and the family as they respond to disruptions in health is the key responsibility of paediatric nurses.
    > Strategies that target responses to disruptions in health include family advocacy, disease prevention and health promotion, health teaching and, importantly, coordination of care.
    > Cultural factors influence the way in which children, young people and their families respond to disruptions in health.
    > Respectful health-care responses to cultural diversity include cultural awareness, acceptance and the provision of spiritual and cultural support.

Learning activities

3.1 Describe the major stress-related factors for a hospitalised child.

3.2 What responses to separation are expected? Discuss in relation to the developmental stage of the child.

3.3 Explain the potential reactions you will encounter in response to injury and pain:
- for an infant
- for a toddler
- for a school-aged child
- for a child older than 12.

3.4 What reactions can siblings have to the hospitalisation of their brother or sister?

3.5 What reactions can parents or caregivers have to the hospitalisation of their child?

3.6 What strategies can the paediatric nurse implement to ameliorate the effect of hospitalisation on the child and family? Include the siblings in your answers.

Further reading

The heavy burden of health problems experienced by the Aboriginal and Torres Strait Islander peoples of Australia, and especially their children and young people, can be overwhelming. The paediatric nurse may feel at a loss to know how their role can make a difference. We suggest the following website, as it provides examples of many successful initiatives that promise hope and resolution: <www.ama.com.au/2013-ama-indigenous-health-report-card-good-news-stories>.

References

Ainsworth, MDS, Blehar, MC, Waters, E, & Wall, S 1978, *Patterns of attachment: A psychological study of the strange situation*, Erlbaum, Hillsdale, NJ.

Australian Government 2013, National Aboriginal and Torres Strait Islander Health Plan 2013–2023, Commonwealth Government, Canberra.

Bandura, A 1977, *Social learning theory*, Prentice Hall, Englewood Cliffs, NJ.

Blackman, JA, Gurka, MJ, Gurka, KK & Oliver, MN 2011, Emotional, developmental and behavioural co-morbidities of children with chronic health conditions, *Journal of Paediatrics and Child Health*, 47(10), pp. 742–7.

Botello-Harbaum, M, Nansel, T, Haynie, DL, Iannotti, RJ & Simons-Morton, B 2008, Responsive parenting is associated with improved type 1 diabetes-related quality of life, *Child: Care, Health and Development*, 34, pp. 675–81.

Bowlby, J 1951, *Maternal care and mental health*, World Health Organization, Geneva.

——1969, *Attachment and loss. Volume 1: Attachment*, Basic Books, New York.

——1988, *A secure base: Clinical applications of attachment theory*, Routledge, London.

Carson, B, Dunbar, T, Chenhall, RD & Bailie, R 2007, *Social determinants of Indigenous health*, Allen & Unwin, Sydney.

Department of Health 1989, *National Aboriginal Health Strategy*, Commonwealth Government, Canberra.

Eksi, A et al. 1995, Psychological adjustment of children with mild and moderately severe asthma, *European Journal of Child and Adolescent Psychiatry*, 4(2), pp. 77–84.

Erikson, EH 1968, *Identity youth and crisis*, WW Norton, New York.

Falvo, D 2013, *Medical and psychosocial aspects of chronic illness and disability*, 4th edn, Jones & Bartlett Learning, Boston.

Gurney, JG et al. 2003, Endocrine and cardiovascular late effects among adult survivors of childhood brain tumors: Childhood Cancer Survivor Study, *Cancer*, 97(3), pp. 663–73.

Hadgkiss, E, Lethborg, C, Al-Mousa, A & Marck, C 2012, *Asylum seeker health and wellbeing*, St Vincent's Health Australia, Sydney.

Helgeson, VS, Honcharuk, E, Becker, D, Escobar, O & Siminerio, L 2011, A focus on blood glucose monitoring: Relation to glycemic control and determinants of frequency, *Pediatric Diabetes*, 12, pp. 25–30.

Hysing, M, Elgen, I, Gillberg, C & Lundervold, AJ 2007, Chronic physical illness and mental health in children: Results from a large-scale population study, *Journal of Child Psychology and Psychiatry*, 48, pp. 785–92.

—— 2009, Emotional and behavioural problems in subgroups of children with chronic illness: Results from a large-scale population study, *Child: Care, Health and Development*, 35(4), pp. 527–33.

Ievers, CE, Drotar, D, Dahms, WT, Doershuk, CF & Stern, RC 1994, Maternal child-rearing behavior in three groups: Cystic fibrosis, insulin-dependent diabetes mellitus, and healthy children, *Journal of Pediatric Psychology*, 19, pp. 681–7

Lambert, V, Coad, J, Hicks, P & Glacken, M 2013, Social spaces for young children in hospital, *Child: Care, health and development*, 40(2), pp. 195–204.

Little, M, Jordens, CFC, Paul, K & Sayers, E-J 2002, Survivorship and discourses of identity, *Psycho-Oncology*, 11(2), pp. 170–8.

Luyckx, K, Seiffge-Krenke, IS, Schwartz, SJ, Goossens, L, Weets, L, Hendrieckx, C & Grovend, C 2008, Identity development, coping, and adjustment in emerging adults with a chronic illness: The sample case of type 1 diabetes, *Journal of Adolescent Health*, 43(5), pp. 451–8.

Meijer, SA et al. 2000, Social functioning in children with a chronic illness, *Journal of Child Psychology and Psychiatry*, 41, pp. 309–17.

Melnyk, BM et al. 2004, Creating opportunities for parent empowerment: Program effects on the mental health/coping outcomes of critically ill young children and their mothers, *Pediatrics*, 113(6), pp. e597–607.

Morawska, A, Calam, R & Fraser, J 2014, Parenting interventions for childhood chronic illness: A review and recommendations for intervention design and delivery, *Journal of Child Health Care*, viewed 18 June 2014, http://www.ncbi.nlm.nih.gov/pubmed/24486817.

Newman, BM & Newman, PR 2011, Is there a sensitive period for attachment? In BM Newman & PR Newman, *Development through life: A psychosocial approach*, Wadsworth/Cengage, Belmont, CA, pp. 166–238.

Northern Sydney Local Health District Aboriginal Health Services 2013, *Aboriginal Health Services Plan 2013–2016*, viewed 1 June 2014, www.nslhd.health.nsw.gov.au/AboutUs/publications/Documents/Aboriginal%20Health%20Service%20Plan%202013-2016%20Final.pdf.

Park, H & Walton-Moss, B 2012, Parenting style, parenting stress, and children's health-related behaviours, *Journal of Developmental and Behavioral Pediatrics*, 33(6), pp. 495–503.

Pinquart, M & Shen, Y 2011, Behavior problems in children and adolescents with chronic physical illness, *Journal of Paediatric Psychology*, 36(9), pp. 1003–16.

Small, L 2002, Early predictors of poor coping outcomes in children following intensive care hospitalisation and stressful medical encounters, *Paediatric Nursing*, 28(4), pp. 393–8.

Smith, BA & Kaye, DL 2012, Treating parents of children with chronic health conditions: The role of the general psychiatrist, *Focus*, 10, n.p.

Streisand, R, Swift, E, Wickmark, T, Chen, R & Holmes, CS 2005, Pediatric parenting stress among parents of children with type 1 diabetes: The role of self-efficacy, responsibility, and fear, *Journal of Pediatric Psychology*, 30(6), pp. 513–21.

Svavarsdottir, EK & Orlygsdottir, B 2006, Comparison of health-related quality of life among 10- to 12-year-old children with chronic illnesses and healthy children: The parents' perspective, *Journal of School Nursing*, 22(3), pp. 178–85.

Svensson, B, Bornehag, CG & Janson, S 2011, Chronic conditions in children increase the risk for physical abuse – but vary with socio-economic circumstances, *Acta Paediatrica*, 100(3), pp. 407–12.

Turkel, S, Pao, M 2007, Late consequences of pediatric chronic illness, *The Psychiatric Clinics of North America*, 30(4), pp. 819–35.

Werner, E & Smith, R 1992, *Overcoming the odds: High-risk children from birth to adulthood*, Cornell University Press, New York.

4 Research in the paediatric setting

Donna Waters

Learning objectives

In this chapter you will:

- Explore your understanding of the terms 'research', 'evidence' and 'evidence-based practice'
- Be introduced to the core principles of human research ethics and research governance
- Develop your knowledge of how these core principles apply to research conducted in the paediatric setting
- Reflect on how you can use this knowledge in your work as a paediatric nurse to support evidence-based practice for children and young people, and encourage their partnership in research.

Introduction

Members of the Australian public have a right to assume that the practice of every health professional is based on the best available **evidence** from **research**, and that this evidence is informing the safety and quality of their care. Parents and carers of children and young people extend this assumption to health-care decisions made on behalf of those in their care. The tenet of using the best available evidence for decision-making is so self-evident and fundamental to health care that standards relating to quality, safety, research and evidence-based practice can be found in the competency standards of all health disciplines.

> **Evidence**
> Contextualised knowledge from research (external) and other (internal) sources
>
> **Research** A systematic and rigorous process for the creation of new knowledge

Research and evidence are intimately linked in nursing and health care, but each makes a slightly different contribution. We can broadly distinguish research as a systematic process for deriving new knowledge, and evidence as the knowledge that is produced. However, evidence from other sources is also used to inform health and treatment decisions. The experience of the clinician, the context of the health-care environment and information about the specific values and priorities of the person or group receiving care ultimately shape decisions about how the evidence is used. Sometimes these sources of knowledge are referred to as external evidence (from research) and internal evidence (related to the persons or setting).

Evidence from research (which we term research evidence) offers new ways of delivering care in paediatrics, for treating ill-health or disease, and for maintaining the wellbeing of families. Research evidence also offers knowledge about what is most important to children, young people and their families, and informs decisions about paediatric workforce needs and research priorities. A natural question that arises when discussing research and evidence relates to what needs to happen with the new knowledge gained from research. Often it is enough to simply add new findings to the paediatric knowledge base, but sometimes the results of research are so powerful that consideration must be given to whether the results should be used to implement a change in practice. Research then becomes the evidence used for practice improvement.

It is sometimes assumed that, as a health professional becomes more experienced in their specialty, their knowledge of research will increase by association. But it takes years to train to be a nurse, and more years of practical experience and education to become a specialist in a field such as paediatrics. If you think of research as another specialty, you can more easily understand that specialist training is also required to become a successful researcher. Further, a different set of skills is needed for clinicians and other health professionals to apply research to the clinical or practice setting.

This first part of this book has discussed the context of paediatric nursing in Australia, and concludes with a discussion of the particular challenges researchers face when conducting research with children and young people. In this chapter, we begin by clarifying the language of research and evidence for nursing. We discuss special considerations for conducting ethical research with children and young people. Finally, we look at how you can support children and young people to become more involved in research and gain influence in setting research priorities. But first, read Case Study 4.1, to which we will refer later in the chapter.

Case study 4.1: Benefit versus harm

Cystic fibrosis (CF) is a common genetic condition in Australia, with approximately one in every four people carrying a mutation of the CF gene. The condition affects a number of organs, including the lungs, pancreas and liver. Because many children and young adults with CF also have pancreatic insufficiency, malnutrition and deficiencies of the fat-soluble vitamins (A, D, E and K) are common. Vitamin E deficiency has been associated with peripheral neuropathy, osteomalacia and inflammation.

You are a paediatric nurse working in the CF out-patients clinic and while you are weighing a 5-year-old boy, the parent shares that he has been approached by a member of a research team (a gastroenterologist) who is conducting a study to look at vitamin E and peripheral nerve dysfunction in children with CF. The study information sheet and consent form the parent shows you states that the child will be required to undergo nerve conduction studies and electromyography on two occasions over the next 12 months, before and after entering a randomised controlled trial of high-dose vitamin E supplementation.

The parent asks you, 'What is the benefit of this research to my child?' and 'Would you allow your child to be part of this study?'

How would you answer?

What is research?

In Chapter 1, we defined some common terms used in the reporting of population statistics. In this chapter, we define terms used in health research and ethics. Somewhat confusingly in research, you will find that people use the same words in different ways, depending on their disciplinary training or geographical background. For example, the term 'knowledge translation' is used extensively in the United States and Canada to describe the process of moving what we have learned from research through to application in health care and practice settings. But you will also see this process referred to as knowledge transfer, research/knowledge diffusion and dissemination. In the United Kingdom and Europe, the term 'evidence implementation' includes research utilisation and evidence transfer. Collectively, these terms refer to a process that is now branded as 'implementation science', or the study of approaches and methods used for evidence transfer or knowledge translation.

Generating knowledge through research

Research is a systematic and rigorous process used for the generation of new knowledge. Researchers choose from a range of **methodological** approaches

> **Methodology**
> The research approach, activities, sample, methods, measures and analyses required to logically follow the steps of the research process to answer the research question – for example, phenomenology
>
> **Method** The application of a common process, tool or technique to collect research data – for example, an in-depth interview with a young person recently diagnosed with epilepsy
>
> **Answerable research question** A clearly articulated and focused research or practice question that is framed to maximise the efficiency and effectiveness of searching literature in order to answer the question
>
> **Research design** The detailed outline or plan of how the research will proceed – for example, a proposal to explore the lived experience of young people diagnosed with epilepsy (a qualitative study). The design includes plans for funding and timelines

and select **methods** to find the answer to a focused and **answerable research question**. In general, an answerable question will define a **p**opulation, person or problem; an **i**ntervention or issue; a **c**omparison group (if used); and have clearly defined **o**utcomes. The **t**imeframe or type of study may also be included. It is common to see questions written in this PICO(T) format.

The systematic and rigorous process of research proceeds through a series of standard steps, but what happens at each step will vary, depending on the theoretical and methodological approach chosen by the researcher. The steps are:

- Define the problem.
- Pose an answerable research question.
- Search the literature to see what is already known.
- Develop a **research design** and choose an appropriate method.
- Gain ethical approval and funding (if required).
- Conduct the study.
- Analyse the results to answer the question.
- Disseminate the results.

Imagine that you are following the steps of the research process to answer a question about effective post-operative pain management in infants. Then think about this same question applied to an adult post-operative setting. The difference in **p**opulations will likely influence your choice of theoretical perspective and application of methodology and method. At each step, you will need to think in a different way about how to answer this question, considering the type of surgery children and adults have, how they are managed post-operatively, the medications that are used for pain (the **i**ntervention), how pain is measured (the **o**utcome) and so on. The process for gaining ethics approval and consent would also be different, but the steps of the research process remain the same. Before we move on, let's be sure that we have a good grasp of research language and how it might be applied to a research question.

What is evidence-based practice?

We have distinguished research as a systematic and rigorous process for deriving new knowledge, and evidence as the knowledge that is produced from research.

We have also acknowledged the contribution of evidence from internal sources in health and treatment decisions. In reality, there are many research questions that simply have not yet been answered, and many for which research exists but may not be of sufficient quality to allow us to confidently answer the question. These are important issues in the generation of evidence from research. The evidence derived directly from research is also called research evidence or external evidence.

Possibilities for using evidence from research can also be impacted from the delivery or demand side (Figure 4.1). For example, good-quality research may exist to answer our question, but the health-care environment may prevent us from acting upon the evidence. This could occur when a health service has insufficient staffing or other resources to change practice, or is unable to offer a new treatment because of cost. Other possibilities are that the child, young person or family simply does not accept the treatment choices offered by the evidence, or that clinicians and other stakeholders are unable to support a practice change. Figure 4.1 illustrates that the success of using evidence in practice relies both on the generation of evidence (the research supply side) as well as the delivery (the demand side).

One less palatable possibility should be mentioned. This is where good-quality evidence from research exists and is well disseminated and possible to implement, but for whatever reason a health professional chooses to ignore it. An example of this occurred in Bristol in the early 1990s, when a consultant

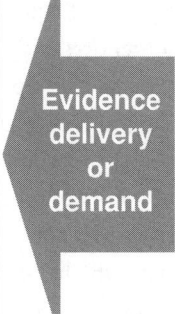

FIGURE 4.1 *Possibilities for generating and using research evidence*

anaesthetist exposed very poor outcomes from cardiac surgery at the Bristol Royal Infirmary (Savulescu, 2002). The hospital had refused requests to investigate three paediatric surgeons who six years later were found guilty of serious professional misconduct. The actions of this so-called whistleblower not only significantly improved the subsequent mortality rates of children having heart surgery in Bristol, but also established basic principles and practices for what is now known as clinical governance across the United Kingdom, Australia and New Zealand.

Evidence as contextualised knowledge

Earlier, we described evidence as contextualised knowledge from research and other sources, and Figure 4.1 showed that a number of possibilities exist for generating and using evidence. But evidence also comes from many other internal sources, the most important of which is the intrinsic cultural and ethical values and preferences of children, young people and their families. Rather than ignoring internal evidence, synthesis of this knowledge with external evidence from research is what permits us to deliver personalised, high-quality and safe care to children and young people in a contextually appropriate way.

It is well known that recommendations for **evidence-based practice** are made with reference to a series of steps (see Table 4.1). Some of these steps are consistent with the research process, but there is a major area of divergence when it comes to the 'doing' of research or the 'using' of evidence. The evidence-based practitioner derives questions directly from their practice. How often have you had a thought like: 'This child keeps pulling their bandages off. I wonder whether there is another dressing I could use to keep the wound covered?' Clearly you cannot immediately set up a randomised controlled trial to test two different types of dressing to help you answer this question. But what you can do is focus your question (*ask*), conduct a search of the research literature (*access*), determine the quality and appropriateness of the literature you find (*appraise*), answer your question and *apply* your new knowledge to your practice, and then *assess* or evaluate whether the change has made a difference. Sometimes you see the five 'As' of evidence-based practice written as **a**ssess the problem or patient, **a**sk the question, **a**cquire the evidence, **a**ppraise it, then **a**pply it to practice.

Regardless, we know that health care is not delivered in a vacuum, and it is in the implementation stage of evidence-based practice that contextualised

> **Evidence-based practice** The application of the best available evidence to the practice setting

TABLE 4.1 *The research process and evidence-based practice*

A RESEARCHER	AN EVIDENCE-BASED PRACTITIONER
• Asks a research question	• Asks a practice question
• Conducts a review of literature	• Conducts a review of literature
• Develops a research design	• Determines the quality of evidence from the literature
• Determines the best method to use	
• Gains ethical approval and funding (if required)	• Summarises the results
	• Answers the question
• Conducts the research study	• Applies results or implements practice changes
• Analyses the results	
• Answers the question	• Evaluates the impact or effectiveness of change
• Disseminates (publishes) the results	

knowledge from other sources most significantly impacts upon the process. There are always going to be a number of competing factors, and every health care encounter will be slightly different because each child and family is different. Similarly, a young person might exercise their right to choose to ignore your advice, regardless of how strong the evidence might be for a particular recommendation. The complex interplay of research evidence with clinician contribution (or lack of such contribution due to experience), and patient and family preference, takes place within the context of a clinic, hospital, home or community – all of which, of course, are also moderated by economic, environmental, social and political context.

While nurses generally accept evidence-based practice, basing practice on evidence is definitely not easy. The US Agency for Healthcare Research and Quality (AHRQ) is often quoted for stating that it may take as long as one or two decades for original research to reach routine clinical practice (AHRQ, 2001). Considering the internal and external factors influencing the implementation of evidence in paediatrics, we clearly have a lot of work still to do.

Reflection points 4.1

- As with any new language or jargon, research language can be intimidating and confusing for someone who is not used to it. Do you believe nurse educators and academics are adequately preparing paediatric nurses for using research?

- 'Research' and 'evidence' are terms that are often used interchangeably, but in fact their meanings are perceptibly different. Do you think the careless use of these words has had any impact on how nurses working in neonatal and paediatric care settings feel about research?
- Evidence can be derived from research (external evidence) or from other sources (internal evidence). What impact might the geographical location, setting or health-care environment have on our ability to use evidence?
- Evidence-based practice is usually presented as a series of five steps, consisting of asking a question, accessing evidence, appraising the quality of the evidence, applying results in practice and assessing or evaluating the effect of the change. Which of these five steps do you think would be the most challenging in paediatric nursing practice, and why?

Researching with children and young people

Before we begin this section, we return again to the language of research. As health professionals, we are privileged to have the opportunity to conduct research with the children, young people, families and carers with whom we come into contact. But this is a privilege, not a right. You will sometimes see or hear researchers refer to research 'in' people or research 'on' people, but how can this be? No researcher, however esteemed, has the right to assume ownership over the rights of another adult or child. The ethics of research include the principles of respect for people and their rights, beneficence and justice, and therefore presume that we conduct research with people and not 'on' them. At a time when not all children receive even basic human rights, it is important to understand that the principles of research and research governance founded in the Nuremburg Code (see Research ethics section that follows) are intended to be applied fully and globally.

Human research and ethics

Human research includes any research that is conducted with or about people, their data, or their tissue. While the process (that is, the steps) of research is largely the same whenever and wherever it is conducted, the paediatric setting presents some specific challenges related to the ethical conduct of human research. Children and young people have various developmental capacities for understanding their involvement in health-care decisions and research, and are nominated as a vulnerable group under Australian ethics guidelines. Further, research with children and young people raises many questions about the ethics of consent and the possibility of conflicting values when parents or carers are giving consent for research participation on behalf of children and young people. This is why offering rewards for participation in paediatric research is rarely regarded as appropriate during consent, and why rewards should never be offered to prevent children withdrawing from a study (RACP, 2008).

The future will present even greater challenges for human research ethics as personal data are collected, shared and stored through social media networks, and banks of human DNA and tissue are progressively accrued through prenatal and newborn screening programs. Further, improved technologies increasingly permit leftover blood or tissue obtained from clinical or screening procedures to be stored for future research, offering enormous potential for genetic and biomedical research. While the Australian National Statement on Ethical Conduct in Human Research (NHMRC, 2007b) provides guidance to human research ethics committees and others, access to specimens stored in human bio-banks will continue to raise important ethical questions into the future. It is increasingly common for research consents to include 'opting in', which gives implied consent to use data or samples for research conducted into the indefinite future. Opting out involves a person actively refusing permission for their sample to be stored and/or used for further research. There remains a great deal of speculation about appropriate opt-in and opt-out procedures with children and young people, and parents are often unaware of their rights and responsibilities around consenting or opting out (Giesbertz et al., 2012). Mechanisms for allowing the young person's autonomous affirmation of consent when they either have capacity or reach the statutory age of consent need to be built into the research design.

Research ethics

The ethics of human research are based on three fundamental principles, which broadly attest that any risks from the research will be outweighed by the contribution of the research to improving health and health care and, that the dignity, privacy and wellbeing of the research participant will be protected at all times. It is difficult to discuss health ethics without reference to history. While codes and guidelines for the ethical conduct of research certainly existed prior to World War II, a lack of mechanisms for monitoring and reporting meant that unethical experiments were rarely exposed. Following the war, a formal investigation into experiments performed by the Nazis culminated in the Nuremberg Trials and became a pivotal point for the development of a universal written code of medical ethics known as the Nuremberg Code of 1947. Interestingly, the first of the 10 principles in the Code relates to the giving of voluntary consent by the human subject. While we now refer to this as the principle of autonomy, at the time, the Code technically precluded children or any other person unable to give direct *voluntary* consent from participation in research (Davidson & O'Brien, 2009).

> **Autonomy**
> Respect for human beings – a fundamental principle of human research ethics. This principle refers to respect for the privacy, confidentiality, customs, perceptions and cultural sensitivities of research participants, and recognises the value and intrinsic right of individuals and collectives to make decisions about participation in research

The Declaration of Helsinki was developed during a general assembly of the World Medical Association in Helsinki in 1964. The Declaration attempted to reflect the major principles of the Nuremberg Code within the specific context of biomedical research. The Declaration has been revised several times, most recently in 2013, and is available online. A range of international organisations have since developed and published guidelines for the ethical conduct of health and biomedical research, including the Council for International Organisations of Medical Sciences (CIOMS) and the World Health Organization (WHO). Australian guidelines have been developed jointly by the National Health and Medical Research Council (NHMRC), the Australian Research Council (ARC) and the Australian Vice-Chancellors' Committee (AVCC). These are published as the National Statement on Ethical Conduct in Human Research 2007 (or National Statement), and were last updated in March 2014 (NHMRC, 2007b). All guidelines developed since the Nuremberg Code specifically outline sections relating to research with vulnerable groups, which include children.

Another pivotal point in the history of human research ethics followed investigation of an experiment commenced in 1932 with African American men who had contracted syphilis. The Tuskegee Experiment (named after the Alabama town where the study was conducted) ran for almost 40 years, and is infamous for denying study participants full information about their disease and access to treatment when this was available (Jones, 1993). The Belmont Report was commissioned by the US Congress in 1974 and, in addition to investigating the Tuskegee Experiment, attempted to further clarify and articulate principles from the Nuremberg Code and Declaration of Helsinki for the conduct of research involving humans. Specifically the report attempted to delineate what we might today call basic research (laboratory or benchtop experimentation) from clinical or applied research conducted with people.

There is documentary evidence dating back to the nineteenth century showing that children in paediatric hospitals and orphanages were being researched 'on', and children and young people were certainly among those experimented on under the guise of medical research during World War II. During the 1960s, parents of mentally disabled children who were institutionalised at the Willowbrook School in New York were forced to consent to their children being infected with hepatitis during vaccine development experiments (Link, 2005). Australia also features among examples of unethical practices, with Dr William McBride, an obstetrician in Sydney, found guilty of falsifying research data in the early 1990s (Purchase, 2004).

Core principles of research ethics

The National Statement organises the discussion of ethical values in research around the central principle of respect for human beings. While this guideline maintains the three fundamental ethical principles of research contained in the Belmont Report (respect for persons, beneficence and justice), reference is also made to research merit and integrity. The broader ethical values of altruism, contribution to societal or community goals, respect for cultural diversity, and nationally specific values are included in a companion document to the National Statement, entitled *Values and Ethics: Guidelines for Ethical Conduct in Aboriginal and Torres Strait Islander Health Research* (NHMRC, 2003).

Research merit and integrity

The principles of respect for persons, beneficence and justice exist under the assumption that any research of poor scientific merit will be unethical. Any child, young person or adult has a right to expect that before their participation in a study is considered, the proposed research has a clear and answerable aim or question, is informed by current research evidence, uses an appropriate design and method, can actually be completed and the results reported (remember the steps of the research process), and will be conducted or supervised by researchers with appropriate paediatric experience and training within a safe and appropriately resourced environment. The role of human research ethics committees is discussed later, but for now we can say that it is also expected that any research involving humans will be reviewed at some level by the ethics committee of the institution at which the study will be conducted. The ethics committee has a role in monitoring **research governance** processes.

> **Research governance** The processes by which institutions establish, conduct and oversee the ethics, quality and safety of human research. This includes establishing and operating institutional human research ethics committees (HRECs) and monitoring individual researcher accountabilities for the ethical design and scientific rigour of their studies. Australian institutions must also ensure that any research for which they are responsible complies with the Australian Code for the Responsible Conduct of Research and the National Statement on Ethical Conduct in Human Research

Human research ethics committees require sufficient evidence of the scientific merit of a study for a decision to be made about the balance of actual or potential risks for the participant against the stated aims of the research. There is an expectation that the proposal will demonstrate that the research will be sufficiently feasible (that it can actually be completed) and scoped (to produce a reliable result) in order to make a meaningful contribution to knowledge. The Australian Code for the Responsible Conduct of Research (NHMRC, 2007a) explains the specific role of institutions and researchers in promoting research integrity, and offers advice on managing departures from best practice such as research misconduct.

With regard to specific considerations for children and young people, research governance principles focus on whether the research method is appropriate for the age and developmental maturity of the intended sample of children, and whether the researchers have the appropriate training and experience to work with children and young people in the context of their research question. An important aspect of the research design will be to describe how children and young people will be approached for participation (recruited to the study); whether the facility or environment in which the study is to be conducted is appropriate to their needs; any potential impact on the child's family or community, such as may occur in school-based research; and a clear description of how researchers will judge the capacity of their potential participants to understand the project and its risks, and give their consent to participate.

Autonomy and respect

The principle of respect recognises that individuals have an intrinsic human value and the right to make autonomous or collective decisions about participation in research. This respect includes valuing the interactions human beings have with each other through common beliefs, customs, perceptions and culture, as well as individual rights to privacy and confidentiality. For children and young people, these interactions extend to relationships with parents and carers, and include the responsibilities of parents and carers to protect children and young people with diminished developmental capacity to make autonomous decisions. In addition to ethical considerations applicable to all humans, the National Statement also identifies specific participants who are considered vulnerable within the context of research. Vulnerable participants include pregnant girls and women and the human foetus; children and young people; people in dependent or unequal relationships; people highly dependent on medical care who may be unable to give consent; people with a cognitive impairment, intellectual disability or mental illness; people who may be involved in illegal activities; Aboriginal and Torres Strait Islander peoples; and people in other countries (NHMRC, 2007b). It is noteworthy that, in addition being named as a vulnerable group in their own right, children and young people may be represented in any or all of these other vulnerable groups.

The National Statement respects the different developmental capacities of children and young people to be involved in decisions about participation in research in two ways: first, the guidelines do not specify exact ages at which consent may or may not be given; and second, the guidelines are flexible around decisions about a child's level of maturity and subsequent capacity to understand the complexities of the proposed research. Apart from suggesting responsiveness to a child's developmental capacity to understand their involvement in research, the National Statement proposes that even young children 'should be engaged *at their level* in discussion about the research and its likely outcomes' (NHMRC, 2007b: 50). Therefore, while an infant clearly cannot participate in this discussion, an older child may be able to understand and ask questions, and may be deemed mature enough to give fully informed and free consent.

Consent in paediatric research

Obtaining consent for participation in research is central to respect for persons. Free and informed consent implies a voluntary decision that is not influenced by coercion, pressure or inducement (Davidson & O'Brien, 2009). When a child is unable to give free and informed consent, parents or guardians are asked to make a judgement based on their interpretation of the child's best interests and the level of risk to be endured for the sake of others. Parents and children are also both at risk of the sometimes subtle coercion that may exist when a favourite nurse or doctor asks them to join a research project.

Australian states and territories each have specific legislation around the age at which minors are deemed to have capacity to consent to treatment (RACP, 2008), but this may not apply directly to participation in a research project. Paediatric research participants can be grouped into three broad categories for discussion of consent for participation in research; however, as the National Statement suggests, it is inappropriate to define individual maturity by age or assume that the complexity of the research is beyond the understanding of the child. It is clear that infants are unable to give free and informed consent, so only parental consent is required. Children may have the capacity to understand the nature of the research and may consent to participate. However, children are still considered vulnerable, and their research participation will require the additional consent of one parent. Finally, mature children and young people capable of understanding the risks and benefits of their participation in research may give sole consent and parental consent may be waived.

In general, consent from children and young people should be gained in the following circumstances:

- For a child or young person, consent may be obtained when they have the capacity to make the decision with additional consent from *either* one parent, guardian or primary caregiver (or any organisation or person required by law).
- For a young person, sole consent may be given as long as the ethics review body is satisfied that the young person is mature enough to understand the relevant information; the research involves no more than low risk; and the research will be of benefit to the group of young people to which the participant belongs, or the young person is estranged or separated from parents or guardian, or it would be contrary to the best interests of the young person to seek parental consent (NHMRC, 2007b: 51).

Exceptions to these general rules can occur when an ethical review body may decide that the nature of the research requires the consent of both parents, or where vulnerabilities might exist in aspects of the life of a young person that are unrelated to their understanding of consent. For example, this might include developmental aspects of accepting risk and burden for moral or altruistic reasons, social immaturity or homelessness. Researchers must therefore take the capacity of each individual child or young person into consideration during the process of consent. The project and all risks should be explained in developmentally appropriate language and with consideration to what is important and valued by the child and their family. This respect for children and young people is fundamental to recognising the intrinsic value of human beings and their capacity to make autonomous decisions about participation in research, including rights to privacy and confidentiality. These basic rights are declared in the World Medical Association's Ottawa Declaration on the Rights of the Child to Health Care, adopted in 1998 and amended in 2009 (WMA, 2009).

In addition to involvement in health and medical research, children and young people also have significant representation in educational research. You may already be aware that the National Statement has a provision that permits parents to give **standing parental consent** to research conducted within the educational setting. Schools may, for example, seek standing parental consent at the beginning of a school year for their child's involvement in research, provided that the research is deemed to be of benefit to children of a similar age and does not compromise learning or involve disclosure of sensitive personal or family relationship and/or potentially identifiable information.

> **Standing parental consent** Enables parents to give consent to their child's involvement in one or more research projects about which they have been informed on the understanding that they may withdraw consent for their child's participation for any individual project or withdraw standing consent at any time

You may see the word 'assent' used in discussions about the participation of children and young people in research. Assent relates to a child agreeing to participate in research without the giving of free and informed consent. It has certainly happened that parents have given consent on behalf of a child who has refused to assent. In this case, it is clearly inappropriate to proceed. In general, both parental and child assent are required for participation in research – except, of course, in the case of infants or where clear possibilities of benefit from the research are demonstrated to the parent. This leads to the next of the three fundamental ethical principles, beneficence, which attests that any risks from the research will be outweighed by the contribution of the research to improvements in health and health care.

Beneficence in paediatric research

The ethical principle of **beneficence** relates to the balancing the risk of benefit and harm in research. In general, researchers are responsible to ensure that their research design minimises any actual or potential risk to participants. Where there are minimal or no likely direct benefits to research participants, the researcher must demonstrate that the risk of participation is lower than would be ethically acceptable when there are likely benefits (NHMRC, 2007b).

> **Beneficence** The act of benefiting others, or contributing to the greater good. In research ethics, beneficence relates to actions taken to remove or reduce any risk or harms associated with the research

Harm In research, harm can be perceived or real. Harm may be physical (such a pain or injury) or psychological (such as feeling guilty, upset or humiliated). Social harm relates to damage of relationships within social networks. Economic and legal harm relates to the imposition of costs or legal prosecution as a result of participation in research

Beneficence is also demonstrated by participants of a research study when they undertake an estimate of their personal level of risk against the risk of not contributing towards improvements in health or health care that may result from the research. Non-maleficence (or doing no **harm**) is another term used in the discussion of benefit versus harm in research. The idea of potential harm to a research participant is balanced by the notion that any perceived or real harm or risk to be suffered will be outweighed or exceeded by the benefit accrued by the individual on behalf of the greater good. In the context of research ethics, a risk is anything that has the potential for harm, discomfort or inconvenience.

Discomfort is a less serious form of risk that can also be physical or psychological, and can be perceived or real. When looking at the difference between methodologies and methods earlier, we gave an example of conducting research with young people being interviewed for their lived experience of being diagnosed with epilepsy. A young person might become psychologically distressed or uncomfortable talking about their experiences, but they are unlikely to suffer long-term harm. There is often a level of inconvenience associated with participation in research. This is especially relevant for parents or carers of children and young people, who may need to take time away from work or family, or who incur financial or emotional costs connected with their child's participation in research. In our example, it may or may not be appropriate to conduct these in-depth interviews in the young person's own home, or in a neutral environment close to psychological support and counselling if needed.

A related concept to ensuring that the research design provides the best possible approach to maintaining the emotional, psychological and physical safety of participants is that of maintaining the best interests of the child or young person. This includes many of the principles we have already discussed, such as respect of a child's right to refuse to participate, the capacity of the child to understand the research and give consent, and for refusal to be overridden by the parent's judgement if this is deemed to be in the best interests of the child or young person. An example clearly demonstrating the failure of researchers to maintain the best interests of children comes from the well-known case of Dr Wakefield and his fraudulent claims of a link between the measles, mumps and rubella (MMR) vaccine and the appearance of autism and bowel disease (Godlee et al., 2011).

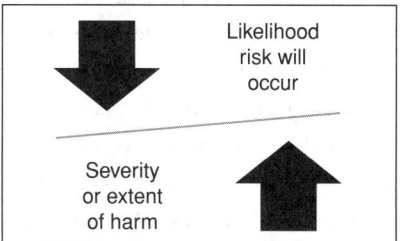

FIGURE 4.2 *Balancing the risk of harm in research participation*

It is generally accepted that the level of risk to which children and young people are exposed through participation in research should be lower than that for adult research participants. However, the assessment of risk is different for everyone, and it is important to remember that risk can be actual or perceived. Risk is the potential for harm, discomfort or inconvenience to occur. The assessment of risk is also about weighing the relative probabilities associated with the likelihood of risk occurring, and the severity or extent of harm that may result if the risk occurs (Figure 4.2). Knowing the probability and severity of risk is one of the ways in which children, young people and their parents or guardians can judge the extent to which they are at risk from participating in research, and researchers and ethics committees can determine how these risks might be minimised and managed.

Human research ethics committees will generally allocate research to a category of risk to determine the level of ethical review required. Research of 'low or negligible risk' refers to types of research in which the actual or perceived risk is gauged to be no greater than discomfort (low) or inconvenience (negligible). In the United States, the term 'minimal risk' is used to denote risk that is no greater than what a child might expect to encounter in everyday life – a child might expect to fall off a bike, for example. However, as Davidson and O'Brien (2009) suggest, a single blood test on a calm infant performed by an experienced venepuncturist using a topical anaesthetic can present an entirely different level of risk when the infant becomes distressed.

Now let's revisit Case Study 4.1 to determine how you might answer the questions posed by the parent of your young patient with CF. To reiterate, you are a paediatric nurse working in the CF out-patients clinic and while you are weighing a 5-year-old boy, the parent shares that he has been approached by a member of a research team (a gastroenterologist) who is conducting a study to look at vitamin E and peripheral nerve dysfunction in children with CF. The patient information sheet and consent form the parent shows you states that the child will be required to undergo nerve conductions studies and electromyography on two occasions over the next 12 months, before and after entering a randomised controlled trial of high-dose vitamin E supplementation. The parent has asked you: 'What is the benefit of this research to my child?' In brackets after each point below are the ethical principles to consider:

- The child and parent have a five-year relationship with a member of the research team, who is also the child's gastroenterologist (coercion?).
- The child has a chronic childhood disease and may have participated in many paediatric research studies during their five years of life (justice?).
- The child may end up being randomised to either the treatment (vitamin E) or placebo (no treatment) arm of the randomised controlled trial (respect for persons and autonomy?).
- Is the child willing to participate in the study, undertake the testing and take more pills (assent and consent?)?
- Nerve conduction studies can be painful (potential for harm?).
- The child and/or parent will need to make at least two extra trips to the hospital for testing, and attend the pharmacy to pick up the medication (inconvenience?).

We will return to your considered response to the parent after we look at the ethical principle of justice.

Justice in paediatric research

Justice is an integral part of all ethical research because this principle is concerned with fairness and equity. Consideration of justice starts with the experience of researchers within the paediatric setting and their ability to focus the research question and design of the study to be consistent with the way children and young people feel comfortable in the world. For example, has the research been designed to maximise chances of participation? Is the process of recruitment fair? Will all children and young people benefit equally from the results? We see examples of research inequity and injustice frequently in the Australian context. Paediatric research translated to care and treatment in the large metropolitan hospitals and clinics may remain largely unknown and unseen in smaller rural and remote facilities. There are also many sub-groups within the Australian paediatric population that we know to be excluded from both participation in and the benefits of research and new discoveries.

- The child's gastroenterologist is an active and experienced researcher who has already contributed significant research evidence to improving the care of children with CF.
- The study has been approved by a human research ethics committee, and the information sheet and consent form clearly state the risks (discomfort) of the nerve conduction studies, describe the randomisation and the possibility that the child may allocated to the placebo arm of the trial.
- High-dose vitamin E is unlikely to be harmful to this child if he is allocated to the treatment arm of the trial.
- The child is likely to experience some discomfort during the testing and the parent will be inconvenienced by two additional trips to the hospital (unless the visits can coincide with routine clinic visits).
- The results of the research are likely to be influential in the future management of fat-soluble vitamin deficiency in CF and, if findings are positive, may potentially reduce or prevent the effects of future peripheral nerve dysfunction.

FIGURE 4.3 *Formulating an answer to a question about participation in research*

Fairness also relates to the burden of the research, as previously discussed. For example, is the inconvenience caused to children and their parents reasonable compared with the actual benefit that an individual child might gain? Is the participation of children and young people indispensable to the conduct of the research, or could the questions be answered by the recruitment of adult participants only? Within the context of autonomy and beneficence, the principle of justice is deeply embedded in decisions around whether it is justifiable to involve children and young people in research when they may not benefit directly, particularly when considering the issue of maturity to give free and informed consent and the age-related development of altruism (Eisenberg et al., 1991). Now let's return to our case study, and the question of whether you would allow your child to be part of the vitamin E study.

One way to answer this question would be determine what might constitute an acceptable level of risk for the child, given their age and diagnosis. As an informed, research-aware paediatric nurse, your 'thought bubble' might look something like the one shown in Figure 4.3.

Reflection points 4.2

- Recognition of autonomy and respect in human research ethics values the intrinsic rights of a human being to hold individual and collective beliefs, perceptions, customs and culture. These principles also imply that the

design and scope of paediatric research will respect the individual capacity of children and young people to make their own decisions. What steps can you take to ensure that power relationships between health professionals, parents, children and young people do not impact on their consent decisions for participation in research?
- Research that exposes a child's genotype permits the early identification and treatment of disease, but also potentially impacts on the future choices of the whole family. These may include access to employment, life or health insurance. There is also a possibility of creating unexpected relationship stress around paternity or family-planning issues that may arise. What other potential risks of genotyping can you identify for the child or young person and their family?
- In research ethics, the principle of justice requires that any potential benefits or burdens from the research are distributed fairly among all age, gender, social, economic, cultural and ethnic groups. Think about research in which you may have been involved in and consider whether this research was 'just'.

Research monitoring and participation

In this final section of the chapter, we will look at the function and role of human research ethics committees (HRECs) in monitoring ethics and research governance in paediatric research. We will also discuss how you can use your knowledge about research, evidence and research ethics to support research-based practice for children and young people, and encourage their participation and partnership in Australian paediatric research.

Human research ethics committees

The ethical review of research conducted within institutions is assessed relative to the level of risk. The National Statement (NHMRC, 2007b) recommends that any research that is perceived to have anything more than a low level of risk must be reviewed by an appropriately constituted HREC. As discussed above, low risk is defined as whenever the actual or perceived risk is no greater than a level of discomfort. Negligible risk describes research in which there is no foreseeable risk of harm or discomfort, but it is recognised that any participation in research is likely to cause some inconvenience. Many institutions have provisions for the approval or exemption of low- and negligible-risk research, often through the formation of a sub-committee of the HREC.

The role of the institutional HREC is to give guidance to the institution and its researchers through a judgement on whether the proposed research meets the requirements of the National Statement. No research that is judged to present any risk to participants may commence until approval from the HREC is received, and often full funding of the research is withheld until evidence of HREC permission is presented. The National Statement (NHMRC, 2007b) gives guidance for processes of research governance and ethical review, including recommendations for the operations and membership of institutional HRECs. In other words, the HREC helps researchers, reviewers and funders of research to identify their responsibility and accountability for ethical research, and provides criteria for reviewing and monitoring the ethics, quality and safety of research projects.

As we have already identified, the National Statement on Ethical Conduct in Human Research (NHMRC, 2007b) and the Australian Code for the Responsible Conduct of Research (NHMRC, 2007a) collectively dictate processes for research governance that enable institutional HRECs to undertake ethical review. The National Statement outlines procedures for the establishment of HRECs, including their resourcing, composition and procedures. At a minimum, membership of HRECs includes two laypersons (a man and a woman) described as having no affiliation with the institution and not currently engaged in medical, scientific, legal or academic work.

Contribution to research

We began the section on research with children and young people by encouraging you to think about children and young people as partners in research. While HRECs have long been mandated to include representative laypersons in their membership, it has taken research funders and teams much longer to organise systems and processes for consulting members or groups with whom they are researching. There is still much work to be done to ensure fair adult representation in research, and even more to promote the representation and active involvement of children and young people in prioritising research topics and funding.

Research engagement with children and young people can be planned through ward-based 'patient committees' or during external events such as conferences and camp activities associated with support groups and charities – for example, Children with Disability Australia, CanTeen, the Raising Children Network, Asthma Australia or the Starlight Foundation. A range of these organisations (and also some state and territory Health Departments) conduct formal training in consumer representation. In this context, a consumer representative may be a young person who perhaps has a long experience of paediatric health and health care, and who has undergone participation in research studies. Young people with a chronic illness or disability are often chosen as candidates for representation on health or hospital committees.

It would be remiss to complete this chapter without discussing the potential 'over-researching' of specific paediatric groups. Children and young people – particularly those with chronic childhood illnesses or disabilities who spend a large part of their lives engaging with hospitals, clinics and other health services – become a captive audience for paediatric researchers. One only needs to look at the paediatric research literature to see which groups of children and young people are most often targeted. The three fundamental principles of research ethics relate to protecting the dignity, privacy and wellbeing of research participants. The paediatric researcher must consider the profile of their intended patient population, whether their research is fair and just for this group, and the possibility that over-researching or research fatigue may impact upon their sample recruitment, retention and possibly the quality of data – thus affecting the quality and outcomes of their research. The research design must also offer an explicit and easy way for children and young people to say 'no' if they do not wish to participate, or wish to withdraw from the study.

Partnering in evidence implementation

There are many models and frameworks for implementing research findings into practice. You may have heard about the PARIHS Model (Rycroft-Malone et al., 2013) or the Knowledge to Action (KTA) framework (Graham et al., 2006), for example. Regardless, evidence-implementation models always propose the initial development of an implementation plan. In the clinical research context, children and young people can be involved in the implementation of research that will inform their care in at least two practical ways:

- Members of the implementation team ask children and young people to identify potential barriers to implementing research evidence into practice change.

- Children and young people who will be affected by the change in treatment or health care are engaged as **champions** to promote the acceptance, implementation and maintenance of the change.

Partnering in research

Practical ways of involving children and young people in the design, conduct and monitoring of research are less well developed. There are beginning expectations from government funding bodies such as the NHMRC to achieve and report on the engagement of consumer representatives (as defined earlier), but these expectations are variously applied and monitored. As discussed earlier, active training for consumer representation is already undertaken by a number of community-based organisations and charities representing adults, and some have extended this training to young people.

> **Champion** In research or evidence implementation, a person (inclusive of health professionals) who will lead and maintain support for a cause or a course of action. A champion must be fully committed and adequately resourced with the appropriate knowledge and time to undertake this role

An example of an online resource for Australian researchers seeking to engage participants in health research can be found in a collaboration between the University of Western Australia (UWA) and the Telethon Institute for Child Health Research, called Involving People in Research. Involving People in Research formed following concerns over the use of health information in data-linkage research, and prompted the release of the first NHMRC Statement on Consumer Participation in 1998 (NHMRC, 2002). This UWA organisation now provides a range of resources to support consumer and community participation in health research, as well as funding for senior-level champions and dedicated staff positions for involving people in research. In addition to a series of online fact sheets and publications for researchers and the community, Involving People in Research also offers a plain-language, practical guide for establishing participation in health and medical research known as the *Green Book* (McKenzie & Hanley, 2008). While not so directly related to research participation, the NSW Commission for Children and Young People offers another useful online resource called *Taking PARTicipation Seriously*, and recently published a paper exploring the effectiveness of peer research as a tool for campaigning for the rights of young people and providing an avenue through which their voices can be heard (Segal & Randall, 2013).

A range of other models and methods are used by local government, psychology, the arts and social sciences for involving young people and their communities in decision-making. These hold possibilities for direct application to increasing engagement in health research. Successful examples of learning and innovating with children and young people should not be excluded just because they fall outside the immediate health context.

Participating for success

Several barriers to implementing models and strategies for participation in health research have been identified. Imbalances of power and lack of control over the funding and design of research programs are commonly cited. Historically, academic institutions and health services are hierarchically structured and difficult enough for adults – let alone children and young people – to access and navigate (Fielden et al., 2007). Minority communities experience institutional racism, along with privilege and power challenges in their relationships with academic organisations (Andrews et al., 2012). The Australian Indigenous experience of health research, for example, has been challenging in terms of processes and outcomes (Kendall et al., 2011). Gaining the trust of family and community stakeholders is another frequently identified roadblock to success, as well as securing commitment to the extra time, money and effort required from health and academic institutions, and consumers, to truly partner in research (Allen et al., 2010; Shalowitz et al., 2009).

An obvious start to successful participation in research is ensuring that family and community engagement is planned within the socio-political and economic context in which health care and treatment is to be delivered. Other key factors for the successful engagement of children, young people and their families as partners in health research include:

- early participation in prioritising and planning the research (including identification of need, scoping of the program and the extent of stakeholder involvement)
- support for the formation of partnerships (Allen et al., 2010) and adequate training of stakeholders and consumers (Andrews et al., 2012)
- clear processes for deciding stakeholder capacity for collaboration, managing conflict and expectations, establishing norms for decision-making (Allen et al., 2010) and planning for ending the engagement when the research is complete, and
- agreeing the desired rewards or outcomes for all members and organisations involved.

> **Reflection points 4.3**
>
> - The interests and needs of children and young people participating in research differ from those of adults. How do Australian human research ethics committees represent and respect these needs and interests?
> - The National Statement on Ethical Conduct in Human Research lists six core values for research with Aboriginal and Torres Strait Islander peoples. These are reciprocity, respect, equality, responsibility, survival and protection, and spirit and integrity. What other cultural values do you believe are important in designing research with Aboriginal and Torres Strait Islander children and young people?
> - Children and young people can be involved in the design, prioritisation and implementation of research that will inform their care by being part of research or evidence implementation teams. Think about some of the other ways in which children and young people can be involved in research that relates to them.

Applying new knowledge to practice

In this chapter, we have invited you to explore and expand your understanding of research and evidence-based practice. We have introduced four core principles of human research ethics (research integrity, autonomy and respect, beneficence and justice) and discussed research governance. We used a case study example to illustrate how these core principles apply to research conducted in the paediatric setting and have asked you to reflect on how you can use this knowledge in your work as a paediatric nurse to support evidence based-practice for children and young people and encourage their partnership in research.

While paediatric research is different from nursing care, there are many occasions when the work of a paediatric clinician intersects with that of a researcher. Children, young people and their families have a right to assume that paediatric nursing care is informed by the best available research evidence. This means that professional nursing practice must rely on a foundation of research evidence, and that a paediatric nurse knows how to interpret and use this knowledge in their work. As an evidence-based practitioner, the paediatric nurse must also be able to decide whether new knowledge from research is of sufficient quality to make a useful contribution to the paediatric knowledge base, or whether the impact of the research is such that it presumes a need for change in practice. Evidence implementation and evaluation are quality practice initiatives for improving paediatric clinical care.

Paediatric nurses may also be engaged in leading research or working as part of a research team. Their research may be conducted in a laboratory, ward or community setting, and be developed exclusively with other nurses or – as is more often the case – with other members of the healthcare team. There are virtually no limits to becoming a paediatric researcher, other than specialist training as a paediatric nurse and specialist training as a researcher. Obtaining research funding is always a challenge, but strong partnerships will help to focus the research on issues and questions that are of primary concern to the children, young people and their families with whom you are researching.

Summary

- Research and evidence are intimately linked in nursing and health care, but each makes a slightly different contribution. We can broadly distinguish research as a rigorous and systematic process for deriving new knowledge, and evidence as the knowledge that is produced. However, evidence from other sources is also used to inform health and treatment decisions. The experience of the clinician, the context of the health-care environment and information about the specific values and priorities of the person or group receiving care ultimately shape decisions about how the evidence is used.
- The ethics of human research are based on the fundamental principles of research integrity, autonomy and respect, beneficence and justice. These principles attest that any risks from the research will be outweighed by the contribution of the research to improving health and health care and that the dignity, privacy and wellbeing of the research participant will be protected at all times.
- Obtaining consent for participation in research is central to respect for persons. While Australian states and territories have specific legislation concerning the age at which minors are deemed to have capacity to consent to treatment, this may not apply to participation in research. The age of consent for participation in research is defined by individual maturity. Children may have the capacity to understand the nature of the research, and may give their consent in addition to their parent doing so. Mature children and young people capable of understanding the risks and benefits of their participation in research may give sole consent, with parental consent being waived in these circumstances.

- In the context of research ethics, a risk is anything that has the potential for harm, discomfort or inconvenience. Harm can be perceived or real, physical or psychological. Discomfort is a less serious form of risk. The inconvenience associated with participation in research may seem minimal to the researcher, but it is especially relevant to the parents or carers of children and young people, who may need to take time away from work or family and who may incur financial or emotional costs as a result of their child's participation in research.
- Practical ways of involving children and young people in the design, conduct and monitoring of research are still developing. Active training for consumer representation is already undertaken by a number of community-based organisations, and some charities representing adults have begun to extend this training to young people. There are a range of other models and methods used outside the health context that present possibilities for direct application for increasing engagement in health research.

Learning activity

Imagine a parent has asked your advice about enrolling their 14-year-old daughter, Katy, in a research study about the emotional effects of asthma diagnosed in childhood. The parent is keen to give consent because they think it would be really good for Katy to talk about the challenges she has faced in managing severe asthma, which was diagnosed at 5 years of age. However, Katy says she is sick of being involved in research because it never helps her and she does not want to talk any more about her illness. She just wants to get on with her life.

4.1 Katy is not assenting, nor will she give consent, to be part of the study. Can Katy's parent overrule her consent in this situation? Explain your answer.

4.2 Katy eventually decides to be interviewed for the study, and both Katy and her mother give their consent. During the interview, Katy reveals that she sometimes manipulates her medication in order to provoke an asthma attack. Sometimes she does it because she doesn't want to go school, and sometimes she does it to 'pay her mother back'. Is the interviewer required to disclose this information to the parent?

4.3 In what situations could Katy be considered to have capacity to give sole consent for her participation in this research?

Further reading

The following resource from the Children's Bioethics Centre at the Murdoch Children Research Institute answers frequently asked questions about designing research with children and explores some difficult issues with specific reference to the Australian National Statement. The resource also covers specific types of research, such as genetic and internet-based research.

- Spriggs, M 2010, *A handbook for human research ethics committees and researchers*, 4th edn, Royal Children's Hospital Melbourne, viewed 20 February 2014, https://www.mcri.edu.au/media/62539/handbook.pdf.

Websites

Codes and standards for research ethics and governance referred to during this chapter include the following:

- Nuremberg Code of 1947: <http://history.nih.gov/research/downloads/nuremberg.pdf>
- Declaration of Helsinki: <www.wma.net/en/30publications/10policies/b3/index.html>
- Belmont Report: <www.fda.gov/ohrms/dockets/ac/05/briefing/2005-4178b_09_02_Belmont%20Report.pdf>
- Australian Joint National Statement on Ethical Conduct in Human Research: <www.nhmrc.gov.au/guidelines/publications/e72>
- Australian Code for the Responsible Conduct of Research: <www.nhmrc.gov.au/_files_nhmrc/publications/attachments/r39.pdf>.

There are also specific guidelines for conducting ethical research with Aboriginal and Torres Strait Islander Peoples:

- From the NHMRC: *Values and Ethics: Guidelines for Ethical Conduct in Aboriginal and Torres Strait Islander Health Research*, <www.nhmrc.gov.au/guidelines/publications/e52>
- From the Australian Institute of Aboriginal and Torres Strait Islander Studies (AIATSIS): *Guidelines for Ethical Research in Indigenous Studies*, <www.aiatsis.gov.au/research/ethics>.

Resources for engaging children and young people in health research include:

- *Involving People in Research* and access to the *Green Book*: <www.involvingpeopleinresearch.org.au>

- NSW Commission for Children and Young People, *Taking PARTicipation Seriously*, < www.kids.nsw.gov.au/Publications---resources/Participation-resources/Taking-PARTicipation-seriously>
- Segal, S & Randall, L 2013, *Youth-led research as an advocacy tool* <www.yacvic.org.au/policy-publications/publications-listed-by-policy-area/36-youth-participation/412-youth-led-research-as-an-advocacy-tool>.

References

Agency for Healthcare Research and Quality (AHRQ) 2001, *Translating research into practice (TRIP)-II*, US Department of Health and Human Services, Rockville, MD, viewed 20 February 2014, http://www.ahrq.gov/research/findings/factsheets/translating/tripfac/index.html.

Allen, ML, Culhane-Pera, KA, Pergament, SL & Call, KT 2010, Facilitating research faculty participation in CBPR: Development of a model based on key informant interviews, *Clinical and Translational Science*, 3(5), pp. 233–8.

Andrews, JO, Newman, SD, Meadows, O, Cox, MJ & Bunting, S 2012, Partnership readiness for community-based participatory research, *Health Education Research*, 27(4), pp. 555–71.

Davidson, A & O'Brien, M 2009, Ethics and medical research in children, *Pediatric Anesthesia*, 19, pp. 994–1004.

Eisenberg, N, Miller, P, Shell, R, McNalley, S & Shea, C 1991, Prosocial development in adolescence: A longitudinal study, *Developmental Psychology*, 27(5), pp. 849–57.

Fielden, SJ, Rusch, ML, Masinda, MT, Sands, J, Frankish, J & Evoy, B 2007, Key considerations for logic model development in research partnerships: A Canadian case study, *Evaluation and Program Planning*, 30(2), pp. 115–24.

Giesbertz, N, Bredenoord, A & Delden, JV 2012, Inclusion of residual tissue in biobanks: Opt-in or opt-out? *PLoS Biology*, 10(8), viewed 20 February 2014, http://www.plosbiology.org/article/fetchObject.action?uri=info%3Adoi%2F10.1371%2Fjournal.pbio.1001373&representation=PDF.

Godlee, F, Smith, J & Marcovitch, H 2011, Wakefield's article linking MMR vaccine and autism was fraudulent (editorial), *BMJ*, 342, viewed 20 February 2014, http://www.bmj.com/content/342/bmj.c7452.

Graham, I, Logan, J, Harrison, M, Straus, S, Tetroe, J, Caswell, W & Robinson, N 2006, Lost in knowledge translation: Time for a map? *Journal of Continuing Education in the Health Professions*, 26(1), pp. 13–24.

Jones, J 1993, *Bad blood: The Tuskegee syphilis experiment*, 2nd edn, Free Press, New York.

Kendall, E, Sunderland, N, Barnett, L, Nalder, G & Matthews, C 2011, Beyond the rhetoric of participatory research in Indigenous communities: Advances in Australia over the last decade, *Qualitative Health Research*, 21(12), pp. 1719–28.

Link, K 2005, *The vaccine controversy: The history, use and safety of vaccinations*, Praeger, Westport, CT.

McKenzie, A & Hanley, B 2008, *Consumer and community participation in health and medical research: A practical guide for health and medical research organisations (Green Book)*, viewed 20 March 2014, http://www.twocanassociates.co.uk/perch/resources/files/The%20GREEN%20BOOK%20MAR08.pdf.

National Health and Medical Research Council (NHMRC) 2002, *Statement on consumer and community participation in health and medical research*, NHMRC, Canberra, viewed 20 March 2014, http://www.nhmrc.gov.au/_files_nhmrc/publications/attachments/r22.pdf.

—— 2003, *Values and ethics – Guidelines for ethical conduct in Aboriginal and Torres Strait Islander Health Research*. NHMRC, Canberra, viewed 20 March 2014, https://www.nhmrc.gov.au/guidelines/publications/e52.

—— 2007a, *Australian code for the responsible conduct of research*, NHMRC, Canberra, viewed 20 March 2014, http://www.nhmrc.gov.au/_files_nhmrc/publications/attachments/r39.pdf.

—— 2007b, *National statement on ethical conduct in human research*, NHMRC, Canberra, viewed 20 March 2014, http://www.nhmrc.gov.au/guidelines/publications/e72.

Purchase, I 2004, Fraud, errors and gamesmanship in experimental toxicology, *Toxicology*, 202(1–2), pp. 1–20.

Royal Australasian College of Physicians (RACP) 2008, *Paediatric policy on ethics of research in children*, viewed 20 February 2014, http://www.racp.edu.au/index.cfm?objectid=39396AC9-E30B-7941-0FD53740FF78DBC8.

Rycroft-Malone, J et al. 2013, The role of evidence, context, and facilitation in an implementation trial: implications for the development of the PARIHS framework, *Implementation Science*, 8, p. 28.

Savulescu, J 2002, Beyond Bristol: Taking responsibility, *Journal of Medical Ethics*, 28, pp. 281–2.

Segal, S & Randall, L 2013, Youth led research as an advocacy tool, http://www.yacvic.org.au/policy-publications/publications-listed-by-policy-area/36-youth-participation/412-youth-led-research-as-an-advocacy-tool.

Shalowitz, MU et al. 2009, Community-based participatory research: A review of the literature with strategies for community engagement, *Journal of Developmental and Behavioral Pediatrics*, 30(4), pp. 350–61.

World Medical Assembly (WMA) 2009, Ottawa Declaration on Child Health, viewed 20 March 2014, http://www.wma.net/en/30publications/10policies/c4.

Part 2

Evidence-based Paediatric Nursing Care

This part shifts the focus from setting the context for students of nursing to become more specific about the role of the paediatric nurse, including nursing assessment, nursing care and nursing interventions in paediatric settings. This includes acute care, complex care, care of the child with a chronic illness and childhood mental health care.

5 Recognising and responding to the sick child

Elizabeth Forster and Loretta Scaini

Learning objectives

In this chapter you will:

- Gain an understanding of normal assessment findings in the paediatric patient and those indicating deterioration
- Learn how to recognise a sick or deteriorating child using an appropriate framework
- Develop an understanding of how to respond to a sick or deteriorating child and provide appropriate respiratory and circulatory support
- Learn the elements of paediatric cardiopulmonary resuscitation
- Consider the importance of supporting families and parental presence during paediatric resuscitation

Introduction

As a nurse caring for paediatric patients, it is important that you develop the ability to recognise and respond to a sick infant or child. The ability to do this is so important that a variety of projects have been undertaken, both internationally and throughout Australia, to ensure that nurses working with paediatric patients are able to recognise, respond promptly to and appropriately manage sick and deteriorating infants and children – for example, the Between the Flags program in New South Wales and the Children's Early Warning Assessment Tool (CEWT) in Queensland. These programs aim to support the assessment skills of the clinician working with infants and children. **Paediatric early warning tools** help clinicians to recognise a deteriorating infant or child and trigger an escalation in care to prevent further deterioration and achieve favourable outcomes. This chapter will provide you with beginning understanding and knowledge so that you will be able to recognise and respond to a sick and deteriorating child.

> **Paediatric early warning tools** Tools that assist nurses to recognise signs and symptoms indicating deterioration in paediatric patients; these include triggers and directions for escalations in management, including urgent medical review

TABLE 5.1 *Respiratory and cardiovascular differences in paediatric patients*

PAEDIATRIC RESPIRATORY CHARACTERISTICS THAT INCREASE RISK FOR RESPIRATORY COMPROMISE	
Infants are obligatory nose breathers	Respiratory difficulties if the nares become blocked with secretions.
Narrow airways	Even a small amount of swelling or secretions results in a large increase in airways resistance, impacting on the work of breathing.
Soft, collapsible airways	In newborns, airway cartilage is not fully developed and is thus more susceptible to collapse. Avoid over-extension of the head.
• Submucosal glands in airway larger than in adults	Possible hyperactivity of mucous production.
• Lower pH of airway lining	May be linked to dysfunction of epithelial cells of respiratory tract, impaired mucociliary clearance and viscosity of secretions
Large tongue and adenoids	Lead to an increased risk of airway obstruction. Adenoids are often problematic around 2 years of age.
Horizontal, cartilaginous ribs	The chest wall collapses inwards when the infant increases their work of breathing. This is seen as intercostal, sternal and sub-costal recession, and often results in decreased air entry.
Immature intercostal and accessory muscles	Primarily use the diaphragm to breathe. The lack of type II muscle fibres results in early fatigue of the infant's respiratory muscles. Increased work of breathing results in head bob, see-saw movement between the chest and abdomen.
Less alveolar surface area available for gas exchange	By approximately 8–12 years of age, a child has nine times the alveoli than was present at birth.
Large head and an inability to reposition	Infants have a large occiput that can push the head forward and obstruct the airway. They lack the muscle strength or developmental ability to reposition themselves to aid breathing.
Higher metabolic rate	Greater need for oxygen to support metabolic processes and consequently higher respiratory rates.
Developmental stage of placing objects into the mouth or nose	Upper airway obstruction due to foreign objects is common, and can be life-threatening in toddlers and young children.
PAEDIATRIC CARDIOVASCULAR CHARACTERISTICS THAT INCREASE RISK FOR CARDIOVASCULAR COMPROMISE	
Immature myocardium	Limited ability to increase contractility, making stroke volume relatively fixed. Cardiac output is increased by increasing the heart rate.
70–80 mL/kg blood volume	Low total blood volume – 240 mL for a newborn. Small losses can result in shock.
Ability to maintain blood pressure	Hypotension is a very late sign of cardiovascular compromise. Other signs of compromise are HR, capillary refill, perfusion. Urine output must be observed.
Changes from foetal circulation may continue for several weeks	Undiagnosed congenital cardiac structural defects may present within the first weeks of life.
Increased risk for fluid depletion	Large surface area increases the risk of insensible losses. Reduced ability to concentrate urine during infancy. Larger percentage of total body fluids.
Limited metabolic and physiological reserve	If left unsupported, infants and children may become exhausted from their disease states. This may manifest as a reduction in respiratory rate or slowing of the heart rate. These are indicators that the child is rapidly approaching cardiorespiratory arrest.

Source: Adapted from Santillanes & Gausche-Hill (2008); Walsh et al. (2011).

Clinical signs – warning of deterioration – are often present in the paediatric patient as for as long as six to 12 hours before a catastrophic event. Failure to identify and treat these early warning signs can result in continued clinical deterioration until cardiopulmonary arrest. The poor outcomes associated with paediatric cardiopulmonary arrest emphasise the importance of being able to detect and respond to early signs of deterioration (McLellan & Connor, 2013).

The primary cause of paediatric cardiopulmonary arrest is respiratory in origin, and the second most common cause is circulatory failure. In both situations, the child will display signs of respiratory or cardiovascular compromise prior to deteriorating into cardiac arrest. Timely intervention can treat or stabilise the child, preventing the progress of the condition. Sudden cardiac arrest is extremely rare in paediatrics, and is limited to a small number of uncommon conditions.

Understanding the causes of deterioration in the paediatric patient is important to enhance early recognition of problems. Due to their stage of development, paediatric patients have anatomical, physiological and behavioural differences that underpin their predisposition to develop illness and their ability to respond to the stress of disease. Table 5.1 reviews some of the significant respiratory and cardiovascular differences.

Structured assessment of the paediatric patient

The use of a structured assessment framework can assist in your ability to perform a patient assessment (Munroe et al., 2013). Assessment frameworks can assist clinicians to prioritise assessment of critical systems and ensure all systems are methodically assessed. We will discuss two commonly used assessment approaches here: The **Paediatric Assessment Triangle** and the **Primary Assessment Framework**.

> **Paediatric Assessment Triangle** A tool that can be used to complete a rapid 'hands-off' – approximately 30 seconds – assessment of the paediatric patient. The tool assesses the child's appearance, work of breathing and circulation to the skin
>
> **Primary Assessment Framework** An assessment framework that provides a 'first look' at body systems – for example, respiratory, cardiovascular and neurological. If an abnormality is detected, it should be addressed immediately

The Paediatric Assessment Triangle

Figure 5.1 represents the paediatric assessment triangle (Dieckmann et al., 2010), represents another rapid-assessment framework used to perform an initial assessment and to quickly identify a sick and deteriorating child.

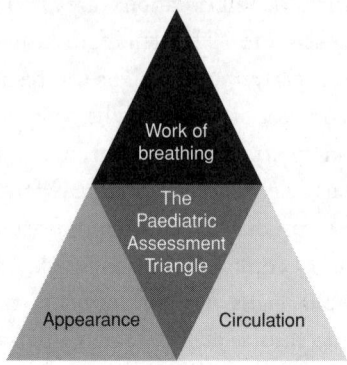

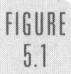 **FIGURE 5.1** *The Paediatric Assessment Triangle*

Source: Adapted from Dieckmann et al. (2010).

The Paediatric Assessment Triangle works via rapid assessment of three components: the child's appearance, work of breathing and circulation to the skin (Dieckmann et al., 2010).

The child's appearance considers:

- *tone* (includes whether the child moves spontaneously, resists being examined, sits or stands (age appropriate)
- *interactiveness* (includes whether the child appears alert and engaged with clinicians/caregivers, interacts with people and environment, reaches for toys, objects)
- *consolability* (includes whether the child stops crying with holding/comforting by caregiver or has differential response to caregiver versus examiner)
- *look/gaze* (includes whether child makes eye contact with clinician, tracks visually)
- *speech/cry* (includes whether the child has a strong cry/uses age-appropriate speech)

The child's work of breathing considers:

- abnormal airway sounds (including snoring, muffled or hoarse speech, stridor, grunting, wheezing
- abnormal positioning (sniffing position, tripoding or preference for seated posture)

- retractions (supraclavicular, intercostal or substernal retractions, head bobbing in infants)
- flaring of the nares on inspiration.

The child's circulation considers characteristic abnormal features such as:

- pallor (white or pale skin or mucous membranes)
- mottling (patchy skin discoloration due to varying degrees of vasoconstriction)
- cyanosis (bluish discoloration of skin and mucous membranes).

The Paediatric Assessment Triangle provides clinicians with a rapid 'hands-off' 30-second assessment that can be completed prior to the hands-on primary survey. It means that lifesaving treatments can be initiated immediately if necessary.

The Primary Assessment Framework

We will now discuss the ABCD, primary survey, or Primary Assessment Framework for assessing the paediatric patient. The Primary Assessment Framework approach to assessment uses an ABCD assessment framework for paediatric patients. Many of the early warning tools established use a variation of the primary survey in guiding the initial assessment of the paediatric patient.

The Primary Assessment Framework is designed to assist to assess and manage clinical deterioration in order of priority. When completing a primary assessment, if life threatening conditions are identified they must be managed prior to continuing with the assessment. The following is a brief description of the primary assessment framework:

A *Airway:* assessed for patency and security
B *Breathing:* work and rate of breathing and the effectiveness of breathing to achieve adequate oxygenation
C *Circulation:* heart rate, skin perfusion and evidence that the body is achieving sufficient adequate blood flow
D *Disability:* mental status and level of consciousness.

You will now be able to use your beginning understanding of the primary assessment framework when you consider Case Study 5.1, which concerns Maggie, an infant with respiratory distress.

Case study 5.1

Infant with respiratory distress

Maggie, a 6-month-old infant, has a three-day history of a respiratory tract infection. She has been admitted to the paediatric ward diagnosed with bronchiolitis (suspected to be Respiratory Syncitial Virus [RSV]). Upon assessment, Maggie is pale and lethargic. She has a moist cough and thick, creamy rhinorrhoea. Her respiratory rate is 48 breaths per minute and she has moderate intercostal and subcostal recession and tracheal tug. Bilateral wheeze can be heard upon auscultation. Her oxygen saturations (SpO2) in room air are 92 per cent. Her heart rate is 154 beats per minute and her temperature is 37.9°C.

Maggie's mother reports that she has been 'not feeding well' over the past few days. Maggie's mother last changed a wet nappy at 5.00 am (six hours ago).

Applying the Primary Assessment Framework
By utilising the Primary Assessment Framework when performing Maggie's assessment, as Maggie's nurse, you are able to collect the data in systematic manner.

› Airway:
  – maintaining own airway – no upper airway noises
  – thick nasal secretions – potential for obstructing nasal breathing
› Breathing:
  – respirations are 48 breaths per minute
  – increased work of breathing evidenced by intercostal and subcostal recession
  – wheeze
  – reduced oxygen saturations in room air: 92 per cent (impaired gas exchange)
› Circulation:
  – heart rate of 154 beats per minute
  – pallor, peripheries cool
  – peripheral pulses present
  – blood pressure 100/52
  – reduced urine output
  – reduced oral intake
› Disability:
  – lethargic
  – responses to voice on AVPU score
  – disinterested in feeding

Recognition of clinical deterioration using a Primary Assessment Framework

You already have a beginning understanding of the elements of the Primary Assessment Framework, and you have applied this to collect assessment data about Maggie in Case Study 5.1. In this section, we will utilise the Primary Assessment Framework to provide you with a systematic and detailed review of a paediatric assessment. In most instances, a rapid assessment should be undertaken to identify the need for emergency care prior to performing a more comprehensive assessment. If, however, immediately life-threatening conditions present during the primary assessment, they must be managed immediately.

A – Airway

In the primary survey, A represents airway assessment. For the paediatric patient, you need to consider whether the patient can maintain their own airway. Is the airway clear or is it obstructed? An inability to maintain a patent airway is immediately life-threatening and needs to take priority in the management of the patient. The child's ability to vocalise or speak provides a rapid assessment of airway patency.

There are a number of anatomical and behavioural developmental factors that increase the paediatric patient's risk for compromised airway. Some of these factors include having a large tongue, a soft floor of the mouth that is easily compressible, a large head and small-sized mid-face (Cullen, 2012a). In a child with a decreased or loss of consciousness, the large tongue could easily obstruct the airway. When artificial support is given, care should be taken to hold masks along the jawline so as not to compress the soft floor of a child's mouth, further contributing to airway compromise. The large head with a predominant occiput can result in the child's neck becoming flexed and obstructing the airway.

The child's upper airway is narrow and cone shaped, with the cricoid cartilage being the narrowest point. This anatomy places the child at increased risk of upper airway obstruction due to swelling associated with infections such as 'croup' (laryngotracheobronchitis).

Another important cause of airway obstruction in young children is a foreign body. Inhalation of small objects, including toys, batteries or pieces of food, can partially or completely obstruct the upper airway.

Characteristics of partial upper airway obstruction may include:

- difficulty breathing with increased work of breathing
- upper respiratory tract noises such a stridor or snoring sounds
- drooling or inability to swallow secretions
- child positioning their neck or head to open their airway
- history of illness or choking on a foreign object
- decreased air entry and impaired oxygenation in severe cases.

Rapidly assessing the child for the cause and degree of respiratory compromise is essential to ensure appropriate management and referral. For example, a child with a partially obstructed airway following anaesthetic may require the application of a simple airway open manoeuvre such as jaw thrust until they are more awake. However, a child with a severe episode of croup may require urgent medical attention.

Children with complete upper airway obstruction will quickly deteriorate into cardiac arrest and require an urgent emergency airway. The management of any child with acute upper airway obstruction is therefore critical. It is important that a doctor who is able to perform a difficult paediatric intubation is notified.

Children at risk of airway obstruction should be observed continuously and never left unattended.

B – Breathing

In the primary survey, B represents breathing – that is, assessment of the adequacy of breathing and therefore oxygenation. In the paediatric patient, this incorporates a variety of assessment parameters, including:

- respiratory rate, which will vary depending upon the age of the infant or child, and the presence of fever or coexisting health conditions (see Table 5.2 for usual paediatric respiratory rates)
- symmetry of chest wall movement
- work of breathing, including the presence of signs such as nasal flaring and head bobbing in infants, recession or retractions, and diaphragmatic movement in conjunction with chest wall movement.

Chest recession or retractions

The assessment of chest recession or retractions is important, as normally there is minimal chest wall movement in the child because they rely upon diaphragmatic abdominal breathing. Therefore, any respiratory issue that causes increased airway resistance results in the generation of increased negative intrathoracic pressure needed to produce inward airflow during inspiration causes recession (Aylott, 2006).

TABLE 5.2 *Respiratory rate parameters for paediatric age groups*

AGE	RESPIRATORY RATE PER MINUTE	CONSIDER AS RAPID	CONSIDER FACTORS THAT MAY AFFECT RESPIRATORY RATE
Newborn (0–28 days)	30–50	>60	Fever
Infant (1–12 months)	20–30	>50	Comorbidities (e.g. congenital respiratory or heart disease)
Toddler (1–3 years)	20–30	>40	Seizure activity
Child (4–11 years)	15–20	>30	Neurological injury PH imbalances Fear, emotional upset, anxiety
Adolescent (12 years and over)	16–18	>24	

Source: Adapted from Gill and O'Brien (2007).

Breath sounds and air entry

Breath sounds and air entry, or the absence of breath sounds, are an important element of breathing assessment in the paediatric patient. Breath sounds can alert the clinician to the nature of the respiratory issue – for example, wheezing indicates fluid in the airways and alveoli, and stridor indicates narrowing, oedema or obstruction of the trachea and upper airway.

Grunting may be heard in infants with severe respiratory distress, and indicates an effort to increase end expiratory pressure during respiration to promote gas exchange (Aylott, 2006).

Oxygen saturation

Oxygen saturations are a measure of the oxygen saturation of haemoglobin, and provide valuable information about the child's oxygenation status. Pulse oximeters are commonly used to measure the oxygen saturation in peripheral blood (Sp02). Normal Sp02 should be greater than 97 per cent in room air (O'Meara & Watton, 2012).

A variety of factors impact on the accuracy of readings in the paediatric patient, including movement, peripheral perfusion and skin pigmentation (Fouzas et al., 2011). This means it is important to look at oxygen-saturation values in conjunction with the general clinical appearance of the child and other assessment data collected.

Table 5.2 shows the respiratory rate parameters for paediatric age groups and factors that may influence respiratory rate.

C – Circulation

In the primary survey, C represents your assessment of the adequacy of circulation in the paediatric patient, and involves assessing:

- heart rate and rhythm
- peripheral pulses and perfusion
- colour
- urine output
- blood pressure.

Assessing paediatric circulation requires an understanding of the way the sick infant or child responds to altered and inadequate circulatory or cardiovascular function. The sick infant or child with cardiovascular compromise will trigger compensatory mechanisms as the body attempts to maintain blood pressure and ensure that vital organs are perfused. A reduced pressure within the circulatory system will trigger the release of catecholamines (adrenaline and noradrenaline) and hormones (angiotensin and antidiuretic hormone) that result in an increased heart rate, vasoconstriction of peripheral blood vessels and retention of sodium and water by the kidneys. These responses enable the sick infant or child to maintain blood pressure and circulation to the heart, lungs and brain. However, if the circulatory compromise is not corrected, these compensatory mechanisms will no longer be able to sustain sufficient perfusion of the vital organs and blood pressure will no longer be able to be maintained. This pre-terminal stage will be evident in a drop in blood pressure and decreased level of consciousness.

Table 5.3 shows the heart rate parameters for paediatric age groups and the factors to consider that may influence heart rate and rhythm.

Heart rate and rhythm

During childhood, the heart rate is faster and the stroke volume continues to increase from birth until 5 years of age. It then stabilises (Top et al., 2011). Normal heart rates and blood pressure values are presented in Table 5.3. During early childhood, cardiac muscle fibres are immature and lack the ability to increase the strength of myocardial contractility. Stroke volume – the volume of blood ejected with each ventricular contraction – is therefore relatively fixed.

In children – particularly infants – cardiac output is increased primarily by increasing the heart rate. The child's dependence on heart rate to manipulate cardiac output makes heart rate one of the most important observations in the

TABLE 5.3 *Heart rate parameters for paediatric age groups*

AGE	HEART RATE BEATS PER MINUTE	CONSIDER AS ELEVATED	CONSIDER FACTORS THAT MAY AFFECT HEART RATE/ RHYTHM	SYSTOLIC BLOOD PRESSURE (MMHG)	DIASTOLIC BLOOD PRESSURE (MMHG)
Newborn (0–28 days)	70–190 Mean 125	At upper end of range and above	Hypoxia, fever	70	30
Infant (1–12 months)	80–160 Mean 120	At upper end of range and above	Comorbidities (e.g. congenital respiratory or heart disease)	75	50
Toddler (1–3 years)	100–110	At upper end of range and above	Dehydration	90–93	55–56
Child (4–11 years)	80–110	At upper end of range and above	Pain	93–103	56–62
Adolescent (12 years and over)	55–90	At upper end of range and above	Fear, emotional upset, anxiety	103	62

Source: Adapted from Top et al. (2011).

paediatric cardiovascular assessment. Observation of trends in heart rate can provide signs of cardiovascular improvement or deterioration. However, while heart rate is a very sensitive sign of cardiovascular status, it is not a very specific sign. The child's heart rate may be increased due to other factors such as temperature, pain or anxiety. Therefore, it is essential to evaluate the heart rate in the context of other clinical observations.

Bradycardia is an important sign of cardiorespiratory decompensation. This may occur in children who have become physiologically exhausted from respiratory or cardiac illness. For infants under 12 months of age, a heart rate of less than 60 accompanied by signs of impaired perfusion will require cardiopulmonary resuscitation.

In the paediatric patient, stroke volume may be evaluated by assessing the volume and strength of pulses, and systemic vascular resistance may be evaluated via assessment of the child's peripheral skin perfusion.

Blood pressure

Normal blood pressure is not a reliable sign of a child's cardiovascular status. Severe cardiovascular compromise and inadequate tissue perfusion can be present despite a normal blood pressure. Performing a paediatric blood pressure assessment is important because hypotension is poorly tolerated and needs to be addressed quickly.

The paediatric patient's compensatory mechanisms in the event of hypovolaemia work towards the maintenance of blood flow to the vital organs despite falling cardiac output due to decreased stroke volume (Hobson & Chima, 2013). The paediatric patient's blood pressure is maintained by increasing heart rate and systemic vascular resistance through peripheral vasoconstriction until shock is severe. A drop in blood pressure is considered a late and preterminal sign (Hobson & Chima, 2013). It is therefore important that early signs of circulatory compromise are detected. Clinicians must utilise heart rate, colour, perfusion, skin temperature, capillary refill times and level of consciousness to ensure that early intervention and circulatory support are initiated. In sick infants, assessing the blood pressure in the upper and lower limbs can provide information about undiagnosed congenital cardiac conditions such as coarctation of the aorta.

Note: The size of the blood pressure cuff is important to ensure accuracy of the measurement. The cuff bladder should encircle 80–100 per cent of the mid-upper arm circumference (National High Blood Pressure Education Program, 2004) Table 5.4 provides a guide for appropriate blood pressure cuff sizes.

Peripheral pulses and perfusion

Pulses should be checked both centrally and peripherally, and evaluated for differences. Marked variation in intensity of pulses may be indicative of blood being directed towards central organs and away from the peripheries. This is a compensatory mechanism that can occur in conditions such hypovolaemia.

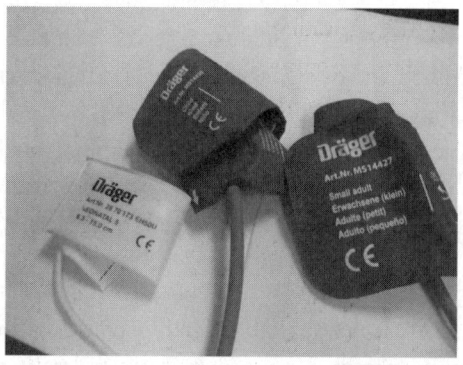

FIGURE 5.2 *Blood pressure cuffs*

TABLE 5.4 *Blood pressure cuff sizes*

	CUFF WIDTH	CUFF LENGTH	MAXIMUM ARM CIRCUMFERENCE
Infant	6 cm	12 cm	15 cm
Child	9 cm	18 cm	22 cm
Adolescent	10 cm	24 cm	26 cm

Source: Adapted from the National High Blood Pressure Education Program Working Group on High Blood Pressure in Children and Adolescents (2004).

The strength and volume of the pulse provide information about stroke volume. A weak or thready pulse, especially if found centrally, is a worrying sign of poor cardiac output. This may be present in a child with severe vasoconstriction and/or impaired cardiac function.

The carotid pulse can be used to assess a central pulse in children. Because infants often have short, chubby necks, the most reliable locations to palpate central pulses in infants are the brachial and femoral arteries. Absent or weak femoral pulses may be inductive of undiagnosed congenital cardiac conditions where upper limb pulses are adequate.

The colour and temperature of skin can reflect the adequacy of peripheral perfusion and provide information about systemic vascular resistance. Skin mottling has been demonstrated to be a reliable measure of skin hypoperfusion and is responsive to changes in peripheral vasoconstriction (Ait-Oufella et al., 2013).

Peripheral vasoconstriction is part of the compensatory response designed to maintain blood pressure during cardiovascular compromise, and is therefore an indirect measure of cardiovascular function. Severe alterations in peripheral perfusion, such as mottling, pale, cold skin and decreased peripheral pulses, are indicative of serious cardiovascular dysfunction.

When assessing skin temperature and perfusion, it is valuable to identify the level of skin involvement so that reassessment for change is possible. For example, the skin may be cool and mottled to the level of the child's knee.

Factors such as low environmental temperatures and fever can also cause peripheral vasoconstriction, resulting in pale or cool skin. Therefore, it is important to apply your assessment finding to the clinical context.

Capillary refill

Capillary refill is often used to assess skin perfusion in the paediatric patient. It refers to the amount of time for the capillary bed to return its colour after pressure has been applied to cause the area to blanche (Pickard et al., 2011). A variety of factors may affect capillary refill time, including:

- *age* (with neonates having an upper limit of three seconds and children having an upper limit of two seconds)
- *environmental, skin and core temperature* – Capillary refill time tends to increase with cooler ambient temperature and decrease with warmer environments such as when radiant heaters are used; skin temperature also affects capillary refill time, and reductions in skin temperature tend to be reflected in an increased capillary refill time; core temperature also influences capillary refill time with each 1°C rise in core temperature, resulting in a shorter capillary refill time (Pickard et al., 2011)
- *duration* of application and *location of pressure* applied.

There is no consensus about the correct duration of pressure application prior to measuring capillary refill time, and the variables range from three to seven seconds, or sufficient time to cause blanching. Recent paediatric studies recommend using your index finger to apply enough pressure to cause the skin to turn pale and applying pressure for five seconds (Crook & Taylor, 2013).

A variety of sites have been used for testing capillary refill, including the forehead, sternum, nail bed of fingers or toes, or pulp or pads of fingertips and heels. The location used may affect the capillary refill time – for example, the capillary refill time at the heel may show a longer time than at the finger, and fingertip capillary refill time is faster than the sternum capillary refill time (Crook & Taylor, 2013).

Urine output

A normal urine output for the child is approximately 1 mL/kg/hour. The normal urine output for an infant is >2 mL/kg/day, which equates to approximately six to eight wet nappies per day. An infant with no wet nappy for more than four to six hours may have a decreased urine output. Weighed nappies can be used to calculate urine output more accurately. If infants have diarrhoea and evidence of dehydration, an indwelling catheter may be needed to accurately assess urine output.

The colour and concentration of the urine also provide information about the child's hydration status. A reduction in urine output with concentrated urine is often associated with hypovolaemia. As part of the compensatory mechanism, increased concentrations of antidiuretic hormone, angiotensin and aldosterone act on the kidney to promote reabsorption of water and sodium into the body and reduce the volume of urine produced. Renal blood flow may also be decreased, resulting in further decreases in urine output.

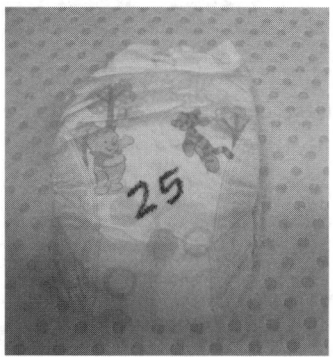

FIGURE 5.3 *Weighed disposable nappy*

It is important to remember that some paediatric conditions that may cause hypovolaemia may have increased urine output – for example, diabetic ketoacidosis, diabetes insipidus and adrenal insufficiency (Hobson & Chima, 2013). In these conditions, urine output may continue to be high despite the child's depleted intravascular volume. Performing a urinalysis and specific gravity can provide more information. During the neonatal period, infants have a reduced capacity to concentrate urine, and may be at greater risk of dehydration.

child with circulatory compromise

Case study 5.2

Robert is a 7-year-old boy who fell from his bicycle yesterday. He sustained a contusion and laceration to his liver. Robert was admitted to the paediatric ward for observation. When you assess Robert, you notice that he looks pale, his heart rate has increased to 140 beats per minute and his peripheral pulse is difficult to feel and thready. You assess his peripheries to be cool up to his elbows. His capillary refill time is three seconds and his respiratory rate is 22 breaths per minute. When you take his blood pressure, it has fallen minimally from 105/55 to 100/54.

Robert is displaying clinical signs of circulatory compromise due to blood loss from his liver injury. His tachycardia and vasoconstriction demonstrate physiological attempts to compensate for the blood loss; however, if Robert does not receive urgent medical treatment he will quickly decompensate into cardiovascular collapse.

D – Disability

The assessment of disability relates to the assessment of the patient's neurological status. It requires a focus on the general appearance, conscious level and responsiveness of the child. Alteration in neurological status may be in response to a primary neurological condition or as a secondary response to other disease processes.

A sick or deteriorating child will often be listless or disinterested in their surroundings, have inappropriate responses to the parents or caregivers, or have a decreased level of consciousness. Reduced level of consciousness in children with respiratory or cardiovascular compromise is a marker for poor cerebral perfusion, and signals the need for urgent cardiorespiratory support.

Muscle and limb tone may provide information about the child's neurological status. Hypotonia may be present in the exhausted or seriously ill child. Abnormal posturing, such as decorticate (upper limb flexion, lower limb extension) or decerebrate (upper and lower limb extension) posturing, is indicative of raised intracranial pressure and serious brain dysfunction (O'Meara & Watton, 2012). Hypertonia or tonic–clonic movements are associated with seizures in children after infancy. Infant seizures are often subtle and easily missed, possibly presenting as apnoeas or subtle movements such as tongue thrusting, lip smacking or bicycling leg movements (Kim et al., 2009).

During illness increased metabolism and disruption to feeding can often cause hypoglycaemia. Hypoglycaemia can result in alterations in neurological status, including jitteriness, hypotonia, lethargy and seizures (DePuy et al., 2009; Hoops et al., 2010). It is important that a blood glucose level is included in the assessment of sick infants and young children (O'Meara & Watton, 2012).

Up to 12 months of age, an infant will have an open anterior fontanel. A tense or bludging fontanel is indicative of raised intracranial pressure: a normal fontanel should be rounded, soft and pulsatile. Performing a paediatric neurological assessment is challenging because of the different cognitive abilities at each developmental stage. In addition to this, there can be significant variations in ability within each developmental stage, making it difficult for clinicians to determine what the child's normal behaviour would be. Psychological factors such as fear of strangers and anxiety often alter a child's behaviour, adding a further challenge to the neurological assessment.

Parents and caregivers are often able to provide valuable information regarding alterations from their child's usual behaviour. When they present with their sick child, caregivers will often report that the child is not their usual self or has been behaving abnormally. Engaging the child's caregivers to assist in neurological assessment is especially important to assist with achieving an accurate assessment.

Changes in pupil size and reactivity can provide important information about the neurological status. In an unconscious child, large and non-reactive pupils are an important sign of life-threatening intracranial hypertension. Small, pinpoint pupils may indicate ingestion or use of narcotic medications (O'Meara & Watton, 2012).

Paediatric neurological assessment tools

Two commonly used paediatric neurological assessment tools, the AVPU and Paediatric Glasgow Coma Scale, will be discussed here to help you gain an understanding of this important aspect of assessing the paediatric patient.

A quick tool that may be used to assess the paediatric patient's level of consciousness is the AVPU (Cullen, 2012a):

A   Alert
V   responds to Voice
P   responds to Pain
U   Unresponsive

This tool is very useful, as it enables the clinician to quickly assess whether the neurological status is normal, slightly abnormal or seriously abnormal. If a child is only responding to painful stimuli, this indicates that the neurological status is seriously abnormal and that the child may no longer be able to protect their own airway.

Medical staff able to intubate the child should be involved in assessing and managing the child. Any child with an altered level of consciousness or mental status needs close and regular monitoring because they are at risk of further deterioration.

The Glasgow Coma Scale (GCS) is also used for the assessment of neurological status. It provides a more comprehensive assessment than the AVPU. The GCS has been modified for infants and children to accommodate for the developmental differences. A GCS of 8 is a serious low score and is associated with the need for clinical interventions to provide airway protection. A GCS of 8 is approximately equivalent to a 'P' on the AVPU scale.

TABLE 5.5 *Glasgow Coma Scale*

PAEDIATRIC GCS	INFANT < 1 YEAR	CHILD 1–5 YEARS
Eye opening 4	Spontaneous	Spontaneous
3	Shouts	Voice
2	Pain	Pain
1	No response	No response
Motor response 5	Spontaneous	Obeys
4	Withdraws	Withdraws
3	Abnormal flexion	Abnormal flexion
2	Abnormal extension	Abnormal extension
1	No response	No response
Verbal response 5	Coos, smiles	Appropriate words, phrases
4	Cries and inconsolable	Inappropriate words
3	Persistent inappropriate crying or screaming	Persistent crying or screaming
2	Grunts, agitated or restless	Grunts or groans
1	No response	No response

Reflection points 5.1

- Early warning tools have been developed to assist clinicians to recognise signs of deterioration in a paediatric patient and trigger an escalation in care, such as an urgent medical review. Consider your clinical experiences in the acute paediatric setting and the early warning tools you have seen or used. What did you find most helpful in relation to the tools? What further learning did they stimulate for you in relation to the care of acutely ill children?
- We have now reviewed two structured paediatric assessment tools: the Paediatric Assessment Triangle and the Primary Assessment Framework for the paediatric patient. What are some of the differences between these approaches? For example, does one approach precede the other?
- The Primary Assessment Framework assesses airway, breathing, circulation and disability. Airway assessment includes history and ability to maintain a clear airway – considering anatomical, physiological and developmental characteristics that increase the paediatric patient's risk for airway compromise, as well as signs of airway compromise, such as inability to speak, manage oral secretions, work of breathing, abnormal breath sounds, posturing in an attempt to open airway and decreased air entry upon auscultation and impaired oxygenation. Why is urgent management of a compromised airway critical in the paediatric patient?
- Breathing assessment incorporates respiratory rate, symmetry of chest wall movement, colour, air entry and breath sound, and signs that indicate

increased work of breathing, including recession or nasal flaring, or head bobbing, and marked diaphragmatic movement in the infant. Oxygen saturation measurements will also complement this data. Why should paediatric nurses look at oxygen saturation readings in conjunction with their complete respiratory assessment?

- The assessment of circulation involves evaluating heart rate and rhythm, peripheral pulses and perfusion, colour and urine output. It is essential to understand the child's normal response and compensatory mechanisms that operate in response to compromised circulatory or cardiovascular function. How might these mechanisms affect heart rate and blood pressure? Why is it important to assess peripheral pulses, perfusion, capillary refill and urine output?
- Disability assessment equates to neurological assessment, and we have reviewed two tools that can assist in this assessment the AVPU and the paediatric Glasgow Coma Scale. If you detected a deterioration in a child's conscious level or responsiveness, what immediate actions would you take?

Case study 5.3: *toddler with neurological compromise*

Angela is a 2-year-old girl who presents to the emergency department being carried by her mother. She had been generally unwell for the previous day and her parents had taken her to the family general practitioner, who had prescribed amoxicillin. This morning, Angela's parents had difficulty waking her. They state that her eyes were rolling back and she was drooling.

Angela is brought into the emergency room to be assessed. Responding to the AVPU method, Angela intermittently opens her eyes when you call her name, consistently withdraws from painful stimuli and makes groaning, incomprehensible noises. Her heart rate is 98, respiratory rate 22, temperature 38.9°C and blood pressure 100/51. Angela has no visible rash and a capillary refill time to two seconds.

Angela displays serious signs of neurological compromise. She needs to be closely monitored and further assessed to ensure that she is able to adequately protect her airway. Angela is later diagnosed with viral encephalitis.

Responding to the sick child

A timely response to the sick child generally requires a team approach. The severity of illness generally will indicate the urgency of treatment. Early warning tools support incorporate the activation of timely responses to clinical assessment findings. This supports the clinician's decision-making and reinforces the need to activate prompt clinical reviews.

Similar to assessment, a structured framework can be used to guide the management of the seriously sick child. Following an A, B, C, D approach, any serious or life-threatening problems must be addressed before continuing with the assessment. For example, if breathing is found to be inadequate, action must be taken to support the breathing before continuing on to assess the circulation.

There has been a significant amount of research into systems that improve the coordination and delivery of emergency care. Often poor communication or inadequate communication systems have been found to create barriers to the effective delivery of timely care. Nurses need to understand the communication processes for individual clinical settings and how to effectively activate a timely clinical review or call for help in an emergency – for example, when and how to initiate a Medical Emergency Team (MET) response.

Paediatric emergency equipment should be available in all clinical areas where children are cared for. As a nurse caring for children, it is important that you are familiar with this equipment and know how to select the appropriate size. There are many resources and algorithms available to assist with paediatric emergency procedures. One example is the Australian Resuscitation Council website (http://resus.org.au).

Respiratory support

Airway and breathing

Respiratory support comprises both airway and breathing support. Some children may require assistance in one of these areas, while others will require both.

Secretions can block the child's airway. Infants primarily breathe through their noses, so suctioning nares that are blocked with secretions can quickly relieve airway obstruction. Oropharyngeal suction can be useful if children are unable to remove oral secretions that pool at the back of the oropharynx. It is advisable to perform oral suction under direct vision to avoid pushing a foreign body back into the airway and causing further obstruction.

Supporting a child's airway can be achieved by effective positioning of the head. For infants, the neutral position optimally opens the airway, while a slightly extended position described as 'sniffing' is used for children over 1 year of age. It is important to avoid neck extension (which would be used in an adult) because this collapses the soft airways, resulting in airway obstruction. Young babies do not have the muscle strength to reposition their heads. Care should be taken when positioning an infant to ensure the head is supported to avoid airway obstruction.

Children at risk of airway obstruction should be observed continuously and never left unattended. In cases where a child has a partially obstructed airway due to swelling or a foreign body, it is prudent to avoid upsetting the child to prevent exacerbating respiratory distress (Fitzgerald & Kilham, 2003). Strategies include leaving a toddler sitting on the parent/caregiver's lap and avoiding unnecessary invasive procedures if possible until someone is present who can confidently manage the airway. Continuous observation and preparation of emergency airway equipment is required because the airway may suddenly deteriorate.

Adrenaline nebulisers may be used to relieve the symptoms of upper airway swelling. The administration of adrenaline causes vasoconstriction to reduce airway swelling, which provides temporarily relief. It is important to monitor these children closely, as the airway obstruction may return as the adrenaline effect wears off. If required, adrenaline nebulisers can be repeated. The use of adrenaline can be very effective in providing time for suitably skilled staff to attend the child. The recommended dose of nebulised adrenaline is 0.5 mL/kg of the 1:1000 solution, up to maximum of 5 mL (Fitzgerald & Kilham, 2003). The dose of adrenaline can be repeated if necessary.

A lowered level of consciousness can result in airway obstruction due to the child's tongue falling back into the oropharynx. Performing a 'chin lift' or 'jaw thrust' manoeuvre lifts the tongue from the posterior oropharynx to open the airway (pemsoft: bag and mask). In an unconscious patient, an oropharyngeal airway can also be used to maintain the airway.

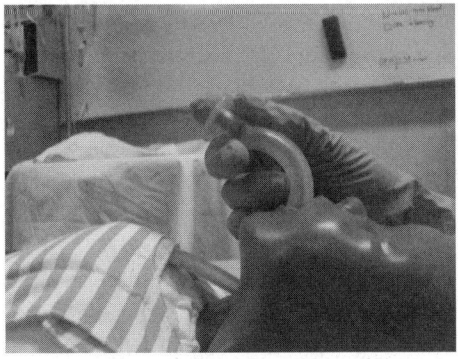

FIGURE 5.4 *Insertion of oral airway*

A small number of children may present to hospital with a tracheostomy tube in situ. Paediatric tracheostomy tubes have a very small diameter and therefore can easily block. Ensuring patency of the tracheostomy tube is an essential element in the airway management of these children. Passing a suction catheter to suction into the tracheostomy tube can both remove secretions and assess the patency of the tube. If the tracheostomy is blocked, a tube change is required. Children presenting to hospital with a tracheostomy tube in situ should have their own supply of appropriately sized tracheotomy tubes with them. Their caregivers will have experience in changing the tracheotomy tube. Consider utilising these resources if required.

> **Clinical tip**
>
> It is important to ensure the oropharyngeal airway is correctly sized by measuring from the centre of the mouth (incisors) to the angle of the jaw. An incorrectly sized guedel airway can obstruct rather than open the airway. The airway should not be rotated in the mouth because this can result in injury to the soft palate. Instead, the airway should be inserted the right way up using a tongue depressor.

Oxygenation

Oxygen should be an early intervention for any sick or deteriorating paediatric patient. For patients with decreased oxygen saturations in room air, oxygen therapy can be applied using a paediatric Hudson mask with a minimum flow rate of 4 L/min. If required, higher percentages of oxygen can be delivered using a paediatric non-rebreathing mask with a reservoir bag. Using an appropriately sized mask and flow rate is important to prevent the retention and rebreathing of carbon dioxide. Nasal prongs can also be used to deliver lower flows of oxygen. Generally, in paediatric patients, the prongs are taped in place using a protective hydrocolloid dressing under the tape to protect the skin.

Circulatory support

Vascular access is important for paediatric patients, and will often be obtained via the insertion of a peripheral cannula upon admission and before problems occur, as the peripheral vasoconstriction that occurs in response to hypovolaemia, for example, can make the already small peripheral veins of an infant or child even more difficult to cannulate. In infants and children, vascular access may be obtained via peripheral veins, including the dorsum of the hand, wrist, forearm and the antecubital fossa, as well as the foot and ankle where the long

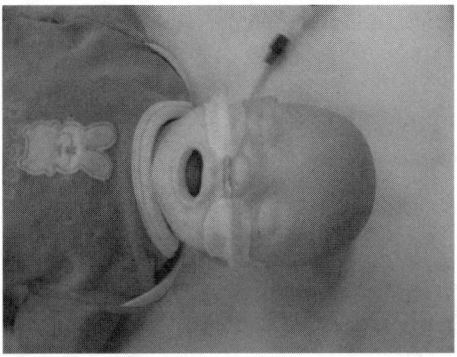

FIGURE 5.5 *Nasal prongs*

saphenous vein may be accessed (ARC, 2010c). In infants, a scalp vein is also sometimes used.

If a child is seriously ill and deteriorating, intravenous access should be attempted for no more than 90 seconds. Failure to obtain access in this time period requires alternative access to be attempted. If a suitably skilled person is available to insert a central venous line, this may be used. Alternatively, the intraosseous route may be used to gain emergency vascular access.

Intraosseous needles are usually used in infants and children up to approximately 6 years of age, as changes to the vascularity of the bone marrow and thickening of the bone after this age make it harder to obtain access. However, if an intraosseous drill is available, the intraosseous route may be used for older children and adults (Cullen, 2012b). The location for insertion of an intraosseous needle in infants and young children is the anterior and medial surface of the tibia, approximately 1–2 cm below the tibial tuberosity (see Figure 5.6) (Cullen, 2012b). The intraosseous route can be used for medications and fluids. Fluids cannot run via gravity, but must be injected or administered via an infusion pump.

Once vascular access has been obtained, fluid resuscitation and/or medications may be administered. If hypovolaemia is suspected as a cause of circulatory compromise, then the administration of an initial 20 mL/kg bolus of a crystalloid solution such as 0.9 per cent normal saline is recommended and the child's response to this initial bolus is then assessed (ARC, 2010a). Further

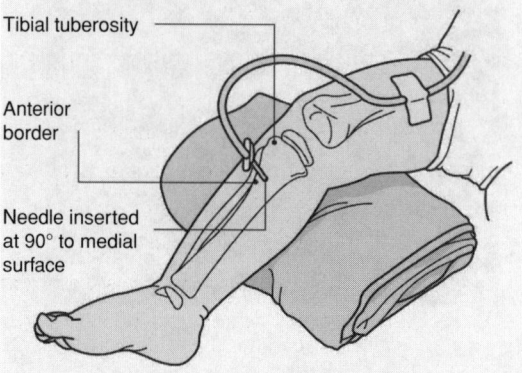

FIGURE 5.6 *Intraosseous cannulation site in children*

Source: Cullen (2012b), used with permission.

boluses of crystalloid solutions or colloids such as 5 per cent albumin may then be ordered by the physician.

A practical method for quickly and accurately administering fluid resuscitation in children is to use 50 mL syringes to draw up and inject the fluid bolus.

Paediatric basic and advanced life support

So far in this section, we have discussed strategies to provide respiratory and circulatory support to the deteriorating child. We will now provide an overview of paediatric cardiopulmonary resuscitation that may be required if the initial measures of respiratory and circulatory support are not successful in averting further deterioration. It is important at this stage to distinguish between **basic life support** and **advanced life support**. Basic life support refers to efforts made to restore or maintain airway, breathing and circulation that do not require adjunct equipment such as airways, masks and so on. Advanced life support involves basic life support with the addition of more invasive measures such as advanced airway management, intubation, intravenous access and defibrillation.

We have already discussed some basic airway support manoeuvres and establishing intravenous access. We will now provide an overview of cardiopulmonary resuscitation and some more invasive respiratory support measures. Table 5.6 provides a summary of the latest guidelines for paediatric cardiopulmonary resuscitation and cardiac compression delivery site and depth, and ratio of cardiac compression to ventilation.

In situations where the infant or child has stopped breathing or respiration is insufficient, the child should be supported by providing bag and mask ventilation. In most cases, this should be provided by using a paediatric self-inflating bag attached to oxygen and with an appropriately sized face mask. A correctly sized mask covers the mouth and nose, and achieves a seal when gently held onto the child's face. To effectively hold the mask, the thumb and index finger form a 'C' around the mask while the other fingers are placed along the jaw line.

When providing bag and mask ventilation, you should observe for rise and fall of the chest. Excessive pressure will result in air being forced into the stomach, which in turn can splint the diaphragm, inhibiting effective air entry. The insertion of a nasogastric tube can be useful to decompress the stomach.

It is worthwhile obtaining paediatric mannequins to be able to practise basic life support with a peer or colleague. Your university clinical laboratory on campus or the clinical educator in the paediatric setting will be able to assist you to engage in this important preparation for paediatric cardiopulmonary resuscitation.

Basic life support Efforts made to restore or maintain airway, breathing and circulation that do not require adjunct equipment such as airways or masks. An example would be being a first responder and performing cardiopulmonary resuscitation in a public area

Advanced life support Incorporates basic life support as well as more invasive measures such as advanced airway management, intubation, intravenous access and defibrillation

Parental presence during resuscitation

Parents may wish to be present during resuscitation. If this is the case, it is very important to have an experienced staff member available to support the family. Some nurses may worry that witnessing resuscitation could be distressing for

TABLE 5.6 *Paediatric cardiopulmonary resuscitation*

CHILD AGE	INFANT <1 YEAR	CHILD 1–8 YEARS	OLDER CHILD >8 YEARS OR ADULT
Pulse check	Carotid, brachial or femoral pulse		
Head tilt position	Neutral position	Slightly extended sniffing position from 1 year For older child, semi- to full-extension head tilt with chin lift	Semi to full-extension head tilt with chin lift
Compression site	Lower half of sternum, below nipple line	Lower half of sternum (calliper method)	Lower half of sternum (calliper method)
Compression delivery method	Pressure with two thumbs or two fingers In the two-thumb technique, hands encircle chest and thumbs compress the sternum	Pressure with heel of one hand	Pressure with heel of both hands
Compression depth	4 cm or approximately one-third depth of anterior-posterior dimension of the chest	4–5 cm or approximately one-third depth of anterior-posterior dimension of the chest	5 cm or approximately one-third depth of anterior-posterior dimension of the chest
Basic life support rescue by one or two rescuers			
Compression:Ventilation ratio	30:2		
ECC rate/minute	Approximately 100 compressions per minute		
Time for one cycle	One compression every 0.6 seconds or almost 2 per second 5 cycles in 2 minutes		
Advanced Life Support rescue by two healthcare rescuers			
Compression:Ventilation ratio	15:2		
ECC rate/minute	75 compressions per minute		
Time for 1 cycle	5 cycles per minute		

Source: Adapted from Australian Resuscitation Council (2010a).

parents; however, a recent Australian study of families whose child required resuscitation in the paediatric intensive-care unit found that parents who did not witness their child's resuscitation experienced greater distress than the parents who stayed (Maxton, 2008).

Family members such as siblings will also need to be supported at an appropriate location and, depending on the circumstances, may be cared for by another family member in the patient lounge or ward play area. In some settings, such as paediatric intensive care units, a nurse or other member of the multidisciplinary team not directly involved in the resuscitation may be available to talk with older siblings who, although not present for the resuscitation, may want to discuss their concerns.

As a nurse caring for paediatric patients, your ability to be able to provide safe care is paramount. Recognising the sick infant or child and responding promptly can prevent deterioration and life-threatening respiratory and circulatory collapse. From your reading and reflection on the case studies in this chapter, you should now be well equipped with the ability to assess an infant or child using appropriate assessment frameworks and tools, be able to detect signs of deterioration and be able to respond quickly and effectively to escalate the need for an urgent medical review of the patient, and provide respiratory and circulatory support if needed to prevent further deterioration.

Summary

- Paediatric patients have distinct developmental, anatomical and physiological characteristics that increase their susceptibility to respiratory and circulatory compromise. Respiratory and heart rates vary according to age, and the assessment of airway, breathing, circulation and disability involves obtaining and evaluating key assessment data within each element of the primary survey in order to detect abnormalities and signs of deterioration that necessitate an escalation in care and medical review.
- Early warning tools such as the Paediatric Early Warning Score (PEWS), the Cardiac Children's Hospital Early Warning Score (C-CHEWS) or Between the Flags may be used in paediatric nursing practice to assist nurses to identify a child who is deteriorating and who warrants an urgent and appropriate response.

- A deteriorating child may require airway and breathing and/or circulatory support, so it is essential that paediatric nurses know how to support the child's airway, provide appropriate oxygenation using appropriate devices (high-flow nasal prong oxygen, masks, or bag and mask ventilation). Circulatory support requires vascular access, either through intravenous or intraosseous routes. If intravenous access is not obtained and there is an urgent need for fluid resuscitation and medications, the intraosseous route is used. Initial fluid resuscitation for hypovolaemia is generally a 20 mL/kg bolus of 0.9 per cent normal saline.
- If initial measures to support respiration and circulation are unsuccessful, then cardiopulmonary resuscitation may be required. The correct head tilt position, appropriate mask, compression site, depth and ratio of compression to ventilation will depend on whether the patient is an infant, child or adolescent, and the number of rescuers. Paediatric nurses need to practise resuscitation skills regularly to ensure their competence in this area.
- Support for the family is integral to effective care for the sick and deteriorating child, and family members should have a designated support person during resuscitation to answer questions, and to provide information and emotional support. Parental presence during paediatric resuscitation can be achieved provided there is adequate support available, but will also be an individual family's choice.

Learning activity

Case Study 5.1 introduced you to Maggie, a 6-month-old infant with suspected RSV bronchiolitis. This learning activity encourages you to explore the nursing assessment and management of Maggie. Read the information below, then answer the questions that follow.

Nasopharyngeal suctioning and bronchiolitis

Nasopharyngeal (NP) suctioning could be very effective to assist Maggie with her breathing. The NP suctioning procedure involves the insertion of a narrow, flexible suction catheter gently into the nasal passage in a similar fashion to a nasogastric tube. The depth of insertion should be no deeper than the distance from the tip of the nose to the tragus of the ear. The suction pressure should be no greater than −120 mmHg, and should only be applied as the catheter is withdrawn. The entire procedure should take less than 15 seconds. Because infants are unable to cooperate, often a second person is required to secure the infant to prevent nasal trauma during the procedure.

High-flow nasal cannulae therapy and bronchiolitis

High-flow nasal cannulae (HFNC) therapy provides respiratory support for infants and children by delivery of warmed and humidified air/oxygen blend at high flow rates. HFNC therapy can be effective in decreasing work of breathing. When it has been used for paediatric patients with bronchiolitis, the need for invasive respiratory support such as intubation and mechanical ventilation has been avoided. It is not clear exactly how it works; however, it is thought that the high flow may provide some continuous positive airway pressure (CPAP), which facilities an opening of the airways to promote gas exchange (Schibler et al., 2011; Beggs et al., 2012).

5.1 Based on your reading in this chapter, what assessment data in the case study indicate that Maggie is experiencing respiratory distress?

5.2 Considering that infants are obligatory nose breathers, and that bronchiolitis results in copious nasal secretions that increase airway resistance and respiratory distress, what nursing interventions could you implement to address this issue for Maggie?

5.3 What is high-flow nasal cannulae (HFNC) therapy, and why is it used in infants with bronchiolitis?

5.4 What additional concerns (other than respiratory distress) are significant for Maggie?

Further reading

- Akre, M et al., 2010, Sensitivity of the Pediatric Early Warning Score to identify patient deterioration, *Pediatrics*, 125, pp. e763–e770. This article provides an overview of the Paediatric Early Warning Score and includes an image of the tool.
- Bressan, S, Balzani, M, Krauss, B, Pettenazzo, A, Zanconato, S & Baraldi, E 2013, High-flow nasal cannula oxygen for bronchiolitis in a paediatric ward: A pilot study, *European Journal of Pediatrics*, 1–8, pp. 1649–56. This

article can be accessed to enhance your understanding of high-flow nasal cannulae oxygen therapy for infants with bronchiolitis.
● Schibler, A, Pham, TM, Dunster, KR, Foster, K, Barlow, A, Gibbons, K & Hough, JL 2011, Reduced intubation rates for infants after introduction of high-flow nasal prong oxygen delivery. *Intensive Care Medicine*, 37(5), pp. 847–52. This article can be accessed to enhance your understanding of high-flow nasal cannulae oxygen therapy for infants with bronchiolitis.

References

Ait-Oufella, H et al. 2013, Alteration of skin perfusion in mottling area during septic shock. *Annals of Intensive Care*, 31(3), viewed 20 March 2014, http://www.annalsofintensivecare.com/content/3/1/31.

Akre, M et al. 2010, Sensitivity of the Pediatric Early Warning Score to identify patient deterioration, *Pediatrics*, 125, pp. e763–e770.

Australian Resuscitation Council (ARC) 2010a, *Guideline 12.2 Advanced life support for infants and children diagnosis and management*, ARC, viewed 27 August 2013, http://www.resus.org.au.

—— 2010b, *Guideline 12.4: Medications & fluids in paediatric advanced life support*, viewed 27 August 2013, http://www.resus.org.au.

—— 2010c, *Guideline 12.6: Techniques in paediatric advanced life support*, viewed 27 August 2013, http://www.resus.org.au.

Aylott, M 2006, Observing the sick child: Part 2a – respiratory assessment, *Paediatric Nursing*.18(9), pp. 38–44.

Beggs, S, Wong, ZH, Kaul, S, Ogden, KJ & Walters, JAE 2012, High-flow nasal cannula therapy for infants with bronchiolitis (protocol), *Cochrane Database of Systematic Reviews*, 2, art. no. CD009609.

Bressan, S et al. 2013, High-flow nasal cannula oxygen for bronchiolitis in a paediatric ward: A pilot study, *European Journal of Pediatrics*, 1–8, pp. 1649–56.

Crook, J & Taylor, RM 2013, The agreement of fingertip and sternum capillary refill time in children, *Archives of Disease in Childhood*, 98, pp. 265–8.

Cullen, PM 2012a, Paediatric trauma: Continuing education in anaesthesia,*Critical Care and Pain*, 12(3), pp. 157–61.

—— 2012b, Intraosseous cannulation in children, *Anaesthesia & Intensive Care Medicine*, 13(1), pp. 28–30.

DePuy, A, Coassolo, K, Som, D & Smulian, J 2009, Neonatal hypoglycemia in term, nondiabetic pregnancies, *American Journal of Obstetrics and Gynecology*, 200(5), pp. e45–e51.

Dieckmann, RA, Brownstein, D & Gausche-Hill, M 2010, The Pediatric Assessment Triangle: A novel approach for the rapid evaluation of children, *Pediatric Emergency Care*, 26, pp. 312–15.

Fitzgerald, D & Kilham, H 2003, Croup: Assessment and evidence-based management, *Medical Journal of Australia*, 179, pp. 372–7.

Fouzas, S, Priftis, KN & Anthracopoulos, MB 2011, Pulse oximetry in pediatric practice, *Pediatrics*, 128, pp. 740–52.

Gill, D & O'Brien, N (eds) 2007, *Paediatric clinical examination made easy*, 5th edn, Churchill Livingstone, London.

Hobson, MJ & Chima, RS 2013, Pediatric hypovolemic shock, *The Open Pediatric Medicine Journal*, 7(Supp. 1), pp. 10–15.

Hoops, D et al. 2010, Should routine peripheral blood glucose testing be done for all newborns at birth? *American Journal of Maternal Child Nursing*, 35(5), pp. 264–70.

Kim, U, Brousseau, D & Konduri, G 2008, Evaluation and management of the critically ill neonate in the emergency department, *Clinical Pediatric Emergency Medicine*, 9, pp. 140–8.

Maxton, FJ 2008, Parental presence during resuscitation in the PICU: The parents' experience. Sharing and surviving the resuscitation: A phenomenological study. *Journal of Clinical Nursing*, 17(23), pp. 3168–76.

McLellan, MC & Connor, JA 2013, The Cardiac Children's Hospital Early Warning Score (C-CHEWS), *Journal of Pediatric Nursing*, 28, pp. 171–8.

Milésien, C, Baleine, J, Matecki, S, Duovais, A & Combonie, G 2013, Is the treatment with high flow nasal cannula effective in acute viral bronchiolitis? A physiologic study, *Intensive Care Medicine*, 39(6), pp. 1088–94.

Moler, FW 2009, In-hospital versus out-of-hospital pediatric cardiac arrest: A multicenter cohort study, *Critical Care Medicine*, 37(7), p. 2259.

Munroe, B, Curtis, K, Considine, J & Buckley, T 2013, The impact structured patient assessment frameworks have on patient care: An integrative review, *Journal of Clinical Nursing*, 22, pp. 2991–3005.

National High Blood Pressure Education Program Working Group on High Blood Pressure in Children and Adolescents 2004, The fourth report on the diagnosis, evaluation, and treatment of high blood pressure in children and adolescents, *Pediatrics*, 114(Supp. 2), pp. 555–76.

O'Meara, M & Watton, DJ (eds) 2012, *Advanced paediatric life support: The practical approach*, 5th edn, Blackwell, London.

Pickard, A, Karlen, W & Ansermino, JM 2011, Capillary refill time: Is it still a useful clinical sign?', *Anesthesia and Analgesia*, 113(1), pp. 120–3.

Santillanes, G & Gausche-Hill, M 2008, Pediatric airway management, *Emergency Clinics of North America*, 26, pp. 961–75.

Schibler, A et al. 2011, Reduced intubation rates for infants after introduction of high-flow nasal prong oxygen delivery, *Intensive Care Medicine*, 37(5), pp. 847–52.

Top, APC, Tasker, RC & Ince, C 2011, The microcirculation of the critically ill paediatric patient, *Critical Care*, 15, pp. 213–19.

Walsh, BK, Hood, K & Merritt, G 2011, Pediatric airway maintenance and clearance in the acute care setting: How to stay out of trouble, *Respiratory Care*, 56(9), pp. 1424–44.

6
End-of-life and palliative care in Australian paediatric care settings

Elizabeth Forster

Learning objectives

In this chapter you will:

- Develop an understanding of the physical and psychological problems experienced by children in end-of-life care
- Develop an understanding of some of the strategies used to address or manage these problems in paediatric end-of-life care
- Consider the importance of communication with the child/young person, parents, siblings and grandparents in paediatric end-of-life care
- Explore ways to support parents, siblings and grandparents in paediatric end-of-life care

Introduction

Although children in Australia enjoy a high life expectancy and high level of wellbeing, paediatric death remains a sad reality for some families, and end-of-life care for children presents an important and challenging area of paediatric nursing practice.

The rate of child mortality in Australia more than halved from 30 to 13 deaths between 1986 and 2006, due to a reduction in the number of paediatric deaths from transport-related accidents; however, the mortality rate stabilised between 2006 and 2010 (AIHW, 2012). Among children aged 1–14 years between 2008 and 2010, the leading causes of death included injury (34 per cent), cancer (17 per cent) and nervous system diseases (11 per cent) (AIHW, 2012).

> **Paediatric palliative care** The multidisciplinary care of the child's physical, psychosocial and spiritual needs, which encompasses the illness trajectory from diagnosis until death and includes end-of-life care. This care and support extends to the child's family
>
> **Paediatric end-of-life care** The multidisciplinary care of the child's physical, psychosocial and spiritual needs, and the care and support of the child's family at end of life and beyond

As a beginning paediatric nurse, it is important that you understand that the terms **paediatric palliative care** and **paediatric end-of-life care** are conceptualised differently, despite some overlap. Paediatric palliative care begins when a disease is first diagnosed, and continues throughout the illness trajectory. It therefore includes, but is not limited to, end-of-life care (Crozier & Hancock, 2012). The majority of paediatric palliative care is delivered by hospital-based or community teams in the last six months of a child's life (Crozier & Hancock, 2012). Paediatric end-of-life care is the care provided to the child and family towards the end of a child's life, and includes care of the child's body and support for the family following the child's death. Although there are distinctions between the two terms, in this chapter they will be used interchangeably.

The World Health Organization (WHO) definition of palliative care for children was developed in 1998 in recognition that paediatric palliative care, although related to adult palliative care, is a distinct and specialised area. The WHO (1998) definition includes the following principles:

- Palliative care for children is the active total care of the child's body, mind and spirit, and also involves giving support to the family.
- It begins when illness is diagnosed, and continues regardless of whether or not a child receives treatment directed at the disease.
- Health providers must evaluate and alleviate a child's physical, psychological and social distress.
- Effective palliative care requires a broad multidisciplinary approach that includes the family and makes use of available community resources; it can be implemented successfully even if resources are limited.
- It can be provided in tertiary care facilities, in community health centres and even in children's homes.

Central to paediatric end-of-life care are the frequent and comprehensive assessment and management of physical and psychological symptoms, facilitating effective and developmentally appropriate communication with the child and family, individualised holistic care with a focus on quality rather than quantity of life, and the involvement of a multidisciplinary team of health professionals (Stayer, 2012).

Paediatric end-of-life care occurs in a variety of contexts, including the acute paediatric setting and the community, in hospice care and in the child's home.

The trajectory or path of a child and family's journey from diagnosis to end-of-life care will vary, and for some families this journey may be as short as a few days or weeks or as long as many years in the case of chronic conditions.

This chapter will provide you with a beginning understanding of some of the common symptoms and concerns for children in end-of-life care and their management, including pain, the management of side-effects of opioids, fatigue, dyspnoea, gastrointestinal disturbances and anxiety. It will also discuss communication with dying children and adolescents, and the importance of family communication and support.

Pain

Pain assessment in children is a complex area requiring keen observation skills and effective, age-appropriate communication. Paediatric pain assessment is discussed in more detail in Chapter 8, and it is recommended that you revise this chapter in relation to the assessment of paediatric pain. In this chapter, paediatric pain management in end-of-life care will be the main focus of discussion. As a foundation for understanding pain management in end-of-life care, it is helpful to review the WHO analgesic ladder.

The WHO analgesic ladder

WHO first introduced the analgesic ladder in the 1980s as a guide for the management of cancer pain. The original ladder had three steps, and was criticised for not recognising the multiple causes of pain (not just disease progression, but side-effects of treatment, psychosocial and so on), being unidirectional/suggesting a one way escalation in pain management for patients, focusing on pharmacological approaches only, and neglecting the importance of psychosocial assessment and other pain-management approaches (Glare, 2011). A more recent article has suggested the following adaptation of the ladder, and includes a fourth step with more complex pain relief strategies, recognition of the need for a step-up and step-down approach to pain relief and the potential need for neurosurgical procedures to relieve pain (Vargas-Schaffer, 2010).

Non steroidal anti-inflammatory drugs (NSAIDs) are found on the first step of the analgesic ladder. NSAIDs are frequently used to manage chronic pain for children in palliative care due to their effectiveness in inflammatory causes of pain; they are also helpful for pain due caused by bony metastases

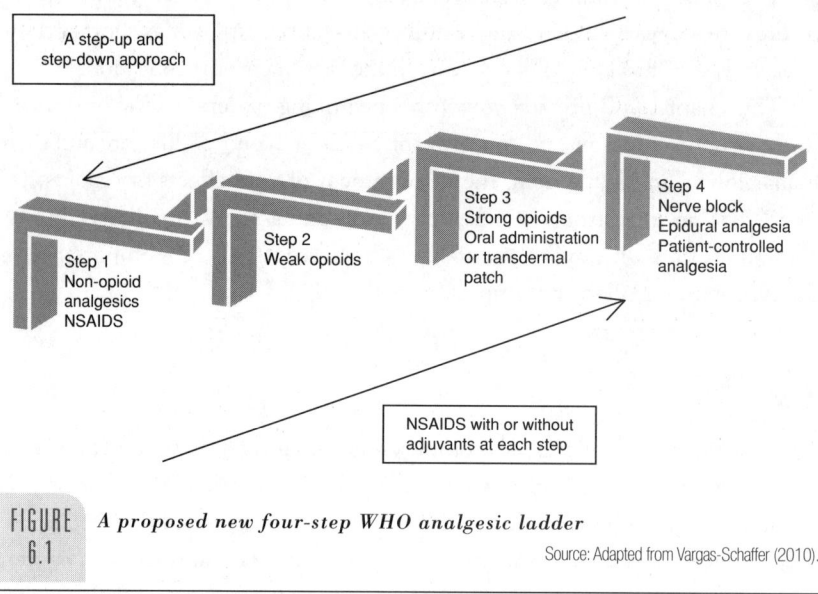

FIGURE 6.1   *A proposed new four-step WHO analgesic ladder*
Source: Adapted from Vargas-Schaffer (2010).

(Dowden, 2014). The WHO ladder then recommends the use of weak opioids such as codeine, then strong opioids such as morphine for severe pain. Although opioids such as morphine remain effective for the management of severe pain, unfortunately they have a variety of side-effects that can increase the suffering of children if not managed promptly and appropriately.

Side-effects of opioids

Although opioids such as morphine can provide good pain relief for moderate to severe pain, there are many side-effects related to their use that may need to be addressed. More common side-effects include constipation, pruritis and nausea and vomiting, and less common ones are urinary retention, respiratory depression and **myoclonus** (Shaw, 2012). Table 6.1 lists some side-effects of opioid analgesia and strategies that may be used to manage these.

As a beginning clinician working in palliative care, you will need to familiarise yourself with the usual doses of medications commonly prescribed in paediatric palliative care. Table 6.2 provides an overview of some of the common opioids prescribed for children in palliative care and their usual starting dosages.

> **Myoclonus**
> Involuntary twitching may occur when high doses of opioids are used, due to an accumulation of metabolites, which have neuro-excitory effects

TABLE 6.1 *Side-effects of opioids and strategies to address these*

OPIOID SIDE-EFFECT AND CAUSE	MANAGEMENT
Constipation Decreased intestinal motility due to opioid	Preventative management with stool-softeners at initiation of opioid treatment.
Pruritis Benign side-effect due to histamine-releasing properties of opioids	Pruritis will usually resolve within a few days, but antihistamines may need to be prescribed by the medical officer.
Nausea and vomiting An initial side-effect of opioids, but may also be linked to constipation	Antiemetic therapies such as Ondansetron or Metoclopramide may need to be prescribed by the medical officer.
Urinary retention An uncommon side-effect of opioids	Try techniques such as running water and Crede's manoeuvre.
Respiratory depression Very rare when appropriate opioid doses and titration are used	Accurate assessment is required to distinguish between a reduced respiratory demand and slowing of respirations that may normally accompany a reduction in pain intensity and true respiratory depression.
	Respiratory depression is usually preceded by a decreased level of consciousness and somnolence.
	Excessive slowing of respiration rate may be managed by rousing the child, slowing the rate of the opioid infusion or administering oxygen.
	Reversal agents such as naloxone should be used cautiously, as they rapidly reverse pain relief, which may lead to severe pain and may result in life-threatening opioid withdrawal.
Myoclonus Brief involuntary twitching that may occur when high doses of opioids are used, or if they are administered over a long period and are due to an accumulation of metabolites which have neuro-excitory effects	Rotating to a different opioid may be a consideration, or the medical officer may need to prescribe benzodiazepines or muscle relaxants.

Source: Adapted from Klick & Hauer (2010); Shaw (2012).

TABLE 6.2 *Starting doses for opioid analgesia*

MEDICATION	DOSE	INTERVAL
Morphine	0.05–0.1 mg/kg/dose	Every 2–4 hours
Intravenous/subcutaneous	0.15–0.3 mg/kg/dose	Every 3–4 hours as prescribed
Oral		Every 1 hour as needed
Oxycodone	0.1–0.2 mg/kg	Every 4–6 hours
Oral		
Fentanyl	0.5–1 µg/kg	Every 1–2 hours
Intravenous	Convert from IV dose	
Transdermal		

Source: Adapted from Klick & Hauer (2010); Shaw (2012).

Non-pharmacological pain relief

In addition to the pharmacological management of pain in paediatric end-of-life care, non-pharmacological strategies have an important complementary role to play. Non-pharmacological pain relief strategies may range from cognitive/behavioural techniques and distraction to strategies involving physical touch, including skin-to-skin contact for infants or massage (Levine et al., 2013).

Cognitive and behavioural techniques encompass a variety of strategies, including guided imagery, hypnosis, relaxation, distraction, storytelling, music and art therapy, and play therapy (Hyde et al., 2012; Monterosso & DeGraves, 2012). These approaches acknowledge that pain involves both physical and psychological elements, and many of these cognitive and behavioural strategies may be helpful in targeting perceptions of pain and therefore contribute to overall pain relief.

Massage is commonly used by parents for a variety of health and discomfort-related problems (for example, infant colic, stress reduction, relaxation, sleep problems and musculoskeletal pain), and is also often used in the health-care setting for relieving discomfort associated with procedures and as a complementary therapy in paediatric cancer (Hughes et al., 2008). A systematic review of the use of massage among patients with cancer, including those in palliative care, has been conducted and found some evidence for its benefit in cancer palliation and supportive care (Ernst, 2009). However, more research is needed, particularly in paediatric palliative care, as this review contains limited paediatric specific studies (Ernst, 2009).

Reflection points 6.1

- Paediatric end-of-life care encompasses the physical, psychosocial and spiritual care of the child, and support for the family leading up to and following the child's death. It may be provided in a hospital or hospice, or at home. How might the setting in which end-of-life care is provided influence your role as a paediatric nurse?
- The WHO analgesic ladder was developed as a guide for the management of cancer pain in the 1980s, but Vargas-Schaffer (2010) suggests a fourth step, and a step-up and step-down approach. Why might a step-down approach to pain management be important for paediatric end-of-life care, especially when this care may be delivered over a long period of time, as in the case of life-limiting conditions?

- Opioids such as morphine remain a commonly used analgesic in paediatric end-of-life care; however, they are also accompanied by many side-effects. Why is the ability to assess and manage these side-effects so important for paediatric nurses working in end-of-life care?
- Non-pharmacological pain-relief strategies may also be used to complement pharmacological pain relief in paediatric end-of-life care. Consider some of the non-pharmacological approaches you have seen used in your clinical practice. How might these be useful in paediatric end-of-life care? Conduct a database search to find out whether any research been conducted using these approaches in paediatric palliative care.

Fatigue

Fatigue is a difficult concept to define, but most agree that it involves both physical and psychological facets. Fatigue remains one of the most common problems experienced by children at end of life (Tomlinson et al., 2011; Ullrich et al., 2010; Wolfe et al., 2000) and has been found to increase as children near death (Tomlinson et al., 2011). In their pioneering study concerning fatigue among children and adolescents with cancer, one group of researchers found that fatigue comprised both physical and psychological symptoms and the descriptions of children and adolescents can be found in Table 6.3.

> **Fatigue** Feelings of tiredness and lethargy; a multidimensional term that includes physical, psychological, energy and sleep facets

Fatigue is a multidimensional problem experienced by dying children, and has been found to be associated with other symptoms such as nausea and vomiting, diarrhoea, nutritional impairment and anaemia, sleep disturbances (especially during hospitalisation) and psychological experiences such as fear, anxiety and sadness (Ullrich et al., 2010). It may also be linked to side-effects of pain and dyspnoea treatments such as opioids and sedative medications (Ullrich et al., 2010).

Paediatric nurses should use valid and reliable tools/scales to assess for fatigue in children. One assessment scale that has been developed and used to measure fatigue among paediatric cancer patients is the Fatigue Scale – Child for 7- to 12-year-olds, which was developed by Hockenberry and colleagues (2003). This scale contains 14 items that are completed by the child using a Likert scale format with total fatigue scores from 0 indicating no fatigue symptoms to 70 indicating high fatigue. More recently, this tool has been reduced to a 10-item scale (Hinds et al., 2010). Children completing the scale rate

TABLE 6.3 *Child and adolescent descriptions of fatigue*

CHILDREN'S DESCRIPTIONS OF FATIGUE	ADOLESCENTS' DESCRIPTIONS OF FATIGUE
Finding it hard to move or run, being not as active as usual	Feeling a wearing away of your body
Feeling like laying around, needing to lie down and wanting to do nothing	Originating in your mind so that if you think you are going to be tired you become tired
Feeling weak or tired, being not able to do much	Being both physical and mental, and when you're physically tired this challenges you mentally
Feeling sad or mad, feeling upset when you are emotionally tired	Feeling not your normal self or up to your normal activity level, and not playing with friends, sport or school
Feeling not able to play or participate in sports and physical activities	Makes you mad, or feel upset when tired and getting mad about it
Physical signs such as difficulty keeping eyes open, having a dull face	Not wanting to be bothered by others
Falling asleep easily and needing to sleep more	Feeling sorry for yourself
	Physical symptoms such as dizziness, nausea, hot and cold flashes
	Feeling sleepy and falling asleep anywhere
	Feeling mentally tired because of having to go through so much
	Not wanting to do anything but lay around

Source: Adapted from Hockenberry-Eaton et al. (1998).

statements such as 'I have been tired', 'My body has felt different' and 'I have been tired in the morning' (Hockenberry et al., 2003: 322).

Fatigue has been described as difficult to treat and manage, although a variety of strategies have been employed in an effort to manage this distressing problem. A small number of studies in paediatric patients undergoing treatment for cancer have investigated exercise for fatigue management; however, the utility of this intervention in end-of-life care is uncertain, due to the child's deteriorating physical condition (Chang et al., 2013). Massage, together with strategies to promote nutrition and energy conservation which have also been used in paediatric cancer studies (Chang et al., 2013), may be more appropriate for children in end-of-life care. Fatigue among children at end of life may be relieved through the management of sedative effects of opioid medications, reducing anorexia, nausea and vomiting, and improving nutrition, and by addressing sleep disturbances and distressing psychological issues such as sorrow and anxiety (Ullrich et al., 2010). The multi-faceted nature of fatigue, and its diverse influencing factors, make it challenging to manage, and further research is needed in paediatric end-of-life care to determine the most effective strategies to combat this problem.

Dyspnoea

Abnormal or difficult breathing is another symptom experienced by children in end-of-life care, and is a cause of distress to both the child and the family (Pritchard et al., 2008).

In children, **dyspnoea** usually occurs due to a combination of:

- increased work of breathing linked to increased airway resistance, decreased lung compliance or decreased muscle strength or abnormality, and
- increased ventilation requirements due to metabolic acidosis, hypoxaemia, anaemia or other physiological states. (Robinson, 2012)

> **Dyspnoea**
> Abnormal or difficult breathing that may include feelings of tiredness, suffocation, air hunger or panic associated with breathing, awareness of the work of breathing and chest tightness

The management of dyspnoea in paediatric palliative care requires a weighing up or balancing of the burden of treatments, which may be quite aggressive and upsetting for the child, versus the more conservative management of symptoms. This needs to be negotiated constantly between health professionals and the child (if appropriate) and parents (Robinson, 2012). In palliative care, the pathophysiological cause of the dyspnoea may not be pursued, and instead the focus will be on the management of the dyspnoea to ensure the child's comfort.

It is important to acknowledge the psychological relationship with dyspnoea and the physiological processes, as this highlights the importance of management strategies that will be targeted towards the child's perceptions, thoughts and feelings about their dyspnoea as well as the underlying physiological processes. A useful way to remember this relationship is to consider how you feel after a long, strenuous aerobic exercise session, where you are struggling to get your breath and feeling a sense of chest tightness or dyspnoea. Because you are not alarmed by this mentally, and understand it is a normal and even desirable response under the circumstances, you feel quite calm as you know it will resolve in a few minutes. However, if you are very ill and you start to experience difficulty breathing, then your cognitive state would likely be quite different: you would likely begin to worry, become fearful and experience a sense of panic. We must consider the cognitive and affective relationship with dyspnoea:

> In addressing the suffering associated with dyspnoea we must consider the fact that the mind is not only an agent through which suffering is experienced or perceived, but it also is an active participant in the physiology of dyspnoea.
> (Hallenbeck, 2012: 849)

Parental perceptions are a vital component of management of dyspnoea in paediatric palliative care, as a child will usually look to their parents to gauge how to interpret most situations. It is very important that parents receive support and education about the possibility that their child may experience breathing difficulties in palliative care, and the importance of remaining calm and reassuring in their child's presence to avoid exacerbating the child's negative perceptions of their dyspnoea, which will in turn worsen their breathing difficulties.

Both non-pharmacological and pharmacological strategies can be used to relieve dyspnoea in children. Non-pharmacological strategies include behavioural interventions such as behaviour modification and techniques to reduce anxiety and controlled breathing techniques. The use of fans to increase circulating air and blow air over a child's face may also be helpful, as some studies using nasal prong flow of air across the nasal passages have achieved relief from dyspnoea in some patients, although the exact mechanism of action is unknown (Abernethy et al., 2010; Robinson, 2012; Ullrich & Mayer, 2007). The main pharmacological strategy for the management of dyspnoea in both adult and paediatric patients is the use of opioids such as morphine. Other strategies may include the use of assisted non-invasive ventilation such as BiPaP or CPAP, but these may not be well tolerated by paediatric patients. They may, however, be used at night and during sleep periods to counteract respiratory muscle fatigue, which may enable a child to have more energy to participate in daytime activities (Robinson, 2012). It is important to consider that parents may not want to have their view of their dying child's face obstructed by the masks used in non-invasive ventilation (Ullrich & Mayer, 2007), and this is another example of balancing the need for treatments and their associated burdens for the child and family.

Gastrointestinal disturbances

There are a variety of gastrointestinal (GI) disturbances that may create unnecessary discomfort for children in palliative care, including constipation, nausea and vomiting. These GI disturbances, as mentioned earlier in this chapter, may be linked to opioid administration. Table 6.1 (earlier in the chapter) lists some strategies to combat these side-effects of opioid analgesia. In relation to constipation, it is important for paediatric nurses to assess the child's risk as well as stool characteristics. A variety of factors, including the use of opioid medications, limited mobility and a deterioration in both food and fluid intake, can place the child in palliative care at increased risk of constipation. The Bristol Stool Form Scale is a useful visual scale for determining the characteristics of the child's stool, and is easy to use for the child and parents because of its visual depictions (Stewart & McNeilly, 2011).

Nausea and vomiting may also be linked to biochemical and vestibular factors, and disturbances in gastrointestinal motility and function, including decreased motility, malignancies, ascites, adhesions and obstructions or neurological disturbances resulting in raised intracranial pressure, which may impact on the chemoreceptor trigger zone (CTZ) of the brain and the vomiting centre in the medulla oblongata (Yates, 2012).

Weight loss and **cachexia** may also occur in paediatric palliative care. Cachexia has its origins in the Greek words *kakos* (bad) and *hexis* (condition), and refers to the loss of appetite, weight and muscle mass that results from an underlying pathological condition, including those seen in palliative care.

> **Cachexia** the loss of appetite, weight and muscle mass that results from an underlying pathological condition, including those seen in palliative care

Nutritional intake may decrease as a child nears end of life, and children will usually be offered small amounts or tastes of foods and fluids as desired, which can be comforting (Crozier & Hancock, 2012). However, sometimes changes such as coughing, gagging and difficulty swallowing may make it difficult and uncomfortable for dying children to eat and drink. Although artificial nutrition and hydration (via nasogastric or parenteral routes) may be considered, these interventions have associated complications, and the palliative care team in partnership with parents will usually weigh up the risks versus the benefits of commencing artificial nutrition (Rapoport et al., 2013). At this stage 'although artificial nutrition and hydration may support biological existence and increase weight, there is no evidence that it improves survival or quality of life in dying children or adults' (Rapoport et al., 2013: 862). Parents, however, will often feel a strong desire to continue to provide nourishment to their dying child, and may be concerned about their child feeling hunger and thirst, and being uncomfortable if adequate nutrition and hydration are not provided (Pritchard et al., 2008; Rapoport et al., 2013). This is an extremely difficult and emotionally painful time for parents, and any decisions concerning whether to implement or forgo artificial nutrition and hydration need to be supported by the palliative care team. Parents need to be reassured that it is normal for appetite to diminish towards end of life, and that their child will likely not feel the desire to eat or drink.

> **Case study 6.1**
>
> Matthew is an 11-year-old boy with acute myeloid leukaemia who is receiving palliative care support after an unsuccessful stem cell transplant. You are visiting Matthew and his family each day at home with the palliative care team. He is surrounded by his parents and younger sister, who is 6 years old. Today you notice that Matthew is struggling to breathe and is quite distressed. Matthew says that he has pain in his stomach and lower back and 'can't breathe'. He spends some time each day sitting out in the recliner chair in the lounge room, which seems to help with his lower back pain. He has not been eating much in the last few days – just a small amount of milk and cereal each day in the morning and a small taste of whatever the family is eating for dinner.

Anxiety

Children and parents have reported experiencing distressing emotional reactions during their experience of terminal illness. These included feeling scared or nervous, dealing with uncertainty, fear of death, thinking about being sick, and questioning: 'Why me?' (Hildenbrand et al., 2011). The reduction of anxiety for children during end-of-life care is important, as it not only creates distress for the child but can have an ongoing impact on parental anxiety and mental health (Jalmsell et al., 2010). Children and their parents may utilise a variety of coping strategies, which either avoid or address these distressing emotional issues (Hildenbrand et al., 2011). Music therapy has been found to promote a sense of calm and relaxation among children in palliative care and their families (Lindenfelser et al., 2012). Communication concerning issues of concern may also be important for reducing anxiety. In a study among adolescents with cancer, participating in a structured, family-centred advance care planning program significantly decreased anxiety among adolescents, but unfortunately increased anxiety among family members (Lyon et al., 2014). The program enabled adolescents with cancer and their families to engage in reflection and discussion about their fears, values, spiritual beliefs and preferences in relation to future treatments and care, as well as palliative care (Lyon et al., 2014). We discuss this program further in the next section.

Communication with children and adolescents

Effective end-of-life care for young people increasingly emphasises the importance of engaging in conversations about dying and advanced care planning because adolescents possess growing cognitive and emotional maturity, which means they understand death and want to be involved in decisions concerning their treatment and end-of-life care (Lyon et al., 2014). Sometimes such conversations may be avoided by health professionals, and leave young people struggling to find ways to communicate their thoughts and feelings about the possibility of their own impending death (Forster, 2012). There are three paediatric advanced care planning models that have been developed with particular target groups of adolescents, including Footprints (designed for patients with muscular dystrophy), the Family-Centred (FACE) Advanced Care Planning for young people with HIV, and FACE-TC, which adapted this model for teens with cancer (Lyon et al., 2014). In their study of 30 adolescents with cancer, participating in advanced care planning conversations significantly reduced the adolescent's anxiety (Lyon et al., 2014). These models were delivered by health professionals who undertook specialised training, and the conversations with the adolescent and family occurred over a number of sessions (Lyon et al., 2009).

Younger children may also want to discuss their worries and fears. Play and art therapy are two strategies that may be used to enable younger children to communicate their worries. Play and art therapy can assist paediatric nurses to understand the problems a child is facing, and help the child to verbalise conscious feelings and thoughts and to act out subconscious feelings and thoughts (Van Breemen, 2009; Walker, 1989). Nurses can also assist parents to engage in play with their child, and by doing so, parents may also gain insights into their child's fears and hopes (Van Breemen, 2009).

For the student and beginning nurse, it is important to aware of the possibility for adolescents and their families to want to discuss their thoughts and feelings about death and end-of-life care, and to be alert to possible cues that indicate this need. Your confidence in responding to such cues and engaging in end-of-life conversations will develop through further training and experience.

In the meantime, being able to listen to young people and their families involving other health professionals when necessary, is important to ensure that any need to discuss these issues is facilitated. By attending family conferences, you will also have the opportunity to observe more experienced health professionals and their communication with children and families in palliative care (Keir & Wilkinson, 2013). This is a good opportunity for you to observe body language and the ways in which experienced health professionals express empathy and engage parents – and, if appropriate, the child – in difficult conversations and respond to intense emotions.

Communication and the family in paediatric end-of-life care

Parents of dying children place great emphasis on the communication with health professionals during their child's illness and around the time of their child's death (Meyer et al., 2006). There may be a tendency among health professionals to avoid communication with parents and family members at this time, and focus on the technical aspects of care (Forster, 2012). However, sensitive and supportive communication is central to the quality of end-of-life care in paediatrics, and can help parents and family members through this overwhelming and devastating time.

Parents caring for their dying child at home may feel quite uncertain about the physical aspects of their child's care, and may struggle to navigate the emotional aspects of facing their child's impending death. In one Australian study, parents described wanting to talk with health professionals about their feelings, but finding that nurses and doctors did not introduce such topics of conversation (Forster, 2012). Therefore, nurses need to find the time to engage with parents about their thoughts and feelings in order to offer their supportive presence. Parents may feel unable to discuss such feelings with friends and in their social circle, and may feel isolated and alone. In addition, with strain upon both parents simultaneously, they may feel unable to fully support each other while going through their own feelings of grief (Moriarty et al., 1996).

It is important that the team of health professionals involved in end-of-life care provides consistent and frequent information to families. The team should also recognise that complex information (even when explained in simple terms) may require repetition, and that parents may need regular meetings in order to be able to make decisions about their child's ongoing care (Crozier & Hancock, 2012).

Siblings

Siblings of the dying child require support and consideration, as they can be impacted in multiple ways during the course of their brother or sister's illness and end-of-life care. Their understanding of the situation will be influenced by their age and development, and this will also guide the strategies employed by nurses and the palliative care team in providing effective support.

Often, siblings have had their usual experiences of family life interrupted and changed due to the illness of their sibling. They may have had to experience being cared for by other family members and friends, they may have been required to take on additional responsibilities and they have, of course, lost time and contact with parents who may have been focused on the care of a sick and dying sibling (Foster et al., 2010). Siblings are also struggling with their own emotional responses to their brother or sister's illness and impending death, and may experience fear, anger, jealousy, shame and guilt, and feel isolated and forgotten (Foster et al., 2010). In their study of 18 siblings aged 9–22 years in New Zealand, Gaab and colleagues (2014) found that siblings wanted to be informed about the impending death of their sibling, and to be included in conversations about symptoms so that they could understand what was happening. These preferences were also balanced by the negative aspects of having this knowledge, as siblings then worried more – for example, that their sibling would go to sleep and not awaken, or that conversations about death and dying were then brought up too much and this made it difficult to live as normal a life as possible. Siblings also engaged in helping behaviours and spent time with their sibling, trying to make them smile and stay positive (Gaab et al., 2014).

Nurses and the palliative care team can support siblings by:

- involving them in discussions about care and treatment throughout their sibling's illness
- enabling siblings to be involved in caregiving if desired
- assigning a social worker to specifically work with siblings
- putting families in contact with relevant sibling support groups
- educating the family about the needs of siblings when a child is sick and dying

- encouraging siblings to continue to be involved in their own interests and pursuits
- helping the family to identify a 'safe adult' in siblings' world to whom they feel they can talk about their feelings and concerns
- referrals to psychologists and counsellors when necessary
- asking siblings about their feelings and experiences. (Jones et al., 2014)

Grandparents

Grandparents often play a central role in supporting parents and families when a child is ill and dying, and therefore also need to be supported at this time and following the child's death. Grandparents have been described as experiencing threefold layers of grief when losing a grandchild, as they are grieving the loss of their cherished grandchild, for their son or daughter who is losing/has lost a child and for themselves (Ponzetti & Johnson, 1991). Grandparents may not discuss their own emotions and inner turmoil because of a need to be strong for their adult child and other grandchildren (Youngblut et al., 2010). It is important for nurses to be aware of grandparents' feelings, and to provide opportunities for them to talk about their feelings and concerns (Youngblut et al., 2010).

Summary

- Although child mortality in Australia has halved since 1986 and stabilised between 2006 and 2010, for some families the death of a child remains a sad reality. The leading causes of paediatric death include injury, cancer and nervous system diseases. These children and their families require specialised end-of-life care that recognises and supports the unique needs of the dying child and their family. Paediatric nurses play a central role in the coordination and provision of this care.
- Paediatric palliative or end-of-life care involves the physical, psychosocial and spiritual care of the child and their family. Its commencement and duration may vary, depending on the child's illness and trajectory, and it may be provided in a variety of settings, including hospitals, community care, hospices and the child's home.
- Children may experience a variety of problems at end of life, including pain, side-effects of opioid medications, fatigue, dyspnoea, gastrointestinal

problems and anxiety. Nurses caring for children at end of life need to be able to assess and identify these physical and psychological concerns, and collaborate with the multidisciplinary team to alleviate these. Research into the effectiveness of management strategies is still needed in paediatric end-of-life care.

- Depending on their development and understanding, children and young people may wish to discuss their fears and worries about dying, and adolescents may like to be involved in advance care planning conversations. The skills to facilitate such conversations will develop with further specialised preparation and experience, and beginning paediatric nurses can observe more-experienced colleagues and increase their awareness of the communication skills used. Being a supportive presence and having a willingness to listen are valuable skills.
- Communication with the dying child's family should be informative, sensitive and provide family members with the opportunity to ask questions, be involved in planning care and management decisions, and disclose fears, concerns and emotions arising from caring for their dying child and their impending loss. Parents may feel isolated and unable to share their feelings with family, friends and even with each other as they struggle with their own feelings of grief. Siblings and grandparents will also need special attention and support as they the loss of their loved one.

Learning activities

6.1 Based on your reading in this chapter, what do you think are the main problems being experienced by our case study patient, Matthew? For each problem you identify, write down why this may be occurring for Matthew.

6.2 What strategies could you use to alleviate these problems for Matthew?

6.3 How would you involve Matthew and his family in your plan of care?

Further reading

- Twycross, A & Stinson, J 2014, Physical and psychological pain relief methods in children. In A Twycross, S Dowden & J Stinson (eds), *Managing pain in children: A clinical guide for nurses and health professionals*, John Wiley & Sons, Chichester, UK, pp. 86–99. This reading provides an overview of a variety of physical and psychological pain-relief strategies and current research evidence concerning their use in paediatric patients. It will provide you with a beginning understanding of pain relief strategies and how they have been used effectively for children experiencing pain.

References

Abernethy, AP et al. 2010, Effect of palliative oxygen versus medical (room) air in relieving breathlessness in patients with refractory dyspnea: A double-blind randomized controlled trial, *The Lancet*, 376(9743), pp. 784–93.

Australian Institute of Health and Welfare (AIHW) 2012, *A picture of Australia's children 2012*, AIHW, Canberra.

Chang, C, Mu, P, Jou, S, Wong, T & Chen, Y 2013, Systematic review and meta-analysis of nonpharmacological interventions for fatigue in children and adolescents with cancer, *Worldviews on Evidence-based Nursing*, 10(4), pp. 208–17.

Crozier, F & Hancock, LE 2012, Pediatric palliative care: Beyond the end of life, *Pediatric Nursing*, 38(4), pp. 198–227.

Dowden, S 2014, Pharmacology of analgesic drugs. In A Twycross, S Dowden & J Stinson, *Managing pain in children: A clinical guide for nurses and health professionals*, John Wiley & Sons, Chichester, UK, pp. 48–86.

Ernst, E 2009, Massage therapy for cancer palliation and supportive care: A systematic review of randomised clinical trials, *Supportive Care in Cancer*, 17(4), pp. 333–7.

Forster, EM 2012, Parent and staff perceptions of bereavement support surrounding loss of a child, PhD thesis, University of Queensland.

Foster, TL, Lafond, DA, Reggio, C & Hinds, PS 2010, Pediatric palliative care in childhood cancer nursing: From diagnosis to cure or end of life, *Seminars in Oncology Nursing*, 26(4), pp. 205–21.

Gaab, EM, Owens, GR & MacLeod, RD 2014, Siblings caring for and about pediatric palliative care patients, *Journal of Palliative Medicine*, 17(1), pp. 62–7.

Glare, P 2011, Choice of opioids and the WHO ladder, *Journal of Pediatric Hematology Oncology*, 31(S1), pp. S6–S11.

Hallenbeck, J 2012, Pathophysiologies of dyspnea explained: Why might opioids relieve dyspnoea and not hasten death? *Journal of Palliative Medicine*, 15(8), pp. 848–53.

Hildenbrand, AK, Clawson, KJ, Alderfer, MA & Marsac, ML 2011, Coping with pediatric cancer strategies employed by children and their parents to manage cancer-related stressors during treatment, *Journal of Pediatric Oncology Nursing*, 28(6), pp. 344–54.

Hinds, PS et al. 2010, Psychometric and clinical assessment of the 10-item reduced version of the fatigue scale-child instrument, *Journal of Pain and Symptom Management*, 39(3), pp. 572–8.

Hockenberry, MJ et al. 2003, Three instruments to assess fatigue in children with cancer: The child, parent and staff perspectives, *Journal of Pain and Symptom Management*, 25, pp. 319–28.

Hockenberry-Eaton, M et al. 1998, Fatigue in children and adolescents with cancer, *Journal of Pediatric Oncology Nursing*, 15(3), pp. 172–82.

Hughes, D, Ladas, E, Rooney, D & Kelly, K 2008, Massage therapy as a supportive care intervention for children with cancer, *Oncology Nursing Forum*, 35(3), pp. 431–42.

Hyde, C, Price, J & Nicholl, H 2012, Neuropathic pain management in children, *International Journal of Palliative Nursing*, 18(10), pp. 476–82.

Jalmsell, L, Kreicbergs, U, Onelov, E, Steineck, G & Henter, J 2010, Anxiety is contagious: Symptoms of anxiety in the terminally ill child affect long-term psychological well-being in bereaved parents, *Pediatric Blood & Cancer*, 54(5), pp. 751–7.

Jones, BL, Contro, N & Koch, KD 2014, The duty of the physician to care for the family in pediatric palliative care: Context, communication, and caring, *Pediatrics*, 133(Supp. 1), pp. S8–S15.

Keir, A & Wilkinson, D 2013, Communication skills training in paediatrics, *Journal of Paediatrics and Child Health*, 49(8), pp. 624–8.

Klick, JC & Hauer, J 2010, Pediatric palliative care, *Current Problems in Pediatric and Adolescent Health Care*, 40(6), pp. 120–51.

Levine, D et al. 2013, Best practices for pediatric palliative cancer care: A primer for clinical providers, *Journal of Supportive Oncology*, 11(3), pp. 114–25.

Lindenfelser, KJ, Hense, C & McFerran, K 2012, Music therapy in pediatric palliative care: Family-centered care to enhance quality of life, *American Journal of Hospice & Palliative Medicine*, 29(3), pp. 219–26.

Lyon, ME, Jacobs, S, Briggs, L, Cheng, YI & Wang, J 2014, A longitudinal, randomized, controlled trial of advance care planning for teens with cancer: Anxiety, depression, quality of life, advance directives, spirituality, *Journal of Adolescent Health*, 54(6), pp. 710–17.

Lyon, ME et al. 2009, Who will speak for me? Improving end-of-life decision-making for adolescents with HIV and their families, *Pediatrics*, 123(2), pp. e199–e206.

Meyer, EC, Ritholz, MD, Burns, JP & Truog, RD 2006, Improving quality of end-of-life care in the pediatric intensive care unit: Parents' priorities and recommendations, *Pediatrics*, 117(3), pp. 649–57.

Monterosso, L & DeGraves, S 2012, Paediatric palliative care. In M O'Connor, S Lee & S Aranda (eds), *Palliative care nursing: A guide to practice*, 3rd edn, Ausmed, Melbourne.

Moriarty, HJ, Carroll, R & Controneo, M 1996, Differences in bereavement reactions within couples following death of a child, *Research in Nursing & Health*, 9(6), pp. 461–9.

Ponzetti, JJ & Johnson, MA 1991, The forgotten grievers: Grandparents' reactions to the death of grandchildren, *Death Studies*, 15(2), pp. 157–67.

Pritchard, M et al. 2012, Cancer-related symptoms most concerning to parents during the last week and last day of their child's life, *Pediatrics*, 121(5), pp. e1301–e1309.

Rapoport, A, Shaheed, J, Newman, C, Rugg, M & Steel, R 2013, Parental perceptions of forgoing artificial nutrition and hydration during end-of-life care, *Pediatrics*, 131(5), pp. 861–9.

Robinson, WM 2012, Palliation of dyspnea in paediatrics, *Chronic Respiratory Disease*, 9(4), pp. 251–6.

Shaw, TM 2012, Pediatric palliative pain and symptom management, *Pediatric Annals*, 41(8), pp. 329–34.

Stayer, D 2012, Pediatric palliative care: A conceptual analysis for pediatric nursing practice, *Journal of Pediatric Nursing*, 27, pp. 350–6.

Stewart, G & McNeilly, P 2011, Opioid-induced constipation in children's palliative care, *Nursing Children and Young People*, 23(8), pp. 31–4.

Tomlinson, D et al. 2011, Chemotherapy versus supportive care alone in pediatric palliative care for cancer: Comparing the preferences of parents and health care professionals, *Canadian Medical Association Journal*, 183(17), pp. 1252–8.

Twycross, A & Stinson, J 2014, Physical and psychological pain relief methods in children. In A Twycross, S Dowden & J Stinson (eds), *Managing pain in children: A clinical guide for nurses and health professionals*, John Wiley & Sons, Chichester, UK, pp. 86–99.

Ullrich, CK et al. 2010, Fatigue in children with cancer at the end of life, *Journal of Pain and Symptom Management*, 40(4), pp. 483–94.

Ullrich, CK & Mayer, O 2007, Assessment and management of fatigue and dyspnea in pediatric palliative care, *The Pediatric Clinics of North America*, 54(5), p. 735.

Van Breemen, C 2009, Using play therapy in paediatric palliative care: Listening to the story and caring for the body, *International Journal of Palliative Nursing*, 15(10), pp. 510–14.

Vargas-Schaffer, G 2010, Is the WHO analgesic ladder still valid?*Canadian Family Physician*, 56, pp. 514–17.

Walker, C 1989, Use of art and play therapy in pediatric oncology, *Journal of Pediatric Oncology Nursing*, 6, pp. 121–6.

Wolfe, J, Grier, HE & Klar, N, 2000, Symptoms and suffering at the end of life in children with cancer, *New England Journal of Medicine*, 342, pp. 326–33.

World Health Organization (WHO) 1998, WHO definition of palliative care for children, viewed 21 January 2014, http://www.who.int/cancer/palliative/definition/en.

Yates, P 2012, Nausea and vomiting in palliative care nursing. In M O'Connor, S Lee & S Aranda (eds), *Palliative Care Nursing A Guide to Practice,* 3rd edn, Ausmed, Melbourne, pp. 167–77.

Youngblut, JM, Brooten, D, Blais, K, Hannan, J & Niyonsenga, T 2010, Grandparents' health and functioning after a grandchild's death, *Journal of Pediatric Nursing,* 25(5), p. 352.

7 Mental health and illness in childhood and adolescence

Jennifer Fraser, Lindsay Smith and Julia Taylor

Learning objectives

In this chapter you will:

- Be introduced to the concept of determinants of child and adolescent mental health
- Gain an understanding of mental disorders and mental health problems experienced in childhood and adolescence
- Become familiar with the importance of positive relationships, experiences and environments to developing adaptive responses to stress and change in children and young people
- Understand that mental disorder in childhood is a dimensional phenomenon
- Learn nursing skills that help promote good mental health and enhance resilience in children and young people

Introduction

The focus of this chapter is the role of the nurse in optimising **child and youth mental health**. An overview of mental disorders experienced during childhood and adolescence is followed by a discussion of mental health promotion for children and young people. The importance of working closely with the parents and families of children and young people disabled by mental illness and the services available to them is emphasised.

Child and youth mental health A state of mental wellbeing in which children and young people can realise their abilities and reach optimal growth and development

The Australian Institute of Health and Welfare (AIHW) conducts a national survey of mental health and wellbeing, providing valuable information on the prevalence of **child and youth mental disorders** in Australia. The AIHW also publishes a list of services that exist for people living with a mental disorder and makes recommendations for services that are needed. The AIHW National Survey included children and adolescents for the first time in 1998, and a new report was scheduled for publication in 2014. However, until the latest report is published, this means that the most comprehensive information available on Australian children and young people's mental health problems comes from data published in 1998. These data revealed that 14 per cent of children and young people between the ages of 4 and 17 years experienced a mental health problem (Sawyer et al., 2000). That is, one in seven children aged 4–17 had mental health problems, 15 per cent of boys and 14 per cent of girls (Sawyer et al., 2000). More recent data are available from individual states in Australia and published by the Australian Bureau of Statistics. These are referred to within the chapter.

Mental health problems and mental disorders

The extent to which children and young people experience symptoms and/or behaviours that cause problems to parents, teachers, peers and society in general varies. Assessment over time is necessary to distinguish the type, frequency and severity of disruption. Many children who are referred for treatment do not have symptoms that meet the criteria for a mental disorder. But this does not mean that the symptoms and behaviour may not meet the criteria at another point in time. The cut-off point between those who receive a formal diagnosis and those who do not is arbitrary. How mental disorders, and mental health and wellbeing, are defined is important:

Child and youth mental disorder A mental disorder, as distinct from a mental health problem, is characterised by a clinically recognisable set of symptoms or behaviours that interfere substantially with social, academic or occupational functioning. Different types of mental disorders consist of a different combination of symptoms that may differ in severity

> Mental health is a state of well-being in which individuals can realise their abilities, can cope with the normal stresses of life, can work productively and fruitfully, and are able to make a contribution to their community ... Conversely, mental health problems can affect perceptions, emotions, behaviour and social well-being. Mental disorders, as distinct from mental health problems, are characterised by a clinically recognisable set of symptoms or behaviours that interfere substantially with social, academic or occupational functioning ... Different types of mental disorders consist of a different combination of symptoms that may differ in severity. (AIHW, 2009: 30)

Recent changes to the way in which children and young people are diagnosed and assessed for mental disorders have been made in the latest version of the manual published for this purpose, the *Diagnostic and Statistical Manual of*

Mental Disorders (DSM). In 2013, the DSM was revised and its fifth edition, DSM-5, published. The new edition saw significant changes that affect the ways in which children and young people are diagnosed and assessed for mental disorders. For children diagnosed prior to the release of DSM-5, no change is made to a diagnosis of mental disorder. Notwithstanding this, changes to the way in which bipolar, ADHD and autism are assessed in children and young people have changed quite significantly.

Disorders are presented in DSM-5 according to age, gender and developmental characteristics. The first section of this chapter focuses on those childhood conditions commonly experienced in health-care settings in which paediatric nurses practise. While not an exhaustive list of the conditions experienced in childhood, they are the conditions that have come under the most intense research and scrutiny during the period leading up to the release of DSM-5. These are Autism Spectrum Disorder (ASD), and Attention Deficit Hyperactivity Disorder (ADHD).

To better understand these changes, the first section of this chapter details selected mental disorders of children and young people. How children's social, behavioural and emotional symptoms are categorised and diagnosed is important to the way in which they are treated. Diagnosis is complex, and the child's development and its trajectory must be considered. For example, some behaviours demonstrated by a 14-month-old infant are acceptable, whereas if the same behaviours continue through to the child's second or third birthday, this may be reconsidered and the behaviours could indicate a mental disorder.

General paediatric nurses in Australia are not responsible for the diagnosis of mental disorders in children, but understanding is crucial. Mental health and wellbeing are essential components of a paediatric assessment. The majority of child and adolescent mental disorders are not seen in paediatric hospitals. When they are, they are usually comorbid with a physical health problem or the result of self-harm. They may also result from a physical health problem (see Chapter 3) and be missed altogether. **Child and youth mental health services** are offered within hospitals and other community settings, but children with mental disorders also present to paediatric services for a range of reasons other than their mental health care. For this reason, it is important to understand disorders of children and young people, and the way in which they are best managed for optimal care in the paediatric environment.

Child and youth mental health services Provide specialist mental health services for children and young people, and assistance to their families or carers

Children's development is a dynamic process. A child's mental health is viewed in the context of their development and maturation overall, rather than being a single element or achievement at only one point in time. It is important to establish those behaviours that are limited and those that are persistent. Focusing on a single aspect at one particular time is of little value in appreciating the complete clinical picture, and often leads to incorrect assumptions. Diagnosis not only occurs over time; it depends on the level of disruption to the child's biopsychosocial development and integration into the wider world – that is, it is a dimensional phenomenon. Cognitive, emotional and psychological development during childhood and the adolescent years occurs in a predictable sequence but is unique to each person. This is taken into consideration when assessing children and young people's mental health.

What mental disorders affect Australian children?

As previously discussed, the most recent publication of national prevalence data for Australia was in 2000 (Sawyer et al., 2000). The method used was to take cases from the clinical ranges of the Child Behaviour Checklist for children (Achenbach, 1991a) and young people (Achenbach, 1991b) as reported by parents of participating children. The measure was of mental health problems and not mental disorders. Mental disorders are diagnosed with more complexity and from more than one source. Data were collected from ages 4–12 and 4–17 to allow for analysis within and between age groups as well as sex. The data indicated high levels of mental health problems for both girls and boys as well as for young people up to the age of 17 years.

The data revealed a prevalence of one in four (26 per cent, or 671 100) Australian children and young people experiencing at least one mental health problem in the preceding 12 months. Rates for girls were higher (30 per cent) than for boys (23 per cent). The breakdown between girls and boys for each of the following disorders was interesting. Overall, 15 per cent reported anxiety, 13 per cent substance abuse and 6 per cent affective (mood) disorders. Of these, the results were 22 per cent, 10 per cent and 8 per cent respectively for girls, and 9 per cent, 16 per cent and 4 per cent for boys. In other words, girls experienced a higher prevalence of anxiety and affective disorders, whereas boys reported more substance abuse disorders.

More recent data have since been published from New South Wales and Victoria (AIHW, 2009). These data were collected using parent or carer reports on the Strengths and Difficulties Questionnaire. Although this may result in

TABLE 7.1 Children scoring 'of concern' on the Strengths and Difficulties Questionnaire, New South Wales and Victoria, 4–12 years (% and 95% confidence intervals)

	NSW (2005–06)		VICTORIA (2006)	
	%	95% CI	%	95% CI
Emotional symptoms	10.6	9.1–12.0	7.8	6.7–8.9
Conduct problems	9.0	7.6–10.4	8.6	7.5–9.7
Hyperactivity	11.4	9.9–13.0	11.1	9.8–12.3
Peer problems	7.5	6.3–8.6	8.4	7.3–9.4
Prosocial behaviour	1.2	0.8–1.7	1.8	1.3–2.3
Total	6.6	5.4–7.7	5.6	4.7–6.5

Note: Children with missing data have been excluded from these results.
Sources: NSW Department of Health (2006), unpublished data; Victoria Child Health and Well-being Survey (2006), unpublished data; AIHW (2009).

either over-reporting or under-reporting by parents, it is still useful in terms of understanding parents' concerns for their children's mental health and wellbeing. For details, see Table 7.1. Hyperactivity was the most prevalent concern, with high proportions of children reported to have emotional symptoms and peer problems.

Attention Deficit Hyperactivity Disorder

Larry

Case study 7.1

A 9-year-old boy, Larry, was admitted to the children's orthopaedic ward three weeks ago for elective surgery. He had a left leg lengthening procedure to correct a congenital anomaly the day after admission. A Taylor Spatial Frame (leg-lengthening mechanism) has been applied and, apart from physiotherapy sessions, he is on complete best rest. Larry's mother Kim attends to his care each day between 7.00 am and 8.00 pm and he sleeps well between his mother's visits. Yesterday, Kim pressed the buzzer several times in succession to gain emergency assistance. Larry was found thrashing around the bed, pulling at his leg-lengthening devise, screaming incoherently and violently responding to his mother's requests to calm down.
Kim is shocked and distressed. The staff are unable to calm him and the psychiatric referral team is called in. Larry is prescribed a paediatric dose of antipsychotic medication and finally settles to sleep. Ongoing care by the psychiatric team is commenced. Following the event, Kim confides that Larry was diagnosed with Attention Deficit Hyperactivity Disorder at the age of 7 and that he was taking medication for about 6 months to treat the symptoms until a few months ago. On the medication, he had been able to concentrate better at school and his academic

> functioning had improved, but Kim disliked the perceived side-effects of the medication and was concerned it would lead to drug addiction in the future. She confides to the nursing staff that she has been following a parenting intervention under the guidance of a psychologist. The program seems to have worked very well with noticeable improvement in Larry's behaviour and emotional regulation. But this makes Kim feel overwhelmed with guilt. Given the success of the program, Kim believes that her parenting style must have caused the condition.

Attention Deficit Hyperactivity Disorder (ADHD) is the most prevalent child mental disorder not only in Australia (AIHW, 2009) but worldwide, with 8–12 per cent of children diagnosed (Biederman & Faraone, 2005). Children present with inattention, hyperactivity and impulsivity and, compared with their normative peers, have poor learning ability, low academic outcomes and social incompetence. There are three sub-types of ADHD: inattentive; hyperactive-impulsive; and combined. Unfortunately, symptoms persist into the adult years in 65 per cent of cases (Biederman & Faraone, 2005).

ADHD is a complex disorder that is difficult to manage well. Nursing interventions to encourage comprehensive evaluations are valuable because management needs to be based on comprehensive neuropsychological and psycho-educational assessments. This not only determines the diagnosis, but also establishes the existence of any potential comorbid conditions (Feldman & Reiff, 2014). Comorbidity is common with this disorder and occurs in as many as two thirds of children with ADHD. Comorbid conditions include learning disabilities, Conduct Disorder, Oppositional Defiant Disorder and anxiety (Biederman et al., 1991). Almost half (45 per cent) have comorbid learning disabilities, placing them at risk for poor educational achievement and potentially low socioeconomic status (Grizenko et al., 2013). Furthermore, poor academic self-concept is associated with the development of anti-social behaviours. Children with the inattentive type of ADHD tend to have the greatest academic failure rates and do poorly at mathematics in particular (Grizenko et al., 2013).

Nursing assessment and interventions

As discussed in Chapter 3, the perspectives of parents and carers, and their willingness to engage in positive health behaviours for the child, determine outcomes. In this case scenario, the nurse has the chance, through crisis, to assist the mother, Kim, to establish the best way forward in managing Larry's symptoms and behaviour (Becker et al., 2009). With Larry as an in-patient in hospital, the paediatric nurse has a window of opportunity to encourage comprehensive evaluations, discuss school advocacy and support services, and reinforce the benefits of changing parenting style and the home environment in ways that may benefit her son (Becker et al., 2009). It is of utmost importance in this case scenario to emphasise that treatment success does not infer aetiology. There are no known causes of ADHD. However, it is common for parents to believe that their parenting was to blame, especially after the success of parenting interventions that modify parenting style. Guilt and shame are also common among parents of children with ADHD, and there appears to be a genetic predisposition with one or both parents often having the same features (Biederman & Faraone, 2005).

Parenting interventions that focus on child behaviour management have proven to be somewhat successful. If implemented correctly, these have been reported to reduce the main symptoms of ADHD in both the short and longer term (Hoath & Sanders, 2002). Importantly, they can improve parenting satisfaction and confidence. At the same time, it is important to emphasise that behaviour management is not as effective as medication, and medication is especially successful in raising the likelihood of academic success and school completion (Grizenko et al., 2013). These outcomes bode well for the child's trajectory into adult life.

The safety and effectiveness of non-stimulant drugs and long-acting methylphenidate and amphetamine medications have been demonstrated in research conducted over the past two decades (Feldman & Reiff, 2014). Parents do remain reluctant to medicate their children for ADHD, despite obvious behavioural and academic improvements when treated by psychostimulants (Grizenko et al., 2013). Longer-term effects of medication for ADHD are not well understood at present. For Larry and Kim, the added burden of a physical disability (one leg has been shorter than the other since birth) would no doubt impact on the way in which they perceive the treatment options for ADHD.

Larry is at a vulnerable stage of development. At 9 years of age, he is likely to be able to recognise cultural and individual differences and may be struggling to come to terms with his problems of inattention, hyperactivity and impulsivity (Erikson, 1968). Impairment in academic performance and social isolation have the potential to interfere with any sense of accomplishment, important to children of his age.

The nurse can assist by recommending:

- comprehensive psychosocial and psychoeducational assessments
- consultation and regular follow-up with a paediatrician for monitoring and modification of medication

- re-engagement with the behavioural parent training program
- support and counselling services, including school support. (Feldman & Reiff, 2014)

> **Reflection points 7.1**
>
> - A high proportion of children and young people – boys and girls – report mental health problems in Australia.
> - Behavioural and emotional changes and changes in function should be referred immediately and appropriately.
> - Ongoing monitoring of the medication regimens is encouraged, and augmentation with behaviour-management strategies recommended.

Autism Spectrum Disorder

Autism Spectrum Disorder (ASD) is a lifelong developmental disability featuring deficits in social communication and social interaction with repetitive patterns of behaviour, interests or activites (APA, 2013). The prevalence rate is estimated to be from 5.7 to 21.9 per 1000, with boys more commonly affected than girls (CDCP, 2014). In the 4th edition of the *Diagnostic and Statistical Manual of Mental Disorders* (APA, 2000), DSM-4, children with ASD were categorised as having one of: autistic disorder; Asperger's Disorder; or pervasive developmental disorder not otherwise specified (PDD-NOS). With the release of DSM-5, these are all now referred to as a single condition, ASD. This is an important change because you will find that, for some children, one of the former categories may still be used. As previously mentioned, DSM-5 relates to diagnoses made since its release in 2013, meaning that children will continue to have a diagnosis of Asperger's Syndrome. ASD also has a severity rating of 1, 2 or 3, depending on how much support the person needs. Some people have mild symptoms while others have more severe and pervasive disability (APA, 2013).

ASD is characterised by the child having difficulties in each of two areas: deficits in social communication; and fixated interests and repetitive behaviours. Deficits in social communication include poor social interaction and limited use of language to communicate. Some children will not speak at all, not respond when spoken to and not join in with others' actions and activities. The second area – fixated interests and repetitive behaviours – can obviously only be observed as the child grows and certain developmental milestones are not met.

Having narrow and intense interests is more obvious as the child goes to school and is expected to become involved in others' interests and games. Sensory sensitivities are also characteristic. The child may choose to only wear one type of fabric, may dislike labels on clothes or have particular bedding preferences. One of the most difficult manifestations is the desire to eat only certain foods with a specific texture or colour.

It is critical to be able to diagnose ASD in early childhood so that early intervention can be implemented. There are a number of successful and evidence based programs available according to the way in which ASD presents in the individual child. Critical decisions about schooling need to be made early, as there needs to be adequate mechanisms of support to optimise learning ability in children with ASD. These decisions should be revised regularly with reflection on the most appropriate context for learning.

Transition to high school – and indeed to adult health and educational services – needs to be carefully planned in advance (Dodd Inglese, 2009).

Benjamin

Case study 7.2

Benjamin, who is 10 years old, was diagnosed with ASD at the age of 6. ASD affects his ability to communicate, his behaviour and his ability to engage with and relate to his peers. Benjamin attends an Aspect school in New South Wales, which provides an individualised program of education for children with ASD. In this learning environment, the specific social and educational needs of children with ASD are catered for. Benjamin's parents are well supported in their community. They are members of a community support group of parents with children with ASD and have access to government assistance to help meet his complex needs. Early diagnosis and multidisciplinary early intervention have assisted Benjamin in developing skills to become as independent as possible in the wider community. The Aspect schoolteachers have recommended that Benjamin attend the Child and Adolescent Mental Health Service for assessment. They are concerned about Benjamin's mental health and wellbeing. Symptoms of anxiety and depression – both common comorbid conditions to a diagnosis of ASD – are impeding his academic progress and limiting his engagement with teachers and peers.

Nursing assessment and interventions

Be sensitive to the way in which Benjamin is experiencing the world. For example:
- listen to parent's concerns and provide accurate information
- acknowledge that the clinic setting is unfamiliar and therefore potentially highly stressful to Benjamin

- if he becomes an inpatient, work closely with his parents to establish structure and routine
- understand the way in which he communicates discomfort and anxiety.
(Dodd Inglese, 2009; Dodd Inglese & Harrison Elder, 2009)

> **Reflection points 7.2**
> - Because nurses will encounter children and young people with ASD across a wide range of services, it is essential to become familiar with what ASD is, understand how to identify children with ASD and to understand how a formal diagnosis is made.
> - Anxiety, depression and dissociative responses to stress are comorbid conditions to ASD.

Externalising disorders: Conduct disorders

Oppositional Defiant Disorder (ODD) and Conduct Disorder (CD)

Case study 7.3: Jack

Jack's mother has an appointment at the GP clinic to see the practice nurse about her son's increasingly disruptive behaviour. She reports that Jack, who is 12 years of age has developed a terrible temper and becomes easily agitated and aggressive for trivial reasons. His anger is especially targeted towards his mother, and she is becoming quite fearful of him for herself and his 7-year-old sister. He had been a happy young child full of energy and fun, but his moods are now unpredictable. In fact, he is quite destructive around the home and at school. He refuses to follow instructions and deliberately sets out to be argumentative. His teachers at school have been calling her to the school two or three times a week for behaviour-management planning in response to him becoming too difficult and disruptive for them to manage. They have suggested that she bring Jack for assessment and treatment.

Jack's disruptive behaviour has escalated to the point where his behaviour is causing problems for his parents, teachers, peers and society in general. Many children are referred for treatment of disruptive behaviour. It is important to have the child assessed and to implement strategies as soon as possible to reverse the conduct problem because severe cases frequently continue to adulthood as Antisocial Personality Disorder or other adult mental health problems (Broidy et al., 2003).

Conduct Disorder (CD) is a formal term used to identify a subset of disruptive children who present with severe and persistent behaviour problems (APA, 2013). Oppositional Defiant Disorder (ODD) is diagnosed when the child is repeatedly argumentative, loses their temper easily and has issues with anger and resentment. These behaviours vary in frequency and severity, and diagnosis tends to be arbitrary. The problems they cause can affect parents, teachers, peers and society in general. CD is much more extreme, and features a child who violates the rights of others, is aggressive and is deliberately cruel to other people or animals.

Until recently, the research conducted in this field was gender biased because of the high rates of conduct disorders found in boys. However, this has now been reversed, and the trajectory for girls' mental health and wellbeing is starting to attract attention. Adolescent onset of conduct disorder in girls shares a similar trajectory towards adult psychopathology and criminal activity as childhood onset CD – that is, that early onset of conduct disorder is associated with a poorer prognosis. On the other hand, adolescent onset of conduct disorder in boys tends to be adolescent limited. That is, they are likely to grow out of their conduct problems (Broidy et al., 2003). This is an important finding because it points to the need to pay more attention to conduct disorder that develops in the adolescent years, especially for girls.

Parenting behaviours associated with conduct problems in children are the use of harsh discipline, a lack of role modelling, positive attention to prosocial behaviour and poor supervision of the child (Loeber & Hay, 1997). Family hierarchy tends to feature the child or children as having more power than the parents, although this deviance may result from the child's condition. Parents may feel that life is easier if they let the child have their own way more often than not (Loeber & Hay, 1997). Community factors that place the child at risk of developing more severe forms of conduct disorder are poorly supervised and impoverished school environments, availability of drugs and weapons, and formation of gangs (Broidy et al., 2003).

Behaviour-modification programs are best commenced as early as possible for the best results (Dadds & Fraser, 2003). Not all children who meet the criteria for conduct disorder will become chronic offenders as adults, but the risk is high. Parents need to be motivated and engaged to contribute to the parenting interventions available. This requires regular feedback and consultation to keep them on track with a tailored program that meets the needs of their child. Institutionalisation and other forms of group-based treatments are not advised due to the strengthening of deviant behaviours through group pressure. Parents may feel that they need respite, but if possible the best approach is to modify their interactions with the child to reduce the severity of the child's conduct problems (Dadds & Fraser, 2003).

Reflection points 7.3

- Family interventions show the most promise of success.
- Disruptive behaviour patterns become more resistant with age.
- Early intervention and prevention are needed.

Risk and protective factors

A number of developmental characteristics or events are associated with the onset of mental problems in children and young people. The worst outcomes result from the cumulative effects of multiple **risk** factors acting on a single child. These risk factors overlap and place the child at risk for both internalising (anxiety and depression) and externalising (CD, ODD) disorders. Thus the same risk factors can be identified for each (McLaughlin et al., 2012). Risk and protective factors are presented in Table 7.2.

Risks
Disturbances to mental health that threaten system function, viability or development

A useful framework for understanding the many risks and protective factors that influence mental heath is an interacting systems approach. Bronfenbrenner's (2001) bioecological model of human development provides a strong framework for this. The bioecological model also provides a useful framework for assessing and treating children who experience mental illness and their families (Taylor, 2003). This perspective has a strong focus on strengthening proximal processes (introduced in Chapter 2) and supportive environments to optimise development. It is important for paediatric nurses to develop a strong nurse–child relationship, and allow time during nursing care for the

TABLE 7.2 *Risk and protective factors for mental health problems in childhood and adolescence*

	RISK FACTORS	PROTECTIVE FACTORS
Child factors	Genetic risk	High intelligence
	Brain damage	Good general health
	Low intelligence	Engaging temperament
	Difficult temperament	Good social skills
	Poor social skills	High self-efficacy
	Low self-esteem	High self-esteem
Parenting and family factors	Poor-quality relationship with parents	Warm and positive relationship with parents
	Insecure attachment style	Secure attachment style
	Harsh, inflexible or inconsistent discipline	Fair, consistent discipline with clear boundaries for behaviour
	Inadequate supervision	Strong involvement with child
	Parental conflict	Domestic harmony
	Parental psychopathology	Good mental health of parents
School factors	Bullying	Strong school culture of support
	Poor resources	Good supervision
Societal factors	Low socioeconomic status	Child's rights upheld
	Discrimination	

Sources: Goodman et al. (2011); Loeber & Hay (1997); McLaughlin et al. (2012); Rutter (2005); Sameroff & MacKenzie (2003); Scott et al. (2011).

relationship to develop. A strong nurse–child relationship is a protective factor against the mental health challenges that can arise for child and youth during health care. Various indicators of the ecology influencing child and youth mental health are presented in Table 7.2.

Internalising disorders: Anxiety and depression

A significant research effort has been conducted to date with regard to risk and protective factors for child and youth mental health. Particular attention has been paid to the influence of maternal depression and to a lesser extent paternal depression on child mental disorders. More research is needed to disentangle the relationships between the complex concepts. Children and adolescents experience anxiety disorders, such as phobias, social phobias and generalised anxiety disorder, in a similar way to adults. Separation anxiety disorder is specific to childhood, and is characterised by extreme anxiety when separated from home or the parent. The child may experience a sense of overwhelming panic. Psychodynamic, behavioural, cognitive and family therapies have demonstrated success in managing anxiety in childhood (Bennett et al., 2013; In-Albon & Schneider, 2007).

There are similar explanations for both child and adult depression. These include loss, learned helplessness, negative cognitions, low serotonin and norepinephrine activity in the brain. Young children are likely to have comorbid separation anxiety, phobias, somatic complaints and behaviour problems. The diagnosis for paediatric depression relies on the ability of the child or their parent to report on the internal affect of the child. Depressed mothers may also over-report depressive symptoms in their child, although a transactional approach to child development suggests that the child's characteristics exacerbate the maternal psychopathology (Sameroff & MacKenzie, 2003). That is, a mother is more likely to be depressed if her child exhibits symptoms of mental health problems. Moreover, a healthy father appears to mediate the relationship between maternal depression and child psychopathology, whereas a child with both parents affected by mental illness is at high risk of childhood depression and other disorders (Goodman et al., 2011)

A number of adverse outcomes may result from childhood mental disorders and poor mental health. These include general suffering, functional impairment, stigma, discrimination and even premature death (McLaughlin et al., 2012). Given the importance of community-based early intervention and prevention approaches to developmental disruption, and children's and young people's mental health and wellbeing, this chapter now focuses on the importance of promoting mental health.

Reflection points 7.4

- Nurses work with children and young people in a range of settings, including mental health and youth justice systems within Australia.
- Promotion of mental health and wellbeing for children and young people has a place in all settings, not only child and adolescent mental health services or the youth justice system.

- Children and young people's mental health problems affect the health and wellbeing of their families and communities.
- A number of developmental factors contribute to the onset of mental disorders in children.

Promoting mental health in children and young people

Case study 7.4: Jason

As a school health nurse in a country high school, you receive a referral from a registered nurse working on the paediatrics ward at the local hospital asking you to make contact with Jason. Jason, a 16-year-old male, is aware of this referral and has agreed to come and see you. The referral form states that Jason has recently been discharged from hospital following an appendectomy. His admission was uneventful; however, during his hospital stay he disclosed to the nursing staff that he had been down lately and had been 'having trouble' at school. Jason's home-room teacher is aware of the referral and comes to see you. Until recently, Jason would have been described as an enthusiastic student. Now he is noticeably withdrawn, increasingly alone at lunchtime and not participating in class activities. There are concerns that Jason is being bullied.

Jason is an only child, and lives with his mother who is a cleaner at the local hospital. His father left the family when he was a baby and Jason has had no contact with him since. Jason and his mother have always been close, but recently Jason has seemed more distant to her.

When you meet with Jason, he spends some time telling you about his life up to this point. As the session progresses, you develop a rapport with Jason, and you see from his body language and conversation that he is becoming more comfortable. You speak to him about the teacher's concerns and give him an opportunity to talk about what he believes has been happening. He says he has always been bullied and it hasn't really bothered him. The boys at school have started to torment him for not joining in contact sports. The town's footy team, for which Jason's father once played, has a long history of winning the regional competition and the community supports the team passionately. Jason shares that he is becoming frightened that these torments will turn violent. Jason's passion in life is dancing. When he is older, he hopes to be able to attend dance classes in the city but at present Jason's mother can't afford the fees and they have no car.

You identify possible supports for Jason, who states that he is close to his aunt and she is aware that he has been bullied at school. You encourage Jason to talk to her if he needs to. You ask Jason whether he feels he is at risk of self-harm, and he says he would never hurt himself. You give Jason the number for Kids Helpline and encourage him to call it at any time if he needs someone to talk to. You end the session by asking Jason what he would like to achieve and whether he would like to talk with you at another time.

Determinants of child and adolescent mental health

Mental health is defined as

> the ability to cope with and bounce back from adversity, to solve problems in everyday life, manage when things are difficult and cope with everyday stressors. Good mental health is made possible by a supportive social, friendship and family environment, good work–life balance, physical health and, in many instances, reduced stress and trauma. (Procter et al., 2014: 4)

This wonderful definition highlights the importance of bioecological factors and how they coalesce to promote an adaptive response to life challenges and **resilience** across the lifespan (Masten, 2014). Recent advances in understanding the determinants of developmental health and neuroplasticity have led to an awareness that much can be done to promote positive mental health in children and youth. Through enhancing early life experiences and strengthening the supportive pathways throughout childhood and adolescence that help develop mental health, many determinants associated with mental illness can be substantially reduced.

Resilience The capacity of a dynamic system (such as a child or family) to adapt successfully to disturbances that threaten system function, viability or development

The majority of children progress into independence and adulthood well. Their mental health is the foundation of their thriving throughout life. They have discovered the keys to adapting to the challenges and stresses that face all children and adolescents. Unfortunately, far too many children are exposed to toxic stress – chronic over-stimulation of the stress-response system – and experience limited or ineffectual support during transition periods. Young people who are at risk of declining mental health frequently lack the opportunity to experience safe and supportive environments where they are loved and secure, and consequently are disengaged from education, family and/or their community (National Scientific Council on the Developing Child, 2012a; O'Donnell et al., 2012; Tomyn, 2013).

Wellbeing measurements, including mental health, have only recently been developed. Such measures are different from biological and epidemiological measures. Wellbeing measures tend to be multifactorial, considering sociological, emotional and even at times spiritual indicators using ordinal and qualitative data. As a result, wellbeing measures can be controversial and often comparison data are not available. The Australian Research Alliance for Children & Youth (ARACY) and the AIHW are at the forefront of developing wellbeing measures. Although both ARACY and the AIHW are yet to publish a specific mental health measure for Australian children and youth, ARACY's Report Card (ARACY, 2013a) aims to report positive measures of wellbeing; however, many available indicators remain 'negative' or 'deficit' measures. The goal for indicators of 'positive family functioning, positive mental health, and social and emotional development is balanced by the realities of the available data, therefore negative measures such as family conflict, suicide rates, psychological distress and violence need to be used' (ARACY, 2013a: 3).

In the Mission Australia Youth Survey (Mission Australia, 2013), young people aged 15 to 19 years ranked the top three issues of concern to them in 2013 and 2012 as coping with stress, school or study problems and body image. Understanding the ecology, and knowing what concerns children and young people, can help guide discussions exploring their mental health and signify where mental health promotion may be required. Paediatric nurses can contribute towards promoting mental health through understanding these key determinants of mental health.

Promoting resilience and positive adaptive responses in children and adolescents

Resilience is defined as 'the capacity of a dynamic system (such as a child or family) to adapt successfully to disturbances that threaten system function, viability or development' (Masten, 2014: 6). It is the application of a systems framework into a functional model. Child and youth mental health is dependent on developing adaptive skills fundamental for resilience. Adaptive skills can be learnt especially well during childhood, while the brain has the most capacity for plasticity. Although the current understanding of the relationship between resilience and mental health is limited, resilience and mental health are weakened when effective adaptive skills are not learnt. Mental health is not the absence of mental illness, and mental health and resilience are not determinants of each other. However, the relationship between mental health and resilience is complex, and further research is needed before we can disentangle these complex interactions. What is important to our work in paediatric nursing is to understand that resilience programs for children and young people have been linked to improved mental health in children and youth (Khanlou & Wray, 2014). The evidence for their use in a variety of settings is growing.

In recent years, ARACY has been conducting extensive research to identify the best evidence for the promotion of child and youth wellbeing. This evidence is summarised in an extensive array of evidence-based summaries and reports available freely online at <www.aracy.org.au>. In a groundbreaking Australian first, ARACY has collated this information and developed a national plan for child and youth wellbeing, The Nest action agenda (ARACY, 2013b). The Nest action agenda strives to provide a framework for promoting child and youth wellbeing, including the mental health of children and young people. Three domains of the Nest applicable to promoting child and youth mental health are:

- being loved and safe
- promoting positive participation, and
- fostering a positive sense of culture and identity.

Being loved and safe

A positive relationship with parents or caregivers is the first step towards children and youth being loved and safe, and maintaining mental health. However, the need for children and youth to be loved and safe is a whole-of-community responsibility. The past failure of Australian institutions involved in child and youth services to protect children and young people from abuse have been documented extensively (see the Royal Commission into Institutional Response to Child Sexual Abuse website, <www.childabuseroyalcommission.gov.au>). The testimonies of child abuse victims provide examples of the magnitude of mental, physical, emotional and spiritual distress that can result from children and youth not being loved and safe in the community. When abuse occurs – in the family or in the community – the shattering of love and safety can pervade the child's life and reduce mental wellbeing substantially. Noble-Carr and colleagues (2013: 19–20) report that young people who experienced abuse

> most often [struggled with] long-lasting emotional pain, disillusionment and a negative view of the world, which sometimes resulted in shutting oneself off from the world ... [they] experienced feeling alone, or even suffering from agoraphobia ... leaving them alone to overcome very negative perceptions of themselves and the world around them.

Their mental health is compromised by the abuse. The first strategy to promote mental health is to foster a loving and safe ecology for children and adolescents in home and in care. This may include early notification and referral of families in need of support. Such nursing action can enhance the nurse–family relationship by demonstrating a commitment to the rights of the child and support future mental health-promotion strategies (see the case study resolution and the responsibility to report child maltreatment section in Chapter 2).

Developing mental health begins during the antenatal period. The wellbeing of parents – particularly mothers – influences the early life experiences of the developing child. Interactions from birth with parents and those around them establish the foundation for mental health (AIHW, 2012). Investing in services that support parents' wellbeing is also an investment in the mental health of children and adolescents. Nurses caring for children also have a role to play in caring for the family. If the child's experience includes maternal/familial deprivation and toxic stress, the healthy development, mental wellbeing and life chances of the child can be adversely affected. The experience that appears to have the most potent influence on promoting mental wellbeing for children and youth, and promotes development of neural pathways and functioning, is being involved in a positive, loving and safe relationship with others from birth and throughout early childhood. Such positive early life interactions are called 'serve and return interactions' (National Scientific Council on the Developing Child, 2012a; Noble-Carr et al., 2013). It is well recognised that children can and do experience mental health problems, and early intervention and support can have a significant positive affect on the development of future mental health (National Scientific Council on the Developing Child, 2012b).

As a result of this knowledge, many schools around Australia put significant effort into developing and maintaining environments that are safe and nurturing in order to foster positive mental health. The Mind Matters program, which is gaining momentum within the Australian high school setting, is a good example of this. Mind Matters involves the implementation of a whole-school program targeted at supporting young people and promoting mental health. It aims to strengthen collaboration between school students, staff, parents and community support agencies by supporting those networks to move towards targeted goals within the specific environment. It provides training for all levels of staff to increase awareness and understanding of the importance of mental health support and promotion for young people (Wyn et al., 2000; see <www.mindmatters.edu.au>). In Case Study 7.4, Jason has some challenges and strengths in being loved and safe. Safe and loving family relationships have provided the support Jason needed in the past to withstand bullying without his self-esteem being undermined. However, promoting Jason's mental health will also require ensuring a safe ecology at school.

Promoting positive participation

During childhood, positive participation is fundamental to positive learning experiences and personal development, having significant benefits such as increased confidence and self-esteem in young people (ARACY, 2013b). Positive family, peer, classroom and community engagement can be encouraged through including children and youth in decision-making, especially in matters that affect their health and any health care they may require (see the section on participation rights in Chapter 2). Participation through technology for social connection and influencing public opinion are newly emerging areas that require further research to determine the relationship to positive mental health outcomes. Marginalised and disengaged young people experience higher rates of social and mental health problems. Youth participation in decision-making and activities that develop personal skills, along with institutions that offer opportunities for positive experiences, have a positive affect on young people feeling valued, and promote mental and social health (ARACY, 2008). Pregnant teenagers and young mums are one example of a group that can be marginalised and at high risk of disengaging from institutions, such as education systems, which can potentially have a positive impact on their mental health. Young mums and their babies are at long-term risk of low educational achievement and low income, which impacts negatively on mental health (AIHW, 2012). There are numerous innovative programs within communities and schools around Australia that aim to keep young mothers engaged in either education or workforce planning and/or participation in order to promote good mental health and increase positive outcomes for these young women and their babies.

Fostering a positive sense of culture and identity

Evidence from resilience and positive youth development research and literature conclusively demonstrates that children and youth develop a positive sense of themselves when they experience positive enduring connections with the people and services around them. Factors found to influence young people's development of a positive sense of identify, purpose and meaning in life are:

- positive, caring connections with others
- opportunities to participate in meaningful activities and/or contribute to their communities (through sport, study, work, youth groups, church groups, music groups, volunteering or caring activities)
- being acknowledged for being good at something

- finding a sense of belonging to a place or group (via family, cultural group, or church), and
- developing hope for the future. (Noble-Carr et al., 2013: 6)

Young people question who they are in relation to those around them, and where they have come from. Strengthening understanding of family and cultural traditions fosters personal awareness and a sense of belonging. Young people who are disconnected from school, education, employment, their family and the community report lower personal wellbeing compared with youth who are connected in meaningful ways (Tomyn, 2013). In modern Australian society, there are many factors that impact on the success of passing on traditional beliefs, and young people not forming a connection with their culture. Maintaining Jason's positive sense of connection to his family, school and community through supporting his passion for dancing and giving him opportunities to participate in this activity may be a way of strengthening his positive sense of identity. The school could explore how Jason could represent it at dancing events previously not engaged in by this community.

Ten practical strategies for promoting child and adolescent mental health

Evidenced-based strategies for promoting mental health of children and youth have been indentified recently through extensive reviews. These strategies can be summarised into a list that provides guidance for promoting mental health through paediatric/child health nursing care in a facility or the community.

1. Be encouraging and focus on strengths, both initially and throughout the care, with a focus on skills development. For example, encourage the young person to identify personal strengths and discuss how these strengths might be used to enhance their mental wellbeing. Identify existing barriers to good mental health and introduce specific skills that may help to avert the potential detrimental impacts of those barriers.
2. Focus your nursing on relationship-building, and be committed to the child or young person and their family needs and wants. Use a communication style that respects the rights of the child and the family, building trust as partners in health care and not simply recipients of your service.
3. Be mindful of, and assess, the expressed needs and wants of the child, young person and their family (if possible) before engaging in mental health support. This engages the young person and helps build a positive sense of self.

Empower children and young people to feel that they are fully participating in the process and decision-making, initially and throughout the care. For example, seek the child's ideas on strategies to implement.

4. Gather information about the child or young person directly from them equally with other sources. Ask what the issue is and why they may be acting the way they are in response. For example, on referral ask the child why they think they are with you and what they would like to achieve. Be collaborative in all care.

5. Focus on outcomes of care, such as developing behaviours that are known to be protective and build resilience. For example, assist the young person to identify existing support networks within their life, and encourage aspiration-building and community engagement.

6. Identify and meet immediate needs such as practical support, safety and access to other services. Be practical in the provision of support by providing concrete acts in response to real needs. For example, provision of school breakfast programs can support both learning and behaviour, leading to building of self-esteem and resilience characteristics.

7. Have multiple gateways into the support service, and be inclusive by reducing eligibility criteria. Universality of service avoids stigmatisation of mental health service. Ensure a quick response to initial referrals and inquiries for service, and follow up on any absence multiple times. Such actions help build trust.

8. Use trusted 'ambassadors' in the local community to support the service – for example, in a school secure key children and young people to be part of the service promotion.

9. Multicultural services are a great starting point, however, they are often unable to adequately meet the specific and complex mental health needs of refugee children and youth. For example, specialist programs and counselling from torture and trauma should be specifically developed for the needs of young refugees, and bicultural and bilingual services should be available through referral. Promoting the mental wellbeing of newly arrived refugees in schools starts with peer-mentoring programs linking young people with others from similar cultural backgrounds and past experiences.

10. Child and adolescent mental health problems are recognised as an indicator that the child/family is in possible need of targeted support to prevent or address child abuse and neglect. The best way to promote mental wellbeing and protect at-risk children is to prevent child abuse and neglect from occurring through providing assistance before family problems

escalate into crises. Identification of needs and early referral can be achieved through adopting the Common Approach to Assessment, Referral and Support – a short checklist completed in the presence of the child and/or family to identify their needs.

These ten practical strategies have been collated from ARACY evidenced-based reports (ARACY, 2006, 2007, 2010) and supported with examples from Julia Taylor's nursing experience.

Resolution

Case study 7.5

Jason agrees to see you again. You plan to gain further insight into Jason's mental health by asking whether there have been any changes in his sleeping, appetite, concentration or ability to enjoy and maintain his usual activities. You also hope to do some self-esteem-building exercises with Jason in future sessions. He gives you permission to discuss the bullying with his teacher, and the teacher plans to address this with those involved.

After four visits, Jason states that he is feeling happier and the bullying has lessened. His relationship with his mother is improving, and he doesn't feel he needs another appointment at present. You encourage Jason to come and see you again at any time if he wants to. You later hear that Jason and a newly formed local dance group are to perform at an upcoming community event.

Summary

- Being loved and safe, having strong relationships, positive experiences and supportive environments, actively participating in community and social activities, and fostering a positive sense of culture and identity all help build adaptive capacity in children and young people.
- Building an adaptive capacity allows the child or young person to manage the transitions and stresses they will experience in childhood and throughout life. This is the foundation of mental health, and a resource for recovery from mental illness.
- Mental health can be promoted most effectively using a strengths approach, enhancing resilience in children, young people and families.
- All nursing interactions have the potential to build on the determinants of mental health.

Learning activity

Watch *Serve & Return* from the Center on the Developing Child, Harvard University (2011). Consider how the 'serve and return' process can be strengthened in your local area through paediatric nursing practice. By enhancing early child development through paediatric nursing practice, you strengthen child and youth mental health.

Further reading

Procter, N, Baker, A, Grocke, K & Ferguson, M 2013, Introduction to mental health and mental illness: Human connectedness and the collaborative consumer narrative. In N Procter, H Hamer, D McGarry, R Wilson & T Froggatt, *Mental health: A person-centred approach*, Cambridge University Press, Melbourne, pp. 1–24. A discussion of the connections between mental health and mental illness at an advanced level, building on the nursing knowledge and skill you have developed by reading Chapter 7.

References

Achenbach, TM 1991a, *Manual for the Child Behaviour Checklist: 4–18 and 1991 Profile*, University of Vermont Department of Psychiatry, Burlington, VT.

—— 1991b, *Manual for the Youth Self-Report and 1991 Profile*, University of Vermont Department of Psychiatry, Burlington, VT.

American Psychiatric Association (APA) 2000, *Diagnostic and statistical manual of mental disorders*, 4th edn (DSM-4), American Psychiatric Publishing, Arlington, VA.

—— 2013, *Diagnostic and statistical manual of mental disorders*, 5th edn (DSM-5), American Psychiatric Publishing, Arlington, VA.

Australian Institute of Health and Welfare (AIHW) 2009, *A picture of Australia's children 2009*, AIHW, Canberra.

—— 2012, *A picture of Australia's children 2012*, AIHW, Canberra.

Australian Research Alliance for Children & Youth (ARACY) 2006, *What interventions are effective in improving outcomes for children of families with multiple and complex problems?*, ARACY, Canberra.

—— 2007, *Working with multicultural youth: Programs, strategies and future directions*, ARACY, Canberra.

—— 2008, *Preventing youth disengagement and promoting engagement*, ARACY, Canberra.

—— 2010, *Working together to prevent child abuse and neglect: A common approach for identifying and responding early to indicators of need*, ARACY, Canberra.

—— 2013a, *The Report Card: The well-being of young Australians*, ARACY, Canberra.

—— 2013b, *The Nest action agenda*, ARACY, Canberra.

Becker, L, Goobic, K & Thomas, S 2009, Advising families on ADHD: A multimodal approach, *Pediatric Nursing*, 35(1), p. 47.

Bennett, K et al. 2013, Cognitive behavioural therapy age effects in child and adolescent anxiety: an individual patient data meta-analysis, *Depression and Anxiety*, 30(9), pp. 829–41.

Biederman, J & Faraone, SV 2005, Attention-Deficit Hyperactivity Disorder, *Lancet*, 366(9481), pp. 237–48.

Biederman, J, Newcom, J & Sprich, S 1991, Comorbidity of attention deficit with conduct, depressive, anxiety and other disorders, *American Journal of Psychiatry*, 148(5), pp. 564–77.

Broidy, LM et al. 2003, Developmental trajectories of childhood disruptive behaviors and adolescent delinquency: A six-site, cross-national study, *Developmental Psychology*, 39, pp. 222–45.

Bronfenbrenner, U 2001, Bioecological theory of human development. In JS Neil & BB Paul (eds), *International encyclopaedia of the social & behavioral sciences*, Pergamon Press, Oxford, pp. 6963–70.

Center on the Developing Child, Harvard University 2011, *Serve & Respond*, https://www.youtube.com/watch?v=m_5u8-QSh6A&list=PL0DB506DEF92B6347.

Centers for Disease Control and Prevention (CDCP) 2014, *Prevalence of Autism Spectrum Disorder among children aged 8 years – Autism and Developmental Disabilities Monitoring Network, 11 sites, US, 2010*, viewed 20 February 2014, http://www.cdc.gov/mmwr/pdf/ss/ss6302.pdf.

Dadds, MR & Fraser, JA 2003, Prevention programs. In C Essau (ed.), *Conduct and oppositional defiant disorders: Epidemiology, risk factors and treatment*, Lawrence Erlbaum, Mahwah, NJ, pp. 193–224.

Dodd Inglese, M 2009, Caring for children with Autism Spectrum Disorder, Part II: Screening, diagnosis, and management, *Journal of Pediatric Nursing*, 24(1), pp. 49–59.

Dodd Inglese, M & Harrison Elder, J 2009, Caring for children with Autism Spectrum Disorder, Part I: Prevalence, etiology, and core features, *Journal of Pediatric Nursing*, 24(1), pp. 41–8.

Erikson, EH 1968, *Identity, youth and crisis*, WW Norton, New York.

Feldman, HM & Reiff, MI 2014, Attention Deficit–Hyperactivity Disorder in children and adolescents, *New England Journal of Medicine*, 370, pp. 838–46.

Goodman, SH et al. 2011, Maternal depression and child psychopathology: A meta-analytic review, *Clinical Child and Family Psychology Review*, 14(1), pp. 1–27.

Grizenko, N, Cai, E, Claude, J, Ter-Stepanian, M & Joober, R 2013, Effects of Methylphenidate on acute math performance in children with Attention-Deficit Hyperactivity Disorder, *Canadian Journal of Psychiatry*, 58(11), pp. 632–39.

Hazell, P 2011, The challenges to demonstrating long-term effects of psychostimulant treatment for Attention-Deficit/Hyperactivity Disorder, *Current Opinion in Psychiatry*, 24, pp. 286–90.

Hoath, FE & Sanders, MR 2002, A feasibility study of Enhanced Group Triple P Positive Parenting Program for Parents of Children with Attention-Deficit/ Hyperactivity Disorder, *Behaviour Change*, 19(4), pp. 191–206.

In-Albon, T & Schneider, S 2007, Psychotherapy of childhood anxiety disorders: A meta-analysis, *Psychotherapy and Psychosomatics*, 76(1), pp. 15–24.

Khanlou, N & Wray, R 2014, A whole community approach towards child and youth resilience promotion: A review of resilience literature, *International Journal of Mental Health Addiction*, 12, pp. 64–79.

Loeber, R & Hay, D 1997, Key issues in the development of aggression and violence from childhood to early adulthood, *Annual Review of Psychology*, 48, pp. 371–410.

Masten, AS 2014, Global perspectives on resilience in children and youth, *Child Development*, 85(1), pp. 6–20.

McLaughlin, KA et al. 2012, Parent psychopathology and offspring mental disorders: Results from the WHO World Mental Health Surveys, *British Journal of Psychiatry*, 200, pp. 290–9.

Mission Australia 2013, *Youth Survey 2013*, Mission Australia, Sydney.

National Scientific Council on the Developing Child 2012a, *The science of neglect: The persistent absence of responsive care disrupts the developing brain*, working paper 12, Center on the Developing Child, Harvard University, viewed 20 March 2014, http://developingchild.harvard.edu.

—— 2012b, *Establishing a level foundation for life: Mental health begins in early childhood*, working paper 6, Center on the Developing Child, Harvard University, http://developingchild.harvard.edu

Noble-Carr, D, Barker, J & McArthur, M 2013, *Me, myself and I: Identity and meaning in the lives of vulnerable young people*, Institute of Child Protection Studies, Canberra.

O'Donnell, M, Nassar, N, Jacoby, P & Stanley, F 2012, Western Australian emergency department presentations related to child maltreatment and intentional injury: Population level study utilising linked health and child protection data, *Journal of Paediatrics and Child Health*, 48(1), pp. 57–65.

Procter, N, Baker, A, Grocke, K & Ferguson, M 2013, Introduction to mental health and mental illness: Human connectedness and the collaborative consumer narrative. In N Procter, H Hamer, D McGarry, R Wilson & T Froggatt (eds), *Mental health: A person-centred approach*, Cambridge University Press, Melbourne, pp. 1–24.

Rutter ML 2005, Environmentally mediated risks for psychopathology: Research strategies and findings, *Journal of the American Academy of Child Adolescent Psychiatry*, 44, pp. 3–18.

Sameroff, AJ & MacKenzie, MJ 2003, Research strategies for capturing transactional models of development: The limits of the possible, *Development and Psychopathology*, 15(3), pp. 613–40.

Sawyer, MG et al. 2000, *Young people in Australia*, Department of Health, Canberra, viewed 4 June 2014, http://www.health.gov.au/internet/publications/publishing.nsf/Content/mental-pubs-m-young-toc.

Scott, KM et al. 2011, Association of childhood adversities and early-onset mental disorders with adult-onset chronic physical conditions, *Archives of General Psychiatry*, 68, pp. 838–44.

Taylor, E 2003, Practice methods for working with children who have biologically based mental disorders: A bioecological model, *Family in Society: The Journal of Contemporary Human Services*, 84(1), pp. 39–50.

Tomyn, A 2013, *Youth connections subjective well-being report – Part A: Report 5.0*, RMIT University, Melbourne.

Wyn, J, Cahill, H, Holdsworth, R, Rowling, L & Carson, S 2000, Mind matters: A whole school approach promoting mental health and well-being, *Australian and New Zealand Journal of Psychiatry*, 34, pp. 594–601.

8 Evidence-based nursing assessments and interventions: The acutely ill child

Nicola Brown

Learning objectives

In this chapter you will:

- Develop your understanding of the evidence-based nursing assessments and interventions used in the care of acutely ill infants and young children
- Develop your understanding of the aetiology, signs and symptoms of key acute illnesses experienced by infants and young children in Australia
- Consider the developmental needs of infants and young children in the planning and implementation of nursing care
- Explore the impact of illness and hospitalisation on infants and young children

Introduction

Children contract infections regularly during early childhood, and are also at risk of injury; thus they can experience episodes of acute illness. For the most part, these episodes are of short duration and resolve with the care of parents at home, sometimes with support from community health care professionals such as a general practitioner. However, in some instances the illness can reach a level of severity that requires nursing care and medical treatment in a hospital setting. Children aged 0–4 years are the most common age group presenting for care in an emergency department (AIHW, 2012). Infants and children are still developing, so they have physiological and anatomical differences from adults that require specialist skills and knowledge. Hospital environments can be challenging for both the young child and their family. For many families, visiting the emergency department with their sick child may be the first time they have ever had to seek acute care from a hospital. It is important that nurses understand this, and that we ensure the child's care is delivered in a way that is supportive and respectful of the individual child and their family.

In Chapter 5, you were introduced to primary assessment of infants and children and recognition of the sick or deteriorating child. In this chapter, we will discuss the more common reasons why children might require hospitalisation, including fever, dehydration and acute respiratory illness, and consider the nursing care required.

Fever in children

Ying

Case study 8.1

Ying is an 18-month-old girl brought to the emergency department by her mother and father. Ying's mother explains that Ying has been vomiting sporadically for 12 hours, and had a brief seizure at home. She is not sure how long the seizure lasted for, but thinks it was less than a minute. Ying's father explains that during the seizure, Ying was staring, had rhythmic clenching of both fists and her body and limbs were rigid.

Ying is pale, sleepy and lethargic. She feels peripherally warm to touch. Her heart rate is 165/min, respiratory rate is 35/min, blood pressure 95/60 and temperature is 39.0°C. Her mouth and lips are dry. Her parents report that she has not kept down any fluids for 12 hours. Each time Ying drinks fluids, she vomits, and she has only passed urine once since the vomiting began.

Fever is a common and normal response to infection; however, the mechanisms by which fever occurs are still not fully understood (Meremikwu & Oyo-Ita, 2009a). What is known is that infection by organisms such as viruses or bacteria can stimulate release of pyrogenic cytokines that stimulate the preoptic area of the hypothalamus via humeral and neural pathways to raise body temperature to a higher level than normal (Ogoina, 2011). At a higher body temperature, it seems that the environment for replication of bacteria and viruses can become unfavourable and that immunological factors in the blood, such as white blood cells, may be enhanced (Blatteis, 2003; Ogoina, 2011). This evidence that fever may be a normal and potentially beneficial response to invasion by pathogens has influenced current practice in the care of children with fever.

> **Fever** In most cases, measurements around 38°C (centrally measured) and higher are regarded as a fever (Forbes, 2013; Meremikwu & Oyo-Ita, 2009a).

Key issues in the monitoring and management of fever in children include definitions of normal body temperature and fever. It is generally accepted that the mean range of normal body temperature is 36.5–37.5°C (Forbes, 2013); however, there is some variation in temperature between individuals and the site of measurement. For example, temperature measurements via the axilla site will be cooler than temperature measurements made via more central sites such as the mouth or tympanic membrane. The variations in range between sites can present an issue when monitoring a trend in temperature over time. It is essential that the site of measurement and the thermometry equipment used are consistent in order to ensure an accurate monitoring of temperature.

The level at which a temperature in an infant or child is defined as a mild, moderate or high fever is less clear. This is complicated by the fact that infants and younger children have more frequent fevers that tend to be higher, last longer and have more rapid temperature increases (Ogoina, 2011). If you read several textbooks, it is likely that you will find considerable variety in the ranges for fever.

The management of fever has not always been based on the best available evidence. The decision to tolerate or treat fever in children has traditionally been controversial. Fever can contribute to the discomfort of illness for children, and can cause anxiety for parents (Walsh et al., 2008) and, as a result, health-care professionals and parents can feel the need to intervene. However, traditional methods of intervening to reduce fever may not be appropriate. Non-pharmacological methods to reduce fever, such as tepid sponging or fans, are not recommended (Meremikwu & Oyo-Ita, 2009b; Watts & Robertson, 2012). If intervention is warranted, then antipyretic medication may be required.

Antipyretic medications

Antipyretic medications are generally considered 'safe' medications, and are widely available without prescription. The use of antipyretic medications such as paracetamol or ibuprofen to reduce fever (Crook, 2010) is not entirely without risk (Meremikwu & Oyo-Ita, 2009b), particularly when the recommendation for dosage is exceeded. For example, overdosing on paracetamol can cause liver damage and overdosing on ibuprofen can lead to renal dysfunction. The action of antipyretic medications is not fully understood, but it is postulated that these medications work by reducing the 'set point' of the hypothalamic control of body temperature (Rang et al., 2011). Aspirin should not be used in children due to concerns about the relationship between the use of aspirin and either influenza or varicella, and

> **Antipyretic medications**
> These include paracetamol or non-steroidal anti-inflammatory medications such as ibuprofen; they are used to reduce fever

the development of Reyes syndrome – a life-threatening illness (Arrowsmith et al., 1987).

> ### Reflection points 8.1
>
> - Even mild episodes of acute illness and fever can make us feel discomfort from pain such as headaches or myalgia.
> - In some cases where children are miserable but without a fever, or with only a mild fever, it can be more appropriate to give a medication such as paracetamol for its analgesic properties and the relief of pain and discomfort than to use it as an antipyretic.

Administering oral medications

For infants and children, the dose of medication prescribed is usually calculated based on weight. In some instances, **body surface area (BSA)** may be used to calculate medications.

> **Body surface area (BSA)** A calculation of the surface area of the human body, expressed in square metres. BSA may be calculated using software or a nomogram. In order to calculate BSA, an accurate weight and height/length of the patient is required

In addition to the usual precautions taken in administering medications to anyone (right medication, right dose, right route, right time, right person), consideration needs to be given to the age and the development of the child. For example, infants are not able to swallow tablets, so wherever possible, a liquid preparation of the oral medication would be preferred. The smaller size of children and the variation in size across age groups means that health professionals need to calculate doses and check prescribed doses of medication carefully. Other challenges in administering medication to children include identifying children who are pre-verbal. It is important that the identity of the child is confirmed, either by the parent or medical identification bracelet, prior to the administration of medications.

Not all oral medications may be available in liquid form. For advice on preparing solid oral medications for administration to infants or younger children, seek advice from a reputable medication information source such as a paediatric pharmacopoeia or a pharmacist.

Administering oral medications to children can be challenging, especially if the child does not want to take the medication or the taste is unpleasant. Some children may be better with a medication spoon, but you may be more comfortable using a syringe – particularly when the child is younger or less cooperative. Wherever possible, nurses should try to make the experience positive.

For practical and comfort reasons, it is wise to sit the child in your lap for administration. It can help to tuck their arm closest to you behind your back and hold the other arm still. Gently administer the oral medication liquid into the mouth, along the inside of the cheek. Administer small amounts, allowing the child to swallow. Administer too much at once, and the child may spit it out. Encourage the child to swallow the medication, and give a lot of positive feedback once the process is complete – even if it was a struggle!

Febrile seizures

Some children will experience a single, brief febrile seizure before the age of 5 years (Reid et al., 2009). Typically, it will be a generalised tonic–clonic seizure, lasting only a minute or two. In most instances, the seizure is caused by a sudden rise in core body temperature. In infancy and early childhood, children are more susceptible to such seizure triggers, as the cerebral cortex is quite excitable, and consequently the threshold for a seizure is lower (Lux, 2010). However, in a few cases, repeated or longer seizures may indicate a more serious condition, such as meningitis or epilepsy (Lux, 2010). If an infant or child has a seizure, it is considered a medical emergency in the first instance.

Studies into the use of prophylactic treatment of febrile seizures do not support the use of anti-epileptic medications or anti-pyretic medications to prevent a fever (Offringa & Newton, 2012), particularly as some of the anti-epileptic medications have undesirable side-effects. More importantly, parents should be advised on the first aid response to a seizure, the risk of recurrence and when to seek medical advice.

For most parents, their child's febrile seizure is their first experience ever of a seizure, and can be a frightening experience for them. It is important that health professionals are sensitive to the distress that parents have experienced, even though the relative risk associated with a simple febrile seizure may be mild.

Dehydration

Dehydration is a common reason for children to require admission to hospital, and a frequent symptom in children presenting to general practice clinics and emergency departments. While children may become dehydrated for a range of reasons, the most common condition causing dehydration is acute gastroenteritis. Dehydration from acute gastroenteritis is one of the leading causes of mortality for children in developing countries (WHO & UNICEF, 2013).

Assessment of dehydration

Underestimating the degree of dehydration and not replacing lost fluids and electrolytes can result in acidosis, electrolyte imbalance, renal damage or death. Initial and ongoing assessment of dehydration is a crucial step in determining required treatment and need for hospitalisation.

Several scales and algorithms have been developed to assess and treat dehydration. Commonly used assessment scales include the World Health Organization (WHO) Scale, the Gorelick Scale and the Clinical Dehydration Scale (CDS) (Pringle et al., 2011). Each scale predicts percentage of estimated weight loss due to fluid loss for different age groups. For example, the WHO and Gorelick Scales are used in children aged 1 month to 5 years, and the CDS is used in children aged 1 month to 3 years. Each scale assesses a range of clinical signs associated with dehydration. In Australia, some modifications of these scales have been developed by expert groups (see Table 8.1).

Essentially, the differences between mild, moderate and severe dehydration are based on changes in the signs of circulation – especially colour, heart rate, activity level, peripheral perfusion, urine output and blood pressure. Early signs of mild dehydration, such as pallor, dry mucous membranes and

TABLE 8.1 *Commonly used scales for assessment of dehydration*

	WHO	CDS	GORELICK	NSW HEALTH
Age group	1 month–5 years	1 month–3 years	1 month–5 years	Not stated
Signs	Condition/level of consciousness	General appearance	General appearance	Lethargy
	Eyes (normal or sunken)	Eyes	Capillary refill	Capillary refill
	Thirst	Mucous membranes	Tears	Mucous membranes
	Skin pinch	Tears	Mucous membranes	Eyes
			Eyes	Breathing
			Breathing	Quality of pulses
			Quality of pulses	Skin turgor
			Skin elasticity	Heart rate
			Heart rate	Urine output
			Urine output	

diminished urine output, are the result of compensatory mechanisms in response to decreased fluid volume. As dehydration becomes moderate, and then severe, signs that the circulation is compromised are more apparent. Signs of moderate to severe dehydration include worsening colour, deterioration in level of consciousness, increasing tachycardia, decreased capillary refill, deterioration in skin turgor and lastly, hypotension. Hypotension in infants and children is considered an ominous sign of severe dehydration that is indicative of hypovolaemic shock.

Gastroenteritis

Viruses are the most common causative pathogen of gastroenteritis in children, particularly rotavirus and norovirus (Kesson et al., 2010; NHMRC, 2013). Health-care service demands arising from rotavirus infections alone in Australia are estimated to be $30 million (Galati et al., 2006). This does not take into consideration the impact of the illness on the community in terms of lost work hours by parents. Since the introduction of the nationally funded rotavirus vaccination program, there has been a significant decline in the rate of hospitalisations for rotavirus infections for children under 5 years of age – an estimated reduction in 7700 hospitalisations per year (Dey et al., 2012)

Viral gastroenteritis causes injury to the small bowel, resulting in low-grade fever and watery diarrhoea (Elliott, 2007). Children can also develop bacterial gastroenteritis, primarily through food poisoning. Children with bacterial gastroenteritis are more likely to have a high fever and bloody stools (NIHCE, 2009). There is an additional risk that bacterial gastroenteritis can progress to a more systemic infection, resulting in sepsis and shock (Elliott, 2007).

Hydration and diet for children with acute gastroenteritis

Oral rehydration therapy (ORT) using commercially developed modified glucose and sodium solutions is one of the safest and most effective methods to treat mild to moderate dehydration caused by diarrhoea and vomiting. In most instances, ORT is used orally, and given in small frequent amounts over several hours, as a 'trial of oral fluids' to see if increased fluid and electrolyte intake via the oral route can result in rehydration, without the need for intravenous cannulation and fluid therapy (Hartling et al., 2006). If vomiting persists or a child refuses to drink ORT, consideration may be given to administering ORT via a nasogastric tube.

For children with moderate to severe dehydration, intravenous fluids may be required. Children with the clinical signs of severe dehydration, including hypotension, may require fluid resuscitation with fluid boluses to ensure adequate circulation (NIHCE, 2009).

An early return to normal diet and the reintroduction of milk is now encouraged for infants and children with acute gastroenteritis once vomiting has subsided. Breastfeeding can continue through the illness period. Evidence suggests that early resumption of diet is associated with a reduction in number of bowel motions, reduced duration of illness and lower weight loss (NIHCE, 2009).

Intravenous therapy

Restoration or maintenance of normal fluid and electrolyte balance is an essential component of care of the sick infant or child. For many reasons, infants or children may be unable to maintain normal intake of fluids because they are sick or because they are being kept nil by mouth. Children with acute illness frequently require intravenous access for a range of reasons, including the administration of fluids, medication, blood products and/or blood sampling. Most often, intravenous access for short-term use is obtained via peripheral venous cannulation. Obtaining and maintaining intravenous access in infants and children can be challenging for many reasons, including the smaller relative size of children's blood vessels, and the fear, anxiety and pain caused by the procedure.

Generally, the site of intravenous cannulation is determined on the basis of the child's history and the type of medication or fluid that is to be administered (Rathnayake, 2012). In most instances, the first site of choice will be the dorsal aspect of the child's non-dominant hand. Other sites that may be considered include the wrist, leg, foot and scalp.

Topical anaesthetics (such as EMLA or amethiocaine) can be applied prior to cannulation to the site(s) of choice to reduce the pain associated with venipuncture, but these generally need to be applied 45 minutes to one hour before cannulation is attempted. Although there is good evidence that topical anaesthetics reduce the pain associated with venipuncture and cannulation (Rathnayake, 2012), some clinicians may elect not to use it as it may cause transient vasoconstriction of superficial vessels. However, results from the first prospective study to compare the success rate of cannulation with or without EMLA found no significant difference in success rate (Schreiber et al., 2013). While these results suggest that EMLA may not reduce the success of cannulation, further studies are required to confirm these findings and reduce clinicians' concerns.

Preparing the child and family for intravenous cannulation

Depending on the age of the child, their capacity to cooperate during cannulation may be limited by their development and their feelings of fear and anxiety. It is important that these factors are taken into consideration when preparing the child and family. In the first instance, parent consent will need to be obtained for the procedure, and details of the approach to the procedure discussed initially with the parent, and then with the child using developmentally appropriate language. It may be necessary to hold the child or their limb during the procedure, and parents should be given a choice about their role in this. At a minimum, children will need their parent close by to provide comfort after the procedure. Partial wrapping of the child's body, leaving the limb intended for cannulation free, can help the parent to hold the child more easily during the procedure.

In addition to topical anaesthetics to reduce the pain of cannulation mentioned earlier, we should consider the use of distraction and other methods to reduce pain. For infants, parent presence, physical comfort and non-nutritive sucking with sucrose or a dummy are simple interventions that may provide comfort during the pain of cannulation. For children, looking at books, blowing bubbles, watching a movie or listening to music are some techniques that can be used.

Reflection points 8.2

- One of the more challenging aspects of caring for children can be communicating our intentions to perform procedures that may cause fear, anxiety or pain. When we plan to talk to children about a procedure like intravenous cannulation, there are a number of issues to take into consideration:
  - their stage of cognitive development
  - their understanding of language – for example, whether their primary language is the same as ours
  - the presence of parents
  - the timing of the information
  - their prior experiences of painful or distressing procedures.

Monitoring the intravenous site and infusion

Intravenous cannulation is painful and distressing for children, and may be technically difficult for clinicians, so protection of a patent cannula is essential. It is important that the child's developmental stage, the condition of their skin, the location of the site and the child's mobility are taken into consideration. The cannula is normally secured at the insertion site with sterile opaque dressing or tape, so that the site can be visualised and monitored for inflammation, leaking and infiltration. Depending on the position of the site and the mobility of the limb, it may be necessary to splint the limb to ensure patency of the cannula. Accessing the intravenous line should be performed using an aseptic non-touch technique (NHMRC, 2010). The site should be checked frequently – up to hourly as required. An intravenous infusion pump is used to ensure the accurate rate of fluids is infused. Administration of intravenous fluids should be accurately recorded in the child's fluid balance chart in addition to other fluid intake and output.

Intravenous fluids: Types and volumes

Infants have higher total body water than older children and adults, and turn over their body water more frequently. In addition, infants have a higher body surface area:mass ratio, and are therefore more susceptible to insensible fluid losses. As a result, accurate and careful calculation of fluid volumes is required. Infants and children are generally prescribed fluids based on body weight. Sometimes their fluids may be calculated based on body surface area. There are different methods for calculating fluid requirements, either based on total daily amounts or hourly amounts.

In addition to different fluid volumes, the types of intravenous fluids used in children are slightly different from those used for adults. Intravenous fluids used for maintaining hydration generally contain a mixture of sodium chloride and glucose. Younger infants have higher energy needs, so they may be prescribed a higher concentration of glucose than older infants and children. For intravenous rehydration fluids, generally 0.9 per cent sodium chloride (with or without glucose) is the fluid of choice.

Acute otitis media (AOM)

Case study 8.2

Lucas

Lucas is a 7-month-old infant brought to the after-hours general practice clinic. Lucas's parents report that he has cried inconsolably for six hours and has little interest in breastfeeds or solids. Lucas appears pale and is peripherally warm. He is noticeably irritable, crying despite being held by his mother. He has profuse nasal secretions and a dry mouth. His parents are concerned that he has not had a wet nappy for six hours. The general practitioner inspects his ears, and notes bilateral inflamed tympanic membranes, with a bulging right tympanic membrane. Lucas has a heart rate of 172/minute, a respiratory rate of 44/minute and his axilla temperature is 39.7°C.

Acute otitis media (AOM) refers to an inflammation of the inner ear, characterised by fluid in the middle ear and pain from inflammation in that area. Many children will have at least one episode of otitis media during early childhood, usually before the age of 2 years (Monasta et al., 2012), and the incidence is higher still in Indigenous children (Yiengprugsawan et al., 2013). Chronic otitis media can lead to hearing loss, affecting language development and educational achievement (Monasta et al., 2012). Children of this age are more likely to develop ear infections, as they have short, horizontal Eustachian tubes that are less likely to drain fluid produced during an upper airway infection. AOM is more likely to occur in households with smokers, in infancy and toddlerhood, in children exposed to more frequent URTI through child-care attendance and in lower SES groups.

The signs of AOM are usually fairly rapid in onset. Most children will initially present as irritable and difficult to settle, and may have loss of appetite and interest in drinking their usual fluids. More definitive signs include fever, earache and sometimes discharge from the ear, if the tympanic membrane ruptures. Many children will have had a recent history of an upper respiratory tract infection (URTI), including a sore throat and rhinitis. A diagnosis of AOM is usually made based on these clinical signs, and confirmed by direct visualisation of the tympanic membrane using an otoscope. Normally, a tympanic membrane is a pale pearl-pink colour. In AOM, the membrane is redder and may bulge from the build-up of fluid in the middle ear.

An earache can be very painful and distressing for an infant or child, and management of this pain is an important intervention. Relief from pain can help the child to settle to sleep, and may improve their intake of oral fluids. In most cases, oral analgesics such as paracetamol or ibuprofen can be used to reduce the pain. Although the main purpose of using either paracetamol or ibuprofen is to reduce pain in this circumstance, these medications can also reduce any fever that is present.

Concerns about the over-use of oral antibiotics in the community have led to the development of evidence-based guidelines to encourage more judicious use of antibiotic therapy in the treatment of AOM. To date, evidence suggests that antibiotics are appropriate for the treatment of children under two years of age with bilateral AOM or for children with both bilateral AOM and a discharge from the ear (otorrhoea) (Morris et al., 2009; Venekamp et al., 2013). If pain persists for longer than 48 hours, antibiotic therapy may be indicated.

Pain assessment

Assessment of pain in children can be challenging. Not only is pain a subjective experience, but language, cognition and previous experience of health care will impact on how infants and children experience and communicate pain to health-care professionals. As pain is subjective, it is can be difficult to assess, and this is one of the reasons why health professionals may not recognise the extent of pain in children.

Ideally, we would like to obtain the child's perspective or judgement of their own pain, yet infants and younger children are not able to do this as they do not yet possess the cognition and/or language to provide reliable or valid reports of pain. Furthermore, some children may deny pain if they have concerns that intervention by health-care professionals may worsen pain or lead to procedures (such as cannulation) that may result in further pain. The three main approaches to the assessment of pain in children include self-report of pain by children or their parent, observation of behaviours, or physiological signs that are known to reflect pain using a standardised pain assessment tool (APAGBI, 2012).

No single pain-assessment tool can be recommended for use in all children. Recent evidence-based practice guidelines for pain management have made recommendations for the use of behavioural and self-report tools in the assessment of pain in children (see Table 8.2).

TABLE 8.2 *Recommended measures for the procedural and postoperative pain assessment based on chronological age*

CHILD'S AGE	MEASURE
Newborn–3 years	COMFORT or FLACC
4 years	Faces Pain Scale – Revised (FPS-R) + COMFORT or FLACC
5–7 years	FPS-R
7 years +	Visual analogue scale (VAS) or numerical rating scores (NRS) or FPS R

Source: Adapted from APAGBI (2012).

Observational and behavioural pain-assessment tools

The signs and symptoms of pain can be similar to fear or distress, and at times it can be difficult for the observer to determine which of these they are observing. This can be particularly challenging in infants and younger, pre-verbal children. For these groups of children, observational and behavioural tools are used for pain assessment. Currently, the COMFORT scale and FLACC scale are most commonly recommended for use as observational and behavioural pain assessment tools.

The COMFORT behaviour scale was initially developed to assess distress in infants in the paediatric intensive-care setting (Ambuel et al., 1992), but has since been validated for the assessment of pain intensity and distress in other age groups, including ventilated adults in intensive care settings (Ashkenazy & DeKeyser-Ganz, 2011), and older infants and toddlers (van Dijk et al., 2000). The scale is based on behavioural and physiological signs. Scores are given for alertness, calmness, respiratory distress, crying, physical movement, muscle tone, facial tension, mean arterial pressure and heart rate.

The FLACC scale is a pain-assessment framework used to quantify pain behaviours in children. It was first developed for use in assessing post-operative pain in infants and children under 7 years (Merkel et al., 1997), and it has since been validated in other studies with similar-aged children (Manworren & Hynan, 2003; Willis et al., 2003), older children and adolescents (Nilsson et al., 2008), children with cognitive impairment (Malviya et al., 2006) and in one study of non-Western children (Bai et al., 2012). The FLACC scale requires the health-care practitioner to assess the degree of tension evident in the face and legs, the level of activity, the extent of crying and how easily the infant or child can be consoled (see Table 8.3).

TABLE 8.3 *FLACC scale*

CRITERIA	SCORE 0	SCORE 1	SCORE 2
Face	No particular expression or smile	Occasional grimace or frown, withdrawn, uninterested	Frequent to constant quivering chin, clenched jaw
Legs	Normal position or relaxed	Uneasy, restless, tense	Kicking or legs drawn up
Activity	Lying quietly, normal position, moves easily	Squirming, shifting back and forth, tense	Arched, rigid or jerking
Cry	No cry (awake or asleep)	Moans or whimpers, occasional complaint	Crying steadily, screams or sobs, frequent complaints
Consolability	Content, relaxed	Reassured by occasional touching, hugging or being talked to, distractible	Difficult to console or comfort

Source: Merkel et al. (1997).

Self-report tools

Self-report tools are commonly used in children over the age of 5 years, who are able to provide a verbal self-report of pain. While many self-report tools have been developed as a way to measure children's self-report of pain, not all are used effectively or consistently, or they lack repeated evaluation data. The self-report tools most commonly evaluated, used and recommended are the Faces Pain Scale – Revised (FPS–R), visual analogue scales (VAS) and numerical rating scores (NRS).

Acute respiratory illness

Jayden

Case study 8.3

Jayden is a 2-year-old boy brought to the emergency department in the late evening by his mother. Jayden's mother explains that he has had a barking cough during the day that has become progressively worse. She is concerned that he seems to be working harder to breathe, even when asleep.

Jayden is pale and sleeping in his mother's arms. As Jayden takes a breath, there is a loud stridor on inspiration and a softer noise on inspiration. You notice that Jayden has tracheal tug on inspiration, and noticeable use of abdominal muscles during respiration. After a few minutes, Jayden rouses and coughs loudly before falling back to sleep.

Acute respiratory illnesses that are characterised by some degree of upper or lower airway obstruction are one of the most common reasons why children in Australia require nursing care and hospitalisation (AIHW, 2012). Essentially, the younger a child is, the narrower their airways are, and thus the more likely they are to develop airway obstruction as a result of the inflammation. The extent to which infants and children become unwell with respiratory illness can vary considerably between individuals, and depending on the cause and site of the obstruction, and sick infants and children can further deteriorate in a relatively short timeframe, as outlined in Chapter 5.

Respiratory tract infections

Respiratory tract infections caused by viruses are a very common event in the lives of children. In most instances, children have a mild illness that resolves within a few days, and some children will develop a severe infection that requires admission to hospital. Symptoms vary, depending on the site and cause of the infection, but in general children are more likely than adults to have symptoms of fever, discomfort and decreased fluid intake.

Croup

Croup (laryngotracheo-bronchitis) is the most common obstructive disorder of the upper airway, usually caused by viruses, such as Para influenza types 1 and 2 (Schomacker et al., 2012; Australian Lung Foundation, 2007). The signs of croup are characteristic – an inspiratory stridor, barking cough, and onset in the evening and at night. In mild cases, these symptoms resolve within a few days. Nonetheless, the symptoms of croup can be frightening for the child and parent.

Croup is usually mild in children, and can be cared for at home, usually after review by a general practitioner. Children with moderate or severe croup require review and close monitoring by health professionals in an emergency department, and may require admission. However, the early use of oral corticosteroids, which can quickly reduce the inflammation in the upper airways and thus reduce obstruction, have significantly reduced both the need to be admitted and the time required for admission in hospital (Dobrovoljac & Geelhoed, 2012; Russell et al., 2004).

Any child with stridor requires close and careful monitoring and assessment, as it can worsen and lead to severe airway obstruction. Furthermore, stridor with drooling and without coughing may indicate the presence of epiglottitis or bacterial tracheitis (Paul et al., 2011; Tibballs & Watson, 2011), conditions associated with acute airway obstruction, which require intubation and intensive care.

It is essential to establish the extent of airway obstruction, as this is the main criterion for determining the degree of severity of illness in a child with croup; thus very careful respiratory assessment is required (see Chapter 5). Children with croup are generally considered to have mild croup when they are interacting normally with parents and their environment. These children may have an audible inspiratory stridor when they are active, but the stridor is absent at rest. When stridor is present even at rest, then children are considered to have moderate croup. More severe croup is characterised by worsening airway obstruction, causing anxiety, sleepiness, marked tachycardia and pallor. Severe airway obstruction is an emergency, and intubation may need to be considered (Fitzgerald & Kilham, 2003; Zoorob et al., 2011).

Children with mild croup require close parental supervision and care at home. Historically, parents have often been advised to reduce stridor by exposing their child to a warm, humidified environment, such as a bathroom with a warm shower running, or steam inhalations. However, there is little evidence that this is effective, and there are also concerns that the use of steam inhalations increases the risk of burns and scalds (Fitzgerald & Kilham, 2003; Zoorob et al., 2011). It is more important to ensure that parents are aware of, and watching for, the signs of increasing airway obstruction.

Medications are the mainstay of treatment for children with moderate and severe croup. The use of corticosteroids such as oral dexamethasone or nebulised budenoside in the management of croup has significantly reduced the length of time required in hospital for children with croup (Russell et al., 2004). Children with moderate and severe croup will generally be prescribed oral or nebulised corticosteroids (Mazza et al., 2008). Some children with mild croup may also be prescribed a single dose of oral corticosteroid (Russell et al., 2004). Nebulised adrenaline may be required to reduce bronchial and tracheal oedema in children with severe croup, and can rapidly reduce the symptoms of croup in 30 minutes (Bjornson et al., 2011). Further doses may be required after two hours.

Bronchiolitis

Respiratory syncytial virus (RSV) is the most common causative virus of bronchiolitis in infants. Despite a high rate of infection, immunity does not last long, and thus repeated RSV infections can occur (Australian Lung Foundation, 2007). The signs and symptoms of bronchiolitis include wheezing, difficult feeding, pallor and respiratory distress.

While most infants have mild bronchiolitis, those who have respiratory distress, hypoxia or cannot maintain adequate fluid intake will require admission to hospital. Treatment is essentially supportive, and may include oxygen therapy, intravenous fluids to maintain hydration or nasogastric feeding. In Chapter 5, Case Study 5.1 discussed the case of Maggie, an infant with bronchiolitis is discussed, and the nursing management is outlined.

Oxygen therapy

As many respiratory infections are viral in origin, often treatment is focused on supportive therapies such as oxygen and hydration. Oxygen therapy is an important intervention to correct or prevent hypoxia in children with acute respiratory illnesses.

Oxygen may be administered via a range of devices, including a face mask, nasal prongs or headbox. The flow rate and concentration of oxygen administered will vary according to the device, and are also influenced by the flow rate of the oxygen through the device, the respiratory rate and the tidal volume of the infant or child (Balfour-Lynn et al., 2009; Frey & Shann, 2003). The age of the child should also be taken into account when choosing a device.

Headbox

Headbox oxygen is most often administered to neonates and young infants, as mobility is reduced with use of a headbox. One of the benefits of headbox oxygen is that it is easier to control the level of FiO_2 in a headbox than with nasal cannula, as it is a more 'closed' system than face mask or nasal cannula. As a result, less room air is drawn in and mixed with oxygen during inspiration (Frey & Shann, 2003). Carbon dioxide build-up may occur, and therefore a minimum flow rate of at least 10 L/minute of oxygen is required (Frey & Shann, 2003).

Face mask

Face mask oxygen is useful where mobility is required, and tends to be preferred by older children than younger children, who may be likely to remove the mask frequently or need to remove the mask for feeding. The level of oxygen varies, but rarely exceeds 40% (Frey & Shann, 2003) and depends on the flow rate of the oxygen and the volume of room air that is drawn in around the face mask during inspiration. A minimum of 4L/minute of oxygen is required to avoid build-up of carbon dioxide.

Nasal prongs

Nasal prongs more often used for low flow rates of oxygen (< 2.5 L/minute) and for longer-term oxygen therapy (Balfour-Lynn et al., 2009). They are particularly useful to ensure continuous oxygen therapy during periods of infant feeding. They may be uncomfortable, as the oxygen can dry the nares and cause irritation. The nares should be observed regularly for drying and irritation. Nasal prongs may also be a strangulation risk to infants and children, and therefore the tubing should be carefully secured on the face and checked regularly.

Humidification

Routine humidification of oxygen is rarely required. In most instances, short-term, low-flow oxygen therapy will not require humidification. Children may require humidification for higher flow rates of oxygen or longer-term oxygen therapy (Balfour-Lynn et al., 2009). It is important that the skin and mucous membranes in and around the mouth and nares are regularly assesses for irritation and dryness, and care is taken to moisten or protect skin as required.

Summary

- Acute viral infections are common in childhood. Although most cause only mild illness, some children will require nursing and medical care in a hospital setting.
- The approach to nursing assessment needs to take into consideration the developmental differences in infants and children.
- Fever, dehydration, hypoxia or pain are common reasons for children to require nursing care and intervention.
- Nursing care needs to consider the age and development of the infant or child, and the needs of the family.

Learning activities

8.1 Clinical practice guidelines (CPG) or evidence-based practice guidelines (EBPG) are often used to guide practice in acute-care settings. These guidelines are developed by expert groups of clinicians and researchers who have systematically reviewed and evaluated evidence for best practice. Following this, the expert groups have determined and then published the best recommendations, information and advice to assist health professionals to assess and intervene in the care and treatment of children with a range of conditions.

In this chapter, you have read several case scenarios of children with different presenting symptoms. Undertake an internet and database search for local and international CPG and EBPG for the care of a child with one of these conditions.
- Read the guidelines. Are they similar or different?
- Do they address all aspects of the condition, including assessment, treatment, nursing care and after care?
- Which expert groups have contributed to their development?
- What level of evidence or literature review has been undertaken in the preparation of the guideline?

8.2 Read the case scenarios for the children in this chapter. For each child, consider your response to the following questions:
- What key assessments and observations would you perform?
- How often would you perform these assessments?
- What changes might indicate that the child's condition is deteriorating?
- What changes might indicate that the child's condition is improving?
- What interventions would you include to meet the child's emotional needs during hospitalisation?

Further reading

- Obtain practice guidelines and policies from your local health service on their approaches to managing acute illness in children.
- Refresh your knowledge of nursing interventions for acute illness using a core nursing textbook.

References

Ambuel, B, Hamlett, KW, Marx, CM & Blumer, JL 1992, Assessing distress in pediatric intensive care environments: The COMFORT scale, *Journal of Pediatric Psychology*, 17(1), pp. 95–109.

Arrowsmith, JB, Kennedy, DL, Kuritsky, JN & Faich, GA 1987, National patterns of aspirin use and Reye syndrome reporting, United States, 1980 to 1985, *Pediatrics*, 79(6), pp. 858–63.

Ashkenazy, S & DeKeyser-Ganz, F 2011, Assessment of the reliability and validity of the Comfort Scale for adult intensive care patients, *Heart & Lung*, 40(3), pp. e44–e51.

Association of Paediatric Anaesthetists of Great Britain and Ireland (APAGBI) 2012, Good practice in postoperative and procedural pain management, *Pediatric Anesthesia*, 22(S1), pp. 1–79.

Australian Institute of Health and Welfare (AIHW) 2012, *Australian hospital statistics 2011–12: Emergency department care*, AIHW, Canberra.

Australian Lung Foundation 2007, *Respiratory infectious disease burden in Australia*, viewed 20 March 2014, http://www.thoracic.org.au/documents/papers/2007_RID_Case_Statement.pdf.

Bai, J, Hsu, L, Tang, Y & van Dijk, M 2012, Validation of the COMFORT Behavior scale and the FLACC scale for pain assessment in Chinese children after cardiac surgery, *Pain Management Nursing*, 13(1), pp. 18–26.

Balfour-Lynn, IM et al. 2009, BTS guidelines for home oxygen in children, *Thorax*, 64 (Suppl. 2), pp. 1–26.

Bjornson, C et al. 2011, Nebulized epinephrine for croup in children, *Cochrane Database of Systematic Reviews*, 16 (2), CD006619.

Blatteis, CM 2003, Fever: Pathological or physiological, injurious or beneficial? *Journal of Thermal Biology*, 28(1), pp. 1–13.

Crook, J 2010, Fever Management: Evaluating the use of ibroprofens and paracetamol, *Paediatric Nursing*, 22(3), pp. 22–6.

Dey, A, Wang, H, Menzies, R & Macartney, K 2012, Changes in hospitalisations for acute gastroenteritis in Australia after the national rotavirus vaccination program, *Medical Journal of Australia*, 197(8), pp. 453–7.

Dobrovoljac, M & Geelhoed, GC 2012, How fast does oral dexamethasone work in mild to moderately severe croup? A randomized double-blinded clinical trial, *Emergency Medicine Australasia*, 24(1), pp. 79–85.

Elliott, EJ, 2007, Acute gastroenteritis in children (Review), *BMJ*, 334(7583), pp. 35–40.

Fitzgerald, DA & Kilham, HA 2003, Croup: Assessment and evidence-based management, *Medical Journal of Australia*, 179(7), pp. 372–7.

Forbes, H 2013, Vital signs. In J Crisp, C Taylor, C Douglas & G Rebeiro (eds), *Potter and Perry's fundamentals of nursing*, 4th edn, Mosby Elsevier, Sydney, pp. 658–702.

Frey, B & Shann, F 2003, Oxygen administration in infants, *Archives of Disease in Childhood – Fetal and Neonatal Edition*, 88(2), pp. F84–F88.

Galati, JC, Harsley, S, Richmond, P & Carlin, JB 2006, The burden of rotavirus-related illness among young children on the Australian health care system, *Australian & New Zealand Journal of Public Health*, 30(5), pp. 416–21.

Hartling, L et al. 2006, Oral versus intravenous rehydration for treating dehydration due to gastroenteritis in children, *Cochrane Database of Systematic Reviews*, 3, pp. CD004390.

Kesson, AM, Benwell, N & Elliott, EJ 2010, Norovirus diarrhoeal disease in infants and children, *Medical Journal of Australia*, 192(2), pp. 108–9.

Lux, AL 2010, Treatment of febrile seizures: Historical perspective, current opinions, and potential future directions, *Brain & Development*, 32(1), pp. 42–50.

Malviya, S, Voepel-Lewis, T, Burke, C, Merkel, S & Tait, AR 2006, The revised FLACC observational pain tool: Improved reliability and validity for pain assessment in children with cognitive impairment, *Paediatric Anaesthesia*, 16(3), pp. 258–65.

Manworren, RCB & Hynan, LS 2003, Clinical validation of FLACC: Preverbal patient pain scale, *Pediatric Nursing*, 29(2), pp. 140–6.

Mazza, D, Wilkinson, F, Turner, T, Harris, C & Health for Kids Guideline Development Group 2008, Evidence-based guideline for the management of croup, *Australian Family Physician*, 37(6), pp. 14–20.

Meremikwu, MM & Oyo-Ita, A 2009a, Paracetamol versus placebo or physical methods for treating fever in children, *Cochrane Database of Systematic Reviews*, 2, n.p.

—— 2009b, Physical methods versus drug placebo or no treatment for managing fever in children, *Cochrane Database of Systematic Reviews*, 4, n.p.

Merkel, SI, Voepel-Lewis, T, Shayevitz, JR & Malviya, S 1997, The FLACC: A behavioral scale for scoring postoperative pain in young children, *Pediatric Nursing*, 23(3), pp. 293–7.

Monasta, L et al. 2012, Burden of disease caused by otitis media: Systematic review and global estimates. *PLoS ONE*, 7(4), p. e36226.

Morris, PS et al. 2009, New horizons: Otitis media research in Australia, *Medical Journal of Australia*, 191(Suppl. 9), pp. S73–S77.

National Health and Medical Research Council (NHMRC) 2010, *Australian guidelines for the prevention and control of infection in healthcare*, Commonwealth of Australia, Canberra, viewed 20 February 2014, http://www.nhmrc.gov.au/_files_nhmrc/publications/attachments/cd33_infection_control_healthcare.pdf.

—— 2013, *The Australian immunisation handbook*, Australian Government, Canberra.

National Institute for Health and Care Excellence (NIHCE) 2009, *Diarrhoea and vomiting caused by gastroenteritis: Diagnosis, assessment and management in children younger than 5 years*, NIHCE, London, viewed 20 February 2014, http://www.nice.org.uk/nicemedia/live/11846/43817/43817.pdf.

Nilsson, S, Finnstrom, B & Kokinsky, E 2008, The FLACC behavioral scale for procedural pain assessment in children aged 5–16 years, *Paediatric Anaesthesia*, 18(8), pp. 767–74.

Offringa, M & Newton, R 2012, Prophylactic drug management for febrile seizures in children, *Cochrane Database of Systematic Reviews*, 4, n.p.

Ogoina, D 2011, Fever, fever patterns and diseases called 'fever' – A review, *Journal of Infection and Public Health*, 4(3), pp. 108–24.

Paul, S, O'Callaghan, C & McKee, N 2011, Effective management of lower respiratory tract infections in childhood, *Nursing Children and Young People*, 23(9), pp. 27–34.

Pringle, K et al. 2011, Comparing the accuracy of the three popular clinical dehydration scales in children with diarrhea, *International Journal of Emergency Medicine*, 4, p. 58.

Rang, HP, Dale, MM & Ritter, JM 2011, *Rang and Dale's pharmacology*, 7th edn, Churchill Livingstone, St Louis, MO.

Rathnayake, T 2012, Intravenous cannulation (paediatric): Clinician information, *[Joanna Briggs Institute] Evidence Summaries*, 1–4.

Reid, AY, Galic, MA, Teskey, GC & Pittman, QJ 2009, Febrile seizures: Current views and investigations, *Canadian Journal of Neurological Sciences*, 36(6), pp. 679–86.

Royal Children's Hospital 2012, *Clinical guideline: Peripheral intravenous device management*, viewed 4 April 2014, http://www.rch.org.au/rchcpg/hospital_clinical_guideline_index/Peripheral_Intravenous_IV_Device_Management.

Russell, K et al. 2004, Glucocorticoids for croup, *Cochrane Database of Systematic Reviews*, 1, CD001955.

Schomacker, H, Schaap-Nutt, A, Collins, PL & Schmidt, AC 2012, Pathogenesis of acute respiratory illness caused by human parainfluenza viruses, *Current Opinions on Virology*, 2, pp. 294–9.

Schreiber, S et al. 2013, Does EMLA cream application interfere with the success of venipuncture or venous cannulation? A prospective multicenter observational study, *European Journal of Pediatrics*, 172(2), pp. 265–8.

Tibballs, J & Watson, T 2011, Symptoms and signs differentiating croup and epiglottitis, *Journal of Paediatrics & Child Health*, 47(3), pp. 77–82

van Dijk, M et al. 2000, The reliability and validity of the COMFORT scale as a postoperative pain instrument in 0 to 3-year-old infants, *Pain*, 84(2–3), pp. 367–77.

Venekamp, RP, Sanders, S, Glasziou, PP, Del Mar, CB & Rovers, MM 2013, Antibiotics for acute otitis media in children, *Cochrane Database of Systematic Reviews*, 1, CD000219.

Walsh, A, Edwards, H & Fraser, J 2008, Parents' childhood fever management: Community survey and instrument development, *Journal of Advanced Nursing*, 63(4), pp. 376–88.

Watts, R & Robertson, J 2012, Non-pharmacological management of fever in otherwise healthy children, *JBI Database of Systematic Reviews and Implementation Reports*, 10(26), pp. 1634–87.

Willis, MHW, Merkel, SI, Voepel-Lewis, T & Malviya, S 2003, FLACC Behavioral Pain Assessment Scale: A comparison with the child's self-report, *Pediatric Nursing*, 29(3), pp. 195–8.

World Health Organization (WHO) & UNICEF 2013, *Ending preventable child deaths from pneumonia and diarrhoea by 2025: The integrated Global Action Plan for Pneumonia and Diarrhoea (GAPPD)*, WHO, Geneva, viewed 20 April 2014, http://www.who.int/maternal_child_adolescent/documents/global_action_plan_pneumonia_diarrhoea/en.

Yiengprugsawan, V, Hogan, A & Strazdins, L 2013, Longitudinal analysis of ear infection and hearing impairment: Findings from 6-year prospective cohorts of Australian children, *BMC Pediatrics*, 13, p. 28.

Zoorob, R, Sidani, M & Murray, J 2011, Croup: An overview, *American Family Physician*, 83(9), pp. 1067–73.

9 Evidence-based nursing assessments and interventions: The acutely ill young person

Nicola Brown

Learning objectives

In this chapter you will:

- Develop your understanding of evidence based nursing assessments and interventions used in the care of acutely ill young people

- Develop your understanding of the aetiology, signs and symptoms of key acute illnesses experienced by young people in Australia

- Consider the developmental needs of young people in the planning and implementation of nursing care

- Explore the impact of illness and hospitalisation on young people

Adolescence
The definition of adolescence can vary considerably. Most commonly, it is considered the period of time between the onset of puberty and the time an individual is legally recognised as an adult – anywhere from 10 to 18 years. However, there is considerable individual variation in development and evidence that final brain development is not complete until the mid-twenties

Introduction

The transition to **adolescence** is a complex and critical period of development. In reality, however, the changes in physical, cognitive and social development during adolescence do not occur at the same time for all adolescents, and therefore it is important to consider the individual adolescent when planning nursing care.

Once children are past early childhood, the frequency of acute infections diminishes. Instead, the reasons for admission to hospital are more likely to be related to acute episodes associated with injury or for chronic conditions. Similar to the infections in younger children, the injuries are often mild and can be managed by parents at home. However, there are times when care and treatment required for the injury or illness result in an admission to hospital.

The nursing care of children and young people with a chronic condition is addressed in Chapter 10. In this chapter, we will focus on the care of young people who need nursing care due to common acute injuries. In addition, the management of young people with appendicitis will also be explored in this chapter, as the peak incidence of this condition occurs in young people.

Key issues for young people during hospitalisation

Injury, illness and periods of admission to hospital can interrupt the life and times of the adolescent to some degree of adversity. Wherever possible, we do our best to minimise the disruption to the life of the young person by avoiding admission and providing ambulatory care in the community when it is appropriate and available to do so. However, some situations do require admission, and when this occurs, ideally a young person is best cared for in an adolescent unit – an environment that understands the unique psychosocial and physical needs of adolescents.

Nurses and other health-care professionals need a good knowledge and understanding of adolescent development, and need to be confident in communicating with adolescents and their families. Unfortunately, adolescents do not always feel that their specific age-related needs are met by health-care services (Hutton, 2008; Jones & Bradley, 2007). Young people have different recreation and social interaction needs than either young children or adults (Hutton, 2010; Jones & Bradley, 2007). In addition, young people can become more self-conscious about their bodies, and may want a greater sense of privacy and control over their environment. However, adolescent-specific services, such as an adolescent ward, are a somewhat rare commodity in health care, and the adolescent is to some extent marooned between paediatric services, which are predominately geared to the care of younger children, and adult services, which are most often used by people over 65 years of age. When adolescent health-care services are not available, then individual needs and consideration of preferences should be taken into account when assessing whether to admit adolescents to either paediatric or adult wards. For example, while it may be appropriate to have the ward lights out and everyone settled to sleep by 8.00 pm for younger children, young people may be more inclined to stay up later at night, and sleep in later in the morning, and may be disturbed by infants who would normally wake during the night.

While still often under the care of parents, young people are beginning to perceive themselves as individuals within a family, and may have different views regarding access to information, care and consent from those of their parents. At the same time, parents are adjusting to the increasing independence of their growing child. Both parents and adolescents need skilled and empathic health-care professionals who are sensitive to the complex and dynamic nature of adolescent–parent relations.

Injuries

In Australia, trauma from injuries is the leading cause of death in young people aged 12–24 years (Eldridge, 2008). Injury is the leading cause of hospitalisation for young people in Australia (AIHW, 2014). In children under 14 years of age, approximately 10 per cent of all admissions to hospital are related to injury (AIHW, 2014). Indigenous children, male children and young people are more likely to die as a result of their injuries (AIHW, 2014). Most commonly, injuries occur in relation to transport, such as motor vehicle accidents (Begg et al., 2007). Young people living in remote areas are more likely to sustain and require hospitalisation for injury (Eldridge, 2008; Harrison et al., 2012).

Self-harm as a result of mental health issues – particularly depression – is an issue in adolescence, and should be considered a factor in any injury incurred in adolescence. High-risk behaviours may indicate that all is not well with the young person (Jones & Bradley, 2007). Hospitalisation for a physical injury may be an opportune time to intervene, or at least assess for a mental health problem. See Chapter 7 for more details regarding mental health.

Head injury

Celine

Case study 9.1

Celine is 12-year-old girl living in a rural farming community. She was transferred by air ambulance to a paediatric tertiary referral centre three days ago following a quad bike accident at low speed. Celine sustained a closed head injury, fracture of the left femur, chest bruising, cuts and grazes. She did not have any loss of consciousness, but is complaining of a persistent headache. Celine is admitted to the high dependency unit.

Most head injuries that occur to children and young people are minor; however, any head injury can result in significant harm. It is therefore important to monitor and assess the child or young person closely after the event. The extent or degree of severity of head injury should determine the initial response. For example, a clear loss of consciousness or confusion is more likely to indicate a severe head injury. However, a person who sustains a head injury and does not lose consciousness initially may still be deteriorating slowly, and requires close initial observation.

Head injuries can be categorised as internal (involving skull or the brain) or external (involving scalp). In Case Study 9.1, Celine's injury involved trauma to the brain and an external laceration of the scalp. The likely severity of the head injury can be estimated according to risk factors (see Table 9.1) that would categorise the injury as high, intermediate or low risk. In the case of Celine, the risk is intermediate (see Table 9.1). The injury occurred at low speed and there was no loss of consciousness at the time of the injury, no vomiting and her behaviour is normal. She does have a persistent headache and a score on the Glasgow Coma Scale (GCS) of 14, and thus requires close observation and ongoing neurological assessment.

Assessment, both at the time of the injury and over time, is a critical element in the nursing management of people who have sustained a head injury. A rapid neurological assessment of level of consciousness can be undertaken using AVPU: is the patient alert, verbal, responding to pain or unconscious? This rapid assessment assists clinicians to assess the severity of the head injury; however, as mentioned above, we should *always* be mindful that it may take several minutes or hours for the full extent of a head injury to become apparent.

In addition to the rapid initial assessment of consciousness, a more in-depth assessment should be performed using the Glasgow Coma Scale (GCS). While a modified GCS is appropriate in children, in young people the standard GCS should be used. In addition to these assessment tools, clinicians should also consider the opinion of parents in neurological assessment. Parents know their children well, and are often the first to notice that all is not well. If a parent is concerned about a change in the behaviour of their child, then we should also be concerned. In addition to changes in behaviour, clinicians should also be alert to any signs of generalised or local seizure activity – clear signs that the injury is severe or worsening. For more details on neurological assessment, please refer to Chapter 5 on recognition of the deteriorating child.

Frequency of neurological assessment and the timeframe for close observation will be determined by the estimated severity of the head injury. Initially, at least hourly neurological and vital observations are required, though these

TABLE 9.1 Risk groups in head injury

	LOW RISK (all features)	INTERMEDIATE RISK (any feature/not low or high risk)	HIGH RISK (CHALICE criteria) (any feature)
HISTORY			
Witnessed loss of consciousness	Nil	<5 minutes	>5 minutes
Anterograde or retrograde amnesia	Nil	possible	>5 minutes
Behaviour	Normal	mild agitation or altered behaviour	Abnormal drowsiness
Episodes of vomiting without other cause	Nil or 1	2 or persistent nausea	3 or more
Seizure in non-epileptic patient	Nil	Impact only	Yes
Non accidental injury (NAI) suspected	No	No	Yes
Headache	Nil	Persistent	Persistent
Comorbidities	Nil	Present	Present
Age	>1 year	<1 year	Any
Mechanism			
Motor vehicle accident (MVA) (pedestrian, cyclist or occupant)	Low speed	<60 km/h	>60 km/h
Fall	<1 m	1–3 m	>3 m
Force	Low impact	Moderate impact or unclear mechanism	High-speed projectile or object
Examination			
Glasgow Coma Scale (GCS)	15	Fluctuating 14–15	<14 or <15 if under 1 year old
Focal neurological abnormality	Nil	Nil	Present
Injury			High-risk features – for example, scalp haematoma in <1 yr of age (see below)
Placement			
Observation area	Anywhere in ED	Acute area in ED	Acute or resuscitation bay
Observations			
• Respiratory rate, oxygen saturations • Pulse, blood pressure • Temperature • GCS, pupillary response and size, limb strength • Pain assessment • Sedation score as necessary	Hourly observations until discharge	Half-hourly observations for four to six hours until GCS 15 sustained for two hours, then hourly observations until discharge. Revert to half-hourly observations/continuous monitoring if signs of deterioration occur	Continuous cardio-respiratory and oxygen saturation monitoring. BP and GCS every 15 to 30 minutes

Notes: High-risk injury: a) penetrating injury, or suspected depressed skull fracture or base of skull fracture; b) scalp bruise, swelling or laceration >5 cm, or tense fontanelle in infants <1 year of age.
Source: NSW Health (2011).

should be more frequent if a higher severity of head injury is suspected. If the head injury is assessed as mild, and observations are normal, most patients are discharged after approximately four hours. If there is concern that the injury is of moderate severity, a longer period of observations and computerised tomography scan (CT) may be required. Children and young people may need to be kept nil by mouth at least initially, pending decisions about further investigations or surgery that may require administration of an anaesthetic.

Not surprisingly, head injuries can be painful; however, clinicians can be concerned about the use of analgesia in patients with head injury – especially analgesics with a known sedative effect. A patient's head injury should not automatically result in the withholding of pain relief (Young et al., 2005b). For mild pain, an oral analgesic (e.g. paracetamol) that does not cause sedation may be appropriate. For more severe pain, consideration may be given to using opioids, but these should be administered with care. The sedative effects of opioids may mask deterioration in level of consciousness due to the head injury. The NSW Clinical Practice Guidelines on management of patients with head injury (NSW Health, 2011) recommend that a sedation assessment is performed in addition to neurological assessments such as GCS to monitor the sedative effect of opioids administered in people with head injury.

Another very important aspect of assessment in head injury is the history of the injury. It is important that clinicians give consideration to whether the severity and location of the head injury accords with the history of the injury that is provided. Sadly, we have to consider that a head injury in a child or young person may be non-accidental. Clinicians need to maintain an open mind to this possibility during assessment. For further details on non-accidental injury and child abuse and neglect, please see Chapter 2.

For young people like Celine, serious injuries incurred in a rural area usually result in retrieval to a city or regional hospital, distant from their home. This can mean additional concerns for young people and their families, who are already frightened or anxious about the extent of the injury sustained. Nurses need to ensure that they support families in this situation. The importance of caring, flexible and understanding health professionals, facilities and resources to enable families to be with their injured child, or to the means for them to stay in contact from a distance are vital. Preparing young people and parents for discharge after head injury is also important. Make sure that parents and young people are clear regarding signs that would require them to return for further assessment.

Children and young people may sustain abrasions or lacerations as a result of the head injury. These injuries may require cleaning and wound closure. If these procedures are likely to cause pain, some thought should be given to analgesia, sedation or even general anaesthetic. The need for tetanus booster should also be considered (Young et al., 2005a).

Musculoskeletal injuries

Musculoskeletal injuries are a frequent reason for children and young people to require hospital care. Musculoskeletal injuries that may occur include strains, sprains, joint dislocations and fractures. For young children, these injuries commonly arises from play activities, while in older children and young people, the injury may arise from sport and recreational activities or from motor vehicle accidents. In both children and young people, attention should be paid to correlation between the injury and the history of how the injury occurred. As mentioned previously, clinicians should always be mindful that an injury may be the result of physical abuse of the child or young person. For further information on child abuse, see Chapter 2.

A fracture of the bone will occur when the force exerted on a bone is greater than the strength of the bone can resist. In younger children, bone formation is still immature. The bones are more porous and the periosteum is thicker, so the bone is compliant and thus less likely to completely break in response to a greater force. For these reasons, younger children and infants will be more likely to have an incomplete fracture, such as a greenstick injury. By early adolescence, the bone is much more dense, and complete fractures are more likely (Benson et al., 2010).

Assessment and management

In the first instance, the fracture is stabilised – at least temporarily – to reduce pain and prevent further damage to bone and soft tissues around the fracture. Early pain assessment and management are important (Young et al., 2005b). In fact, just splinting the affected limb can reduce the pain associated with a fracture; however, oral or intravenous analgesia may also be required (Benson et al., 2010).

Infection control is an important consideration for management of people with an open fracture. The wound should be covered and intravenous antibiotic cover may be considered and prescribed, even prior to surgery. Tetanus prophylaxis may also be requested. Depending on the nature of the fracture, open or closed reduction of the fracture and application of traction or plaster cast under anaesthetic may be required, and therefore preoperative care should be considered.

Frequent and accurate neurovascular observations are an essential component of nursing assessment in the care of people with a fracture. These

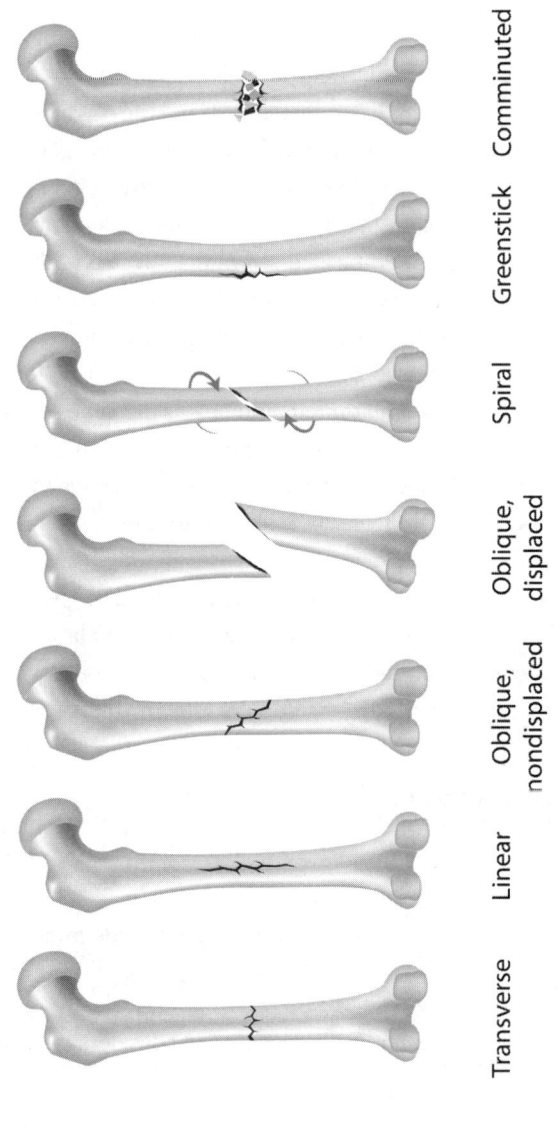

FIGURE 9.1 *Types of bone fractures*

assessments are somewhat easier in young people than younger children, as young people are more likely to understand the questions put to them as part of the assessment. The main components of neurovascular assessment include the five Ps – pain, paralysis, paresthesia, pulses and pallor (Dykes, 1993; Shields & Clarke, 2011; Wright, 2007).

Regular pain assessment should be undertaken, as increasing pain can indicate neurovascular impairment (Benson et al., 2010). We also need to consider whether the pain is from the original injury and the need for appropriate analgesia to be administered as required. The child or young person should be asked to move their limb distal to the injury. Be aware that pain may inhibit movement, so it is important to ensure that adequate analgesia is administered. Sensation, pulses and colour should be assessed in the affected limb and compared with those in the unaffected limb. The limb pulses should be palpated for rate and quality at a site that is distal to the injury, traction or cast. If pulses are absent or unable to be assessed due to a plaster cast, then perform capillary refill assessment. Capillary refill time should be less than two seconds. The colour and swelling of the limb are also important indicators of vascular impairment – a swollen cool, pale or mottled limb is a concerning sign (Dykes, 1993; Shields & Clarke, 2011; Wright, 2007). The limb should be elevated and medical review should be requested.

Prior to discharge, young people and their parents should be given information on the signs of neurovascular impairment. In addition, if a plaster cast is applied, cast care instructions should be discussed, including protection from water, physical damage and the risk of the insertion of foreign objects into the cast.

Abdominal pain

Alicia

Case study 9.2

Alicia is a 15-year-old girl who presents to the general medical practice accompanied by her mother and older sister. Alicia has had abdominal pain for several days, but it has increased in severity over the past 12 hours. During examination, it becomes apparent that the pain is difficult to localise, although it increases when Alicia moves. Alicia has not eaten or had a drink since yesterday. Her mother reports that she has been 'off her food' for a day or two. Her bowel movements have not changed recently.

Alicia has a low-grade fever (37.8°C), a heart rate of 110/minute and blood pressure of 95/55mmHg. The medical officer of not certain of the cause of the pain, but considers that it may be early appendicitis and refers Alicia to the emergency department of her local hospital. The team at the hospital decides that there are reasonable grounds to suspect appendicitis. Alicia is prepared for transfer to theatre for an emergency laparoscopy and possible laparoscopic appendicectomy.

Abdominal pain is a common problem in children and young people. It is often non-specific and difficult to localise, and thus it can be difficult to determine the cause of the pain. It may indicate a range of conditions from mild conditions, such as constipation, to more serious problems due to acute conditions, such as appendicitis or trauma. Symptoms of abdominal pain in younger children are less specific and more difficult to localise, whereas a young person should be able to localise and describe the pain in more detail. However the nature of abdominal pain seems to vary considerably between individuals and conditions.

Historically, clinicians were reluctant to give analgesia to relieve abdominal pain until a diagnosis of the cause of the pain was made. Recent clinical guidelines indicate that there is no evidence to support the withholding of analgesia in young people or children with acute abdominal pain, nor does the use of analgesia impede diagnosis or treatment (National Institute of Clinical Studies Emergency Care Community of Practice, 2008).

Appendicitis

Acute appendicitis is the most common surgical emergency in children and young people, although in some cases appendicitis may be treated conservatively. Approximately 16 per cent of people in developed countries will have an appendicectomy during their lifetime, with the peak incidence between the age of 8 and 14 years (Bradbury et al., 2012). Although it is relatively common in comparison to other abdominal conditions, the causes of acute appendicitis are not fully understood. It may be related to some degree of obstruction of the appendix that triggers an inflammatory response in the mucosa of the appendix. The inflammation may cause venous congestion and diminish arterial blood supply, leading to ischaemia and infarction (Bradbury et al., 2012). If this does not resolve, appendicitis can lead to perforation and sepsis.

There is no definitive test to diagnose appendicitis apart from direct visualisation via laparoscopy – a rather invasive diagnostic tool! Thus clinicians rely on clinical signs and symptoms in deciding whether to proceed to laparoscopy and, if required, appendicectomy, or to wait, watch and observe to see whether the pain decreases or increases, and whether other symptoms develop. In addition to abdominal pain, individuals with appendicitis may have nausea, vomiting, diarrhoea, fever, pallor or abdominal distension (Howell et al., 2010). None of these signs or symptoms is conclusively indicative of appendicitis – they can indicate other conditions such as inflammatory bowel diseases, mesenteric adenitis, pelvic inflammatory disease or ectopic pregnancy, to name just a few.

As some of the symptoms of appendicitis may also be symptoms of gynaecological disorders, it is important to establish whether the young person has commenced menstruation and whether they are sexually active, in order to exclude pregnancy (Royal Children's Hospital, 2013). It is essential that discussions about puberty, sexual activity and any related tests are handled with great tact and diplomacy. Please recognise that the young person may not be willing to disclose their sexual history in front of parents, friends or family. Furthermore, young people may deny that they are sexually active, even when they are.

> ### Reflection points 9.1
> Imagine that you are required to ask Alicia to provide a urine sample for a pregnancy test. Think about who might be present, the environment you may be in, and the words you might use.
> - What will you say to Alicia?
> - What will you do to maintain her privacy?
> - What right does Alicia have to consent to or refuse this urine sample?
> - What right does Alicia have to confidentiality of the results of such a test?

Preoperative care

Adequate preparation for operations is an essential and important role that nurses have in the care of children and young people. For children and young people who require elective procedures, there is often sufficient time to support parents to be the main 'preparers' for the child or young person, or at least for parents to provide the initial explanation to their child about what will happen. Emergency procedures such as the one Alicia required are often a shock to the parent, and they may be unable to take in, process and use the information we provide to explain to their child what is about to occur to an adequate level. In either event, the onus is on medical and nursing staff to ensure that everyone – parents and young person – is clear about what is required and what is likely to occur. Older children and adolescents may have a more sophisticated understanding of the workings of their insides than younger children; however, it is important to remember that the level of understanding can vary considerably between individuals when providing explanations about preoperative procedures and postoperative care.

Apart from psychological preparation, physical preparation is required. This may include nil by mouth for a period of time, showering prior to the procedure and dressing in a theatre gown. These procedures are very familiar to nurses used to caring for adults, but it is important to remember that, for most young people like Alicia, this would be their first experience of surgery. Seemingly strange practices such as the requirement that patients do not wear any underwear to theatre can be unsettling for a young person who is modest and conscious of their body. A young person such as Alicia may become quite anxious once the decision is made to operate, and therefore consideration may also be given to some form of preoperative sedation.

Obtaining informed consent for procedures is an important part of preparation. Details of the legal and ethical issues that arise in obtaining consent are dealt with in Chapter 2.

Postoperative care

The principles of postoperative care are similar for children, young people and adults. The priority of nursing care in the immediate postoperative period is to monitor for any adverse effects of the surgical intervention and/or anaesthesia, including airway obstruction and haemorrhage. Initially, continuous cardiorespiratory monitoring is indicated until the young person rouses and then, once they are awake, frequent assessment of respiratory and cardiovascular status, including heart rate, respiratory rate, respiratory assessment, blood pressure and oxygen saturation is required. The incision site should be observed for excess blood loss.

Pain management is an important component of postoperative care. By the time children reach early adolescence, they are able to describe and quantify pain with greater precision and detail. Pain-assessment tools, including the FACES pain scale or numerical rating scales, can be used with young people. Analgesics should be administered regularly to relieve pain and to facilitate early postoperative ambulation. Patient-controlled analgesia (PCA) is an excellent choice for young people, and can help to give them a sense of control over their postoperative care.

Alcohol poisoning

Ryan

Case study 9.3

Ryan is a 14-year-old boy who has been drinking at a party with a large group of friends. During the evening, Ryan consumed a large quantity of alcohol. Eventually he became disorientated, vomited and eventually passed out. His friends were unable to rouse him. One of his friends called an ambulance, and Ryan was assessed and transferred to the emergency department of the local hospital. On arrival at hospital, Ryan is lethargic, confused and difficult to rouse, responding only to painful stimuli, with a GCS of 11. His pupils are equal and reacting to light. His vital observations include heart rate 115 per minute, respiratory rate 18 per minute, BP 90/50mmHg and SaO2 95 per cent in room air. He smells strongly of vomit and alcohol. Bloods are taken, and the results reveal a blood alcohol level of 55mmol/L.

Approximately three of every four Australian secondary students aged 12–17 years will have tried alcohol, and the rate of alcohol consumption increases with age. By the age of 16 years, approximately 13 per cent of young people report an episode of binge drinking in the past seven days, consuming more than four standard drinks on one day (White & Bariola, 2012). Subsequently, some young people may consume harmful amounts of alcohol, resulting in alcohol intoxication and poisoning, and requiring acute care in a hospital setting.

In addition to the risks associated with alcohol poisoning, younger brains – particularly the hippocampus – are more susceptible to the damaging effects of alcohol than mature adult brains, and this can result in neurocognitive deficits (Squeglia et al., 2009). In the acute period, alcohol is a central nervous system (CNS) depressant. The sedative effects of alcohol, in addition to the risk of vomiting when intoxicated, mean there is a significant risk of respiratory arrest.

Immediate care of the young person with alcohol poisoning begins with maintaining a clear airway. In Case Study 9.3, Ryan is at risk of aspirating vomit, and therefore should be positioned on his side in the recovery position. The next important priority is to monitor level of consciousness. We would expect this to improve over time, as Ryan has stopped ingesting alcohol and the residual alcohol in his blood should be metabolised. Administration of intravenous fluids may be required to maintain hydration and replace fluids lost from vomiting.

Once the initial acute phase has resolved, consideration needs to be given to psychosocial issues. Abuse of alcohol can be an indicator of psychosocial or mental health problems in the young person. Some young people may use substances such as alcohol to deal with feelings of sadness, anxiety or despair. It is important that the young person's mental health and wellbeing are assessed prior to discharge. An admission related to alcohol abuse should be seen as an opportunity to provide education and support for a young person to deal with alcohol abuse and any related psychosocial issues, and refer them to appropriate community-based services.

> *Reflection points 9.2*
>
> People from different ethnic and cultural backgrounds often have different perspectives on adolescence, particularly in relation to social and emotional development. In a country with diverse multicultural populations, such as Australia, there can be a range of views on what might be appropriate behaviour, rules and expectations regarding adolescents. Take a few minutes to think about the following points:
> - What is your ethnic and cultural background?
> - In your family, would Ryan's drinking be accepted or tolerated, or not?
> - How might your background impact on your perception of Ryan's behaviour?
> - If you found Ryan's behaviour confronting, what could you do to ensure that your personal judgement of this behaviour did not impede the care you provided to Ryan?

Summary

- Adolescence is a time of transition for both the young person and their family.
- The health-care needs of adolescents are different from those of young children and adults, and care should be tailored to their needs.
- Young people should be cared for in an environment that is best able to meet their special developmental needs.
- Injury is a common reason for hospitalisation of young people, and some will require admission to hospital for nursing care and medical treatment.
- Injuries may indicate underlying psychosocial and mental health issues in young people.

Learning activities

9.1 Even though the proportion of young people requiring hospital care is substantial, not all hospitals or health-care services provide adolescent-specific services. In recognition of the special needs of children and adolescents, professional and consumer organisations have worked collaboratively to develop guidelines and standards in order to encourage and guide health-care services on how best to meet the special needs of children and young people, including adolescents. One such guideline was developed and published in 2008, and can be accessed online; see Royal Australasian College of Physicians (2008). Once you have read the standards, consider the following questions:
- What age group of young people do you care for?
- What specific facilities or policies are used to support the care and wellbeing of young people in the hospital or ward where you work?
- How could the environment or service in which you work be modified to better meet the needs of young people?

9.2 Read the case scenarios for the young people in this chapter. For each young person, consider your response to the following questions:
- What key assessments and observations would you perform?
- How often would you perform these assessments?
- What changes might indicate that the young person's condition is deteriorating?
- What changes might indicate that the young person's condition is improving?
- What interventions would you include to meet the young person's emotional needs during hospitalisation?

Further reading

- Obtain and review practice guidelines and policies from your local health-care service on their approaches to the care of young people with acute illness.
- Refresh your knowledge of nursing interventions for acute injury, and preoperative and postoperative care, using a core nursing textbook.

References

Australian Institute of Health and Welfare (AIHW) 2014, Safety and security, viewed 28 February 2014, https://www.aihw.gov.au/child-health/safety-and-security/#injuries.

Begg, S et al. 2007, *The burden of disease and injury in Australia 2003*, Australian Institute of Health and Welfare, viewed 21 February 2010, http://www.aihw.gov.au/publications/index.cfm/title/10317.

Benson, M, Fixsen, J, Macnicol, M & Klausdieter, P 2010, *Children's orthopaedics and fractures*, Springer, London.

Bradbury, AW, Forsythe, JLR & Parkes, RW 2012, *Principles and practice of surgery*, Churchill Livingstone, London.

Dykes, C 1993, Minding the five Ps of neurovascular assessment, *American Journal of Nursing*, 193(6), pp. 38–9.

Eldridge, D 2008, *Injury among young Australians*, AIHW, Canberra, viewed 21 February 2014, http://www.aihw.gov.au/publication-detail/?id=6442468094.

Harrison, JE, Berry, JG & Jamieson, LM 2012, Head and traumatic brain injuries among Australian youth and young adults, July 2000–June 2006, *Brain Injury*, 26(7–8), pp. 996–1004.

Howell, JM et al. 2010, Clinical policy: Critical issues in the evaluation and management of emergency department patients with suspected appendicitis, *Annals of Emergency Medicine*, 55(1), pp. 71–116.

Hutton, A 2008, An adolescent ward: 'In name only'? *Journal of Clinical Nursing*, 17(23), pp. 3142–9.

—— 2010, How adolescent patients use ward space, *Journal of Advanced Nursing*, 66(8), pp. 1802–9.

Jones, R & Bradley, E 2007, Health issues for adolescents, *Paediatrics and Child Health*, 17(11), pp. 433–8.

National Institute of Clinical Studies Emergency Care Community of Practice 2008, *Pain medication for acute abdominal pain: A summary of best evidence and information on current clinical practice*, NHMRC, viewed 20 March 2014, http://www.nhmrc.gov.au/_files_nhmrc/file/nics/material_resources/pain_medication_aute_abdominal_pain.pdf.

NSW Health 2011, *Children and infants: Acute management of head injury*, NSW Health, Sydney, viewed 20 March 2014, http://www.health.nsw.gov.au/policies/pd/2011/pdf/PD2011_024.pdf.

Royal Australian College of Physicians 2008, *National Standards for the Care of Children and Adolescents*, http://www.racp.edu.au.

Royal Children's Hospital 2013, Clinical practice guidelines: Abdominal pain, viewed 4 April 2014, http://www.rch.org.au/clinicalguide/guideline_index/Abdominal_pain.

Shields, CJ, & Clarke, S 2011, Neurovascular observation and documentation for children within accident and emergency: A critical review, *International Journal of Orthopaedic and Trauma Nursing*, 15(1), pp. 3–10.

Squeglia, LM, Spadoni, AD, Infante, MA, Myers, MG & Tapert, SF 2009, Initiating moderate to heavy alcohol use predicts changes in neuropsychological functioning for adolescent girls and boys, *Psychology of Addictive Behaviors*, 23(4), pp. 715–42.

White, V & Bariola, E 2012, *Australian secondary school students' use of tobacco, alcohol, and over-the-counter and illicit substances in 2011*, Australian Government Department of Health and Ageing, http://www.nationaldrugstrategy.gov.au/internet/drugstrategy/Publishing.nsf/content/BCBF6B2C638E1202CA257ACD0020E35C/$File/National%20Report_FINAL_ASSAD_7.12.pdf.

Wright, E 2007, Evaluating a paediatric neurovascular assessment tool, *Journal of Orthopaedic Nursing*, 11(1), pp. 20–9.

Young, SJ, Barnett, PL & Oakley, EA 2005a, Bruising, abrasions and lacerations: Minor injuries in children I, *Medical Journal of Australia*, 182(11), pp. 588–92.

—— 2005b, Fractures and minor head injuries: Minor injuries in children II, *Medical Journal of Australia*, 182(12), pp. 644–8.

10 Evidence-based nursing assessments and interventions: The child and young person with a chronic illness

Donna Waters and Helen Stasa

Learning objectives

In this chapter you will:

- Develop an understanding of the aetiology, signs and symptoms of common chronic conditions experienced by children and young people in Australia
- Review evidence-based nursing assessments and interventions for children and young people with common chronic conditions
- Consider the developmental needs of children and young people in planning and implementing nursing care for chronic medical conditions
- Explore some of the challenges young people face in transitioning to adult care

Introduction

As a paediatric nurse, you will frequently care for children and young people with **chronic conditions**. Your initial contact may be at diagnosis or during subsequent treatment (such as for childhood cancers). You may have intermittent contact during the management of an acute illness as part of the chronic condition, as might occur during an exacerbation of asthma or a urine infection in a child with spina bifida. Depending on your role, you may extend your involvement to a clinic, home, school or community – for example, if running a healthy weight program. If you work in one organisation or within one specialty area practice for any period

Chronic condition Any ongoing physical or mental impairment that causes a functional limitation (or health burden), or necessitates the use of a service or care beyond that regarded as routine. The ABS defines a chronic condition as one that has lasted, or will last, for six months or more (ABS, 2009)

of time, you may form long-term relationships with chronically ill children and their families, becoming part of their lives as they grow into young people and adults – or, inevitably for some, until their death.

It is not usual to associate chronic illness with children and young people; however, between 2007 and 2008, 37 per cent of children and young people in Australia had at least one long-term chronic condition. This figure equates to more than 1.5 million future Australian adults (ABS, 2009). Asthma, diabetes and cancer are the most common chronic medical conditions affecting both adults and children in Australia, collectively accounting for 20 per cent of the burden of disease among children aged 0–14 years (AIHW, 2012), but the range of chronic conditions affecting children and young people is much broader than that. There are other neurological, congenital and genetic conditions that significantly impact on the way a child lives, grows and functions within their family and community.

In Chapter 1, we described chronic conditions that affect Australia's children and young people by prevalence – in other words, by measuring how common the condition is within a particular age group or population at any given point in time. We also discussed hospital separation rates as a measure of the burden of illness caused by chronic diseases. In addition, we identified that around 7 per cent of Australian children aged 0–14 years currently experience some type of disability (AIHW, 2012). Disability can be a result of a sensory, intellectual or mental impairment, but it can also result from the treatment or care of common childhood disorders. There is also great deal of variation within and between conditions. For example, the cause of congenital heart disease (CHD) is multifactorial, but approximately 20 per cent of cases are associated with known chromosomal abnormalities such as Trisomy 21 (Down syndrome) (Blue et al., 2012). The early surgical repair of simple structural problems like ventricular and atrial septal defects will effectively 'cure' the condition; however, the success of surgical care and improved survival has effectively ensured that the relatively small group with more complex cardiac lesions are also reaching adulthood. Children with more complex cardiac problems such as tetralogy of Fallot, or repaired transposition of the great arteries, are likely to require ongoing medical management and surgical procedures into their adult lives. Their numbers now exceed those of children with structural heart abnormalities (Khairy et al., 2010).

Whether disease or disability, all chronic conditions have the potential to interrupt normal childhood growth, emotional maturation and social development (see Chapter 3). The hospitalisations, treatments, physical manifestations and psychosocial consequences associated with chronic conditions can have immediate and possible long-term effects. While there are now a large number of online resources, blogs, and chat sites for children and young people with chronic conditions, these can only ever be part of the whole picture. The management of all chronic diseases requires a multidisciplinary team approach, with integration of care and treatment, family support and involvement, and specific self-management education. The physical, emotional, educational and social wellbeing of a child or young person with a chronic illness can easily be overlooked, with the focus being on their disease rather than on the person. The effect on family economic and social functioning is also significant (see Chapter 12).

This chapter discusses the aetiology, signs and symptoms of some common paediatric chronic illnesses you are likely to encounter in your work as a paediatric nurse. While there are a range of associated nursing assessments and interventions associated with these conditions, it is important to understand that evidence from research is constantly changing. Your practice should be based on the most up-to-date clinical practice guidelines and evidence-based recommendations. Further, children and young people with chronic conditions, and their parents and carers, live with these illnesses every day. They are likely to know much more about the condition and its management than you do. Therefore, your care of chronically ill children and young people relies on using the best available evidence from research, but must also include listening carefully to the experience and needs of the whole family. Finally, this chapter will explore the challenges faced by young people with chronic illnesses in leaving the familiar environments and people of the paediatric setting to make the transition to adult health care.

Reflection points 10.1

- Some children and young people living in remote and very remote regions of Australia have limited access to health and support services. What will be the likely impacts on their care and treatment if they also have a chronic condition?
- Children and young people with chronic conditions are often more vulnerable to common childhood illnesses and may become very unwell. What general health-promoting activities would you recommend to a young person with a chronic illness?
- Children and young people with a chronic illness have often spent a lot of time in hospitals and clinics. What impacts do chronic illnesses have on a child's education, and how might you be able to mitigate some of these effects?

Chronic conditions

While it is not possible to explore all chronic conditions that might affect children and young people, this section discusses two of the most common chronic medical conditions of childhood – asthma and diabetes – as well as the most common genetic disorder affecting the Australian Caucasian population – cystic fibrosis (CF). All of these conditions will require ongoing medical or surgical management, health maintenance and education for self-care, as well as significant health professional involvement in successfully transitioning to the adult care environment.

Asthma

The last Australian National Health Survey (2007–08) reported that around 10 per cent, or almost 415 000 Australian children aged 0–14 years had an **asthma** diagnosis (ABS, 2009). This makes asthma the most common long term chronic condition affecting children and young people in Australia and one of the most common causes of hospital admission and visits to a general practice. Although placing considerable burden on the child and family, asthma can be effectively managed with appropriate preventer treatment, avoidance or control of trigger factors and medication. Deaths directly attributable to asthma are now rare (26 deaths between 2008 and 2010), but the underlying causes of this disease are still not well known.

> **Asthma** A chronic lung disease characterised by the presence of both excessive variation in lung function and respiratory symptoms such as wheeze, shortness of breath, cough and chest tightness. Where age or level of development precludes formal lung function testing, diagnosis is based on the presence of respiratory symptoms alone

The National Asthma Council of Australia (NACA, 2014) describes asthma as a chronic lung disease that can be controlled but not cured. Asthma is characterised by chronic inflammation of the airways, airway hyper-responsiveness and intermittent narrowing of the airways caused by bronchoconstriction, congestion, mucus or oedema (or combinations of these) (GINA, 2012). As a paediatric nurse, it is important that you are aware of, and follow, local protocols for the treatment of acute asthma. In general, an asthma diagnosis should be considered in a child who presents with cough, wheeze or difficulty in breathing. A prolonged expiratory phase may be an early sign if wheeze is not present.

The NSW Ministry of Health Clinical Practice Guideline for the Acute Management of Asthma (Ministry of Health, 2012) identifies three common patterns of childhood asthma, with subsequent implications for the management of an acute attack and for ongoing asthma management planning (Table 10.1).

TABLE 10.1 *Common patterns of childhood asthma*

PATTERN	PROPORTION OF CHILDREN WITH ASTHMA AFFECTED	CHARACTERISTICS
Infrequent, intermittent asthma	Approx. 70–75%	• Commonly triggered by upper respiratory tract infection • Acute illness lasts few days to one week, intervals > 6 weeks apart • Symptom-free during interval
Frequent, intermittent asthma	Approx. 20–25%	• Intervals often < 6 weeks apart • Minimal or no symptoms between intervals
Persistent asthma	Approx. 5–10%	• Symptoms on most days including disrupted sleep and exercise intolerance
High-risk asthma	< 5%	• Recurrent presentations • Multiple asthma medication (including admission for intravenous treatment or steroids in past 12 months) • Previous intensive care admission • Re-presentation soon after discharge • Coexistent medical condition • Unresponsive to bronchodilator

In summary, it is likely that, rather than being just one condition, asthma represents a spectrum of conditions with different pathophysiology. while asthma is most often associated with hypersensitivity to allergens – environmental, lifestyle and genetic factors are also thought to play a part in the development of childhood asthma.

Nursing assessment and interventions

An asthma attack may initially present following a period of recurrent or persistent symptoms or, in those already diagnosed, may indicate a need for review of a current asthma plan. Judging the severity of an acute asthma attack is the most important aspect of the initial clinical assessment. Listening to the child and accompanying parent or carer's interpretation of severity is an important part of this assessment. Severity of the attack is measured by oxygen saturation in air, heart rate, ability to talk (if verbal) or cry, accessory muscle use and level of consciousness. Any tachycardia, cyanosis, drowsiness or agitation with moderate to severe accessory muscle use is serious, and requires immediate medical intervention with close observation and review. When stable, a thorough clinical examination with medical history inclusive of a family history of smoking, asthma, eczema or allergic rhinitis should be undertaken. In young children, it is important to exclude bronchiolitis or pneumonia as differential diagnoses, and always to consider the possibility of an inhaled foreign body.

Harriet

Case study 10.1

Harriet is a 13-year-old girl with a history of asthma and is brought into the emergency department by ambulance with severe shortness of breath. On arrival, she is conscious, only able to speak single words and very short of breath (RR 35 bpm). Her saturation on a Hudson mask is 92 per cent. Auscultation of her chest reveals wheeze and decreased breath sounds bilaterally.

Harriet is what some health professionals call a 'frequent flyer'. She has a history of severe asthma and previous intensive-care admission and intubation. She has been short of breath for four hours, and this is worsening. She had been nebulising with salbutamol every hour at home.

Harriet deteriorates, even though given maximal therapy, becoming drowsy, tachycardic (130bpm) and further desaturates (SaO2 90%). Current status is conscious, only able to speak in single words and very short of breath. SaO2 on a Hudson mask is 92%. RR 25; HR 110 bpm, BP 130/80.

The treatment of asthma is individual, and highly dependent on the severity of the attack, but it will usually include a symptom-control medication (such as an inhaled bronchodilator) and a preventer medication (commonly a low-dose corticosteroid or long-acting bronchodilator). Oral steroids and other inhibitor medications may also be used for acute attacks. In severe asthma attacks like Harriet's, bronchodilators (salbutamol, aminophylline or magnesium sulphate) and corticosteroids (hydrocortisone or methylprednisolone) would be administered intravenously as she has had no response to nebulised treatment. Because of her history (high-risk asthma), Harriet is transferred directly to the intensive care unit for continuous cardiorespiratory monitoring and blood gases. Continuous nebulised salbutamol is delivered while intravenous access is established and medications commenced.

Following initial diagnosis or an acute asthma attack, the further management of asthma is guided by the pattern and severity of symptoms. A main aim of asthma management is to ensure that asthma is correctly diagnosed, and that the child or young person can maintain as normal a life as possible without interruption from asthma or the effects of asthma medications (NACA, 2014). For most children, young people and their parents or carers, this aim is facilitated by the shared development of an asthma plan and maintenance of the lowest possible dose of medications to achieve good asthma control and prevent acute attacks. Preventer medications (often low-dose inhaled corticosteroids) are important as these make the airways less sensitive by drying up mucus and reducing swelling, but they need to be taken every day. There are combined forms of reliever and preventer medications that work well for some children and young people.

A definition of good asthma control (NACA, 2014) includes:

- asthma symptoms experienced on less than two days per week and rapidly relieved by bronchodilator medication
- no limitation on activities
- no disruption to sleep or symptoms on waking.

Asthma management plans are individually tailored guidelines that include the tracking of symptom patterns against treatment variations and environmental triggers; advice for managing acute attacks; information about correct medication administration (such as inhaler or spacer technique); and health maintenance (nutrition, immunisation and avoidance of tobacco smoke). Perhaps unsurprisingly, Ellwood and colleagues (2013) have recently reported on the potential protective effects of healthy eating on severe asthma.

The most common causes of poor asthma control are problems with inhaler technique, inappropriate medication dose and type for the age and stage of development, inability of the child or family to follow the asthma management plan recommendations, and exposure to as yet unidentified asthma triggers. The asthma management plan needs continuous review as the child grows and begins to take more responsibility for the monitoring and control of their asthma. For Harriet, entry into adolescence, combined with her unstable (sometimes called 'brittle') asthma, indicates a clear point of review for her plan. If the child or young person agrees, it is useful for their general practitioner, school, child-care or sporting club to have copies of their plan, and asthma first aid protocols are freely available from NACA.

Type 1 diabetes

Type 1 diabetes (T1D) accounts for the majority of childhood cases of diabetes in Australia, and is estimated to account for 10 per cent of all diagnoses of diabetes in this country (AIHW, 2011). The incidence of new cases of T1D increased from 19 per 100 000 in 2000 to 22 per 100 000 in 2009 (AIHW, 2012). This increase occurred mainly before 2005, with rates stabilising at 11 per 100 000 in 2011(AIHW, 2014a). This rising incidence has been attributed to an increasing proportion of people with low-risk human leukocyte antigen (HLA) genotypes. Categorised an autoimmune condition, the exact cause of T1D is unknown, but is believed to be an interaction of genetic predisposition and environmental factors (Craig et al., 2011).

> **Type 1 Diabetes (T1D)** A lifelong autoimmune disease that develops when the immune system is triggered to damage the insulin-producing cells of the pancreas, preventing the normal production of insulin. Diabetes is very uncommon in infants under 1 year of age. Type 1 diabetes typically presents during childhood and adolescence, but can be diagnosed at any age

Type 1 diabetes is currently incurable, and there is no known way to prevent it. In 2008, the prevalence of T1D in children aged 0–14 years was 138 cases per 100 000 population, or approximately one in every 300 children and young people. According to Catanzariti et al. (2009), the mean age of onset of T1D in Australia is approximately 8 years. The incidence of T1D increases with age, peaking during early adolescence and coinciding with puberty. Consequently, children in the 10–14 years age group are 2.6 times more likely to be diagnosed with T1D than children in the 0–4 years age range, and 4.7 times more likely to be hospitalised than those under the age of 5 years (AIHW, 2012).

The pancreas produces a range of enzymes and hormones important for normal digestion and energy regulation. Insulin is produced by beta cells in the pancreas. When beta cells are damaged, insulin is not produced and blood glucose levels become elevated. Glucagon-producing cells also become damaged, leading to a loss of glucagon regulation, even when insulin therapy has commenced. The function of the hormone glucagon is to increase blood sugar when levels become too low.

The typical presentation of T1D includes a pre-clinical phase, a presentation phase (usually when symptomatic), a partial remission (known as the 'honeymoon' phase), followed by a chronic phase requiring long-term insulin replacement. The presenting symptoms of T1D include polyuria, polydipsia, hyperventilation, tiredness, and abdominal pain or vomiting; occasionally, T1D is detected incidentally during the pre-clinical phase. Symptoms and presentation may vary and T1D can easily be misdiagnosed as any of a range of childhood illnesses. When metabolic symptoms are mild, T1D may also be difficult to differentiate from Type 2 diabetes (T2D – see p. 239), particularly in children and young people with signs of insulin resistance (who are generally overweight or obese). If diagnosis is delayed, severe diabetic ketoacidosis will inevitably occur, requiring urgent hospitalisation for rehydration and insulin infusion.

Nursing assessment and interventions

The main aim of management for T1D is balancing blood glucose control with insulin treatment in order to optimise the prognosis of the disease and maintain quality of life, normal growth and psychological wellbeing (Craig et al., 2011). As with all chronic conditions of childhood, regular care by (initially) a paediatric multidisciplinary team is important. Clinicians need to be aware that the comorbidity of psychological disorders, inclusive of eating disorders, is relatively common in children and young people with T1D, and there is a longitudinal association between glycaemic control and some aspects of educational performance and cognitive function. Regular monitoring of height and weight is important both for ensuring normal growth and for early prevention of overweight or obesity. Insulin requirements will change frequently with growth in response to periods of illness and during puberty (Craig et al., 2011). The specialist health-care team works with the child, young person, family and general practitioner to achieve consistent continuity of care in:

- recommending diabetes care and self-management
- initiating required changes in medical management
- undertaking regular reviews and screening for diabetes complications
- advising on 'sick day' management plans
- offering psychological and psychosocial support.

Strategies to improve access to primary health care services are an important aspect of coordinated care for those children and young people living in remote locations. Telemedicine and mobile phone text messaging of blood glucose levels, weight and other information are particularly useful adjuncts to self-management for this group. Children and young people presenting with T1D should be managed in an appropriately resourced ambulatory care section of an in-patient hospital setting (Craig et al., 2011). In-patient management is recommended for children under 2 years of age at diagnosis, those who have significant other medical or social problems, inadequate support or mental health issues, those living in geographically remote locations, and those for whom English is a second or poorly understood language.

The following is an anonymous blog post as it appears in the 'Living with Diabetes' section of the Diabetes Australia website.

Blog post (anonymous 2 May 2010)

I was diagnosed just after I turned 6, three days after my birthday to be precise. I woke up an ordinary morning ... the morning of my birthday party, but I got the chicken pox. I was taken to the doctor, then a nurse, and then I was diagnosed with Type 1 diabetes. My birthday cake was put in the fridge and I was stuck in hospital for a week! I've gone through many diabetic things in my life, like the Humalog pen and Jelly Baby Month Stalls (i've done for 7 years.)[sic] I'M HOPING A CURE IS FOUND SOON FOR ALL THOSE WITH DIABETES, THE HORRIBLE DISEASE THAT FORCES DAILY INJECTION SHOT JUST TO STAY ALIVE AND LIVE AGAIN TOMARROW [sic]!!

Source: <www.diabetesaustralia.com.au/Living-with-Diabetes/Type-1-Diabetes/My-Story/Unknown-author1>.

The Australian *National Evidence-based Guidelines for Type 1 Diabetes in Children, Adolescents and Adults* (Craig et al., 2011) are a reliable and constantly updated collaborative source of evidence for the care of children and young people with T1D. For evidence-based practitioners, recommendations for the care of children and young people with T1D should be from these sources of evidence, rather than from texts, which can quickly become outdated. However, Table 10.2 outlines the mainstay of treatment for T1D internationally. There is increasing evidence from a number of major trials that continuous subcutaneous injection of insulin using an external insulin pump has greater potential to minimise hypoglycaemia and maintain long-term glycaemic control (Craig et al., 2011). However, children, young people and their families need to be willing and motivated to succeed in using this currently quite complex therapy.

TABLE 10.2 *Essential aspects of care for type 1 diabetes*

Blood glucose monitoring	Intermittent capillary testing of blood glucose level (BGL) using a portable meter or continuous glucose monitoring system (CGMS). Many blood glucose meters now have the ability to download and store results to smartphones.	A urine test for glycosylated haemoglobin (HbA1c) shows an average of blood glucose level over the past 10–12 weeks.
Human insulin or insulin analogues (rapid acting)	Intermittent subcutaneous injection or via continuous subcutaneous infusion (insulin pump).	Dose adjusted according to BGL, dietary intake and anticipated exercise, or 'sick days'.

Hypoglycaemia is the most common acute complication of T1D, but this can usually be self-managed by ingestion of a fast-acting carbohydrate such as fruit juice followed by a longer acting carbohydrate (such as a sandwich) if not resolving. However, there may be a reduced awareness of hypoglycaemia symptoms in around a quarter of people who have had T1D for 10 years or more (Craig et al., 2011). Fortunately, severe hypoglycaemia with inability to self-manage is much less common. Severe hypoglycaemia manifests as loss of coordination or consciousness, slurred speech, confusion or fitting. This is an emergency and requires the administration of glucagon (a hormone that raises blood glucose levels). Table 10.3 outlines recognised acute and chronic complications of T1D. Attention to the long-term maintenance of glycaemic control does have the potential to delay or reduce chronic complications such as retinopathy, nephropathy and neuropathy (Craig et al., 2011).

TABLE 10.3 *Common acute and chronic complications of type 1 diabetes*

COMPLICATION	POSSIBLE CAUSE OR EFFECT
Hypoglycaemia due to low blood sugar	• Too much insulin
	• Missed or delayed meals/exercise
	• Reduced symptomatic awareness
Diabetic ketoacidosis due to high blood sugar	• Insulin dose too low or missed
	• Infection or other illness
	• Stress or excitement
Microvascular (longer-term)	• Retinopathy
	• Nephropathy
	• Peripheral neuropathy
Macrovascular (longer-term)	• Cardiovascular
	• Cerebrovascular
	• Peripheral vascular disease
Weight (longer-term)	• Overweight or obese
	• Metabolic syndrome

Type 2 diabetes

Sources for monitoring the national incidence and prevalence of type 2 diabetes (T2D) in younger age groups are only just being established; however, data from two national datasets have recently been combined to prepare one of the first working papers on this subject (AIHW, 2014b). There is evidence to suggest that the incidence of T2D may be increasing among children and young people due to increased levels of obesity and physical inactivity. Between 2002–03 and 2011–12, there were approximately 4000 new cases of T2D among 10–24-year-olds, or an average of nearly 400 new cases per year (AIHW, 2014b). Among young people in Australia, the risk of T2D in 10–14-year-olds rose from an annual average rate of three per 100 000 to eight per 100 000 for those aged 15–19 years. Between 2006 and 2011, the rate of T2D was eight times higher in Indigenous Australians aged 10–14 years and four times higher for Indigenous Australians aged 15–19 years.

The characteristics of T2D are the progressive failure of insulin production and the resistance of body tissues to the action of insulin (insulin resistance). Risk factors are both modifiable and non-modifiable. For example, up to 85 per cent of children and young people diagnosed with T2D in the United States were overweight or obese at diagnosis (AIHW, 2014b). Therefore, modifiable risks include preventing obesity through a healthy diet, weight loss and exercise, possibly inclusive of bariatric surgical procedures (ADC, 2012) Non-modifiable risk factors for the development of T2D in young people include maternal diabetes and genetic predisposition to insulin resistance. As both types of diabetes can lead to range of serious complications involving the blood vessels and nerves, most young people diagnosed with T2D will commence insulin, even though oral glucose-lowering medication is most often the first line of treatment for adults. Clearly, the younger a person at diagnosis, the greater the risk of complications because of longer exposure to the disease. An additional burden on a young person is the need to self-manage this condition for the rest of their life with ongoing potential for interference with full participation in study or the workforce, and disability from the associated comorbidities of diabetes – such as vision impairment, vascular, heart, kidney and nerve damage.

Nursing assessment and interventions

Strategies for the effective management of T2D in children and young people are not as well advanced as they are for adult patients. Some obvious areas of difference in managing the condition in young people include the effect of hormones and puberty, compliance with medication and diet, and complex maturational and psychosocial effects.

As for T1D, the aim of treatment is stabilisation of blood glucose levels and prevention of complications. Optimal management will be through regular self-monitoring of blood glucose levels and insulin therapy as above, with the involvement of (initially) a paediatric multidisciplinary team with specialist skills in endocrinology, diabetes education, dietetics, social work and psychology, as well as effective transition to adult care.

Congenital, chromosomal and genetic disorders

Congenital anomalies are a major cause of hospitalisation in infancy and childhood in Australia; however, the collation and reporting of data specific to the major personal, social, community and economic influences of caring for children and young people with congenital conditions is not routine. Reporting for the Australian Perinatal Statistics Unit, Abeywardana and Sullivan (2008) suggest that hypospadias – a condition characterised by the opening of the urethra on the ventral side of the male penis, is the most commonly reported congenital condition in Australia. The overall rate of hypospadias, regardless of the severity of the condition, is approximately 23.8 per 10 000 births or 46.4 per 10 000 male births.

Congenital anomalies or birth defects Health problems or physical anomalies that are present birth and result in either long-term morbidity or death

Neural tube defects occur in approximately 4.2 per 10 000 births, but again it is estimated that up to 76 per cent of affected pregnancies are terminated or the foetus dies (Abeywardana & Sullivan, 2008). Other congenital anomalies associated with chronic conditions of children and young people include spina bifida, cleft lip or palate, intestinal atresia or stenosis, and limb-reduction deficits.

Trisomy 21, or Down syndrome, is the second most commonly reported condition in Australian children, occurring at a rate of 11.1 per 10 000 live births. However, it is estimated that approximately 64 per cent of foetuses affected by this chromosomal abnormality are either managed by termination or die in utero, making the actual rate for Trisomy 21 closer to double the birth rate at 26.3 per 10 000 pregnancies. Children with **chromosomal birth defects** or abnormalities are born with either an irregular number of chromosomes or with one or more chromosomes that have an irregular structure, such as a duplication or deletion.

A chromosomal birth defect A birth defect caused by an alteration in the number or structure of chromosomes (extra copies or missing copies of specific chromosomes), or having chromosomes with missing or extra pieces. Chromosomes are the genetic structure of a cell that carries DNA

Other common chromosomal conditions in Australia are Klinefelter syndrome (which affects boys), Turner syndrome (which affects girls), and Prader-Willi and Angelman syndromes (McDevitt & Ormrod, 2007).

Single **gene defects** can occur on any of the dominant (non-X-linked) 22 chromosome pairs, as a recessive defect on both chromosome in one of the matched pairs or as problem in a recessive gene on the X chromosome in boys, or in a gene on both (XX) chromosomes in girls. Neurofibromatosis is a common dominant gene defect affecting Australian children, with the mild form occurring in one per 2500 to 4000 live births in Australia. Other single gene defects cause Huntington disease, phenylketonuria (PKU), Sickle Cell Disease, Tay-Sachs disease, thalassaemia, Duchenne muscular dystrophy (which affects boys) and cystic fibrosis (McDevitt & Ormrod, 2007).

> **Gene defects** Mutations or alterations to chromosomes (the genetic structure of a cell that carries DNA) causing abnormalities in the genome. These defects cause genetic disorders which are present from birth (congenital)

Cystic fibrosis

Cystic fibrosis (CF) is the most common life-limiting autosomal recessive genetic condition affecting people of European/Caucasian decent, with an incidence of approximately 1 in every 2800 live births in Australia. On average, one in 25 people carries the CF gene (over one million Australians), but most are unaware they are carriers. The gene responsible for the symptoms of CF, the cystic fibrosis transmembrane regulator (CFTR) protein gene, was discovered in 1989 (Riordan et al., 1989). More than 1500 different mutations of the CFTR have now been identified, which partially explains previously observed variances in the symptomatic and geographic presentation of this condition. Therefore, CF should be seen as a spectrum of illness.

CFTR is a protein that functions as a channel across the membrane of epithelial cells. CFTR controls chloride ion transportation across the cell membrane, thereby controlling the movement of water in and out of the cell. Since water is necessary for the free flow of mucus, the symptoms of CF are largely observed in those organs that rely on lubrication by mucus, including the lungs and gastrointestinal system (intestine, pancreas, gall bladder and liver). Sodium ion transport is also affected. The most common CF mutation in Australia is a deletion in the CFTR protein called $\Delta F508$ (CFA, 2013).

> **Cystic fibrosis (CF)** Caused by mutations in the cystic fibrosis transmembrane conductance regulator (CFTR) protein gene, resulting in abnormal regulation of chloride and sodium transport at the surface of epithelial cells. This results in a multi-system disease characterised by lung and digestive complications

Newborn screening programs (by bloodspot or Guthrie test) have included screening for CF in some regions of Australia since the early 1980s, and there is good evidence of benefits from early diagnosis and intervention (Dijk et al., 2011). Strategies for newborn screening now largely reflect the variable mutation profiles, with tests on neonatal blood spots extended to include a range of non-ΔF508 mutations. In a recent Australian study, the mean age of death from CF between 1979 and 2005 reportedly had increased from an average of 12.2 to 27.9 years for males, and from 14.8 to 25.3 years for females (Reid et al., 2011). The significant survival disadvantage for girls with CF is persistent and largely unexplained, but has been attributed to adolescent compliance and differences in energy expenditure, with higher proportions of female adolescents with CF reported as underweight. The most common cause of death in CF is related to pulmonary complications.

Neonatal screening has contributed greatly to our understanding of this genetic disorder, and to improving the treatment of respiratory and nutritional symptoms of infants with this condition, but there are likely many other factors contributing to improved survival in CF. These include improvements in co-ordinated, multidisciplinary CF centre-based care, availability of bacteria-specific antibiotics, improved physiotherapy techniques for chest clearance, and maintenance of normal growth through nutritional support and pancreatic enzyme replacement therapy (Bell et al., 2008). Screening cohorts have also been entered into registries throughout the world, with the Australian Cystic Fibrosis Data Registry (ACFDR) offering further information on the demographics, clinical features and outcomes of people with CF in this country. While the outlook for children diagnosed with CF was previously bleak, there is now evidence from the ACFDR (CFA, 2013) that 90 per cent of children with CF reach adulthood. While this is clearly an achievement, living into adulthood with a chronic condition like CF introduces other medical, social and psychological challenges, as discussed in Chapter 3, when we were introduced to Ellen, a 16-year-old young woman with CF (see Case Study 3.6).

Nursing assessment and interventions

The ACFDR (CFA, 2013) reports that 65 per cent of the 66 new cases of CF diagnosed in 2012 presented through newborn screening. A significant percentage, however, presented with respiratory (12 per cent) or gastrointestinal (4.5 per cent) symptoms and a small number with meconium ileus at birth. As more than 80 per cent of infants with CF will be diagnosed before they are

3 months of age, it is likely that early contact will be around establishing diagnosis and initiating preventative treatments as recommended by the *Cystic Fibrosis Standards of Care, Australia* (Bell et al., 2008), outlined in Table 10.4.

TABLE 10.4 *Establishing treatment in the newly diagnosed infant with cystic fibrosis*

Access to specialist CF centre or service	• Prompt access to experienced medical, nursing and allied health team
	• Confirmation of diagnosis by sweat test
	• Assessment of pancreatic function and commencement of enzyme replacement therapy if required
	• Salt, electrolyte and vitamin replacement therapy especially in hot, humid conditions
	• Establish regular follow-up appointments
Family education and counselling	• Access to all CF team members for education on management of condition
	• Establish contact with support organisations and people
	• Access to genetic counselling service

There is no cure for CF, so treatment is aimed at managing symptoms to slow organ damage caused by the disease and maintain normal nutrition for growth. As the CFTR gene impacts fluid transport across exocrine cells, the resulting abnormally thick mucus will lead to varying degrees of blockage of ducts in the bronchi, pancreatic ducts and intestines. Blocked mucus in the lungs traps bacteria and causes infection. Pancreatic enzymes required for normal digestion are also blocked in the pancreas, and around 80 per cent of children and young people with CF will require enzyme replacement to help digest their food and maintain normal nutrition. The treatment of CF has improved greatly in recent years and, as for all the chronic conditions of children and young people we have reviewed so far, regular attendance at a major CF centre or clinic facilitates specialist care from a multidisciplinary team that includes respiratory physicians, gastroenterologists, physiotherapists, dieticians, psychologists, pharmacists, social workers and nurses.

Following the initial diagnosis, paediatric nurses will most frequently encounter children and young people with CF in a clinic or hospital. Almost half of all patients attending CF clinics will be admitted to hospital at least once each year, and mostly these admissions will be for a two-week course of antibiotics to treat a respiratory infection (CFA, 2013). Around 10–15 per cent of older children and adults complete their intravenous antibiotic treatments at home once intravenous access and dosages are established. While *Staphylococcus aureus* is the most commonly identified organism causing respiratory infections in younger children with CF, children older than 12 years are more likely colonised with various species and forms of *Pseudomonas*. The medical complications of CF, including reduced lung function, increase with age (Table 10.5). More than 30 per cent of adult patients with CF will have chronic insulin-dependent diabetes and gasto-oesphageal reflux. More than 40 per cent are likely to have osteoporosis due to nutritional comorbidities and long-term medication use (CFA, 2013).

TABLE 10.5 *System complications of cystic fibrosis*

SYSTEM	COMPLICATION OR EFFECT OF DISEASE
Pulmonary	• Infection
	• Haemoptysis
	• Pneumothorax
Gastrointestinal	• Pancreatic insufficiency
	• Gastro-oesphageal reflux
	• Abnormal liver function
	• Cirrhosis or portal hypertension
Endocrine	• Chronic or intermittent insulin dependent diabetes
Other	• Osteoporosis
	• Male infertility
	• Osteopenia

Similar to the other chronic conditions described in this section, children and young people with CF should have a plan for management of acute exacerbations, exercise and medication. Young people may wish to express their preferences for transition to adult care and end of life. The management plan should preferably be in a form that can be shared with family, carers, schools and medical teams. Parents of young children with CF carry the largest burden, however. In addition to the normal routines of raising and educating a child or young person, there are daily responsibilities for physiotherapy, including inhalations and airway clearance, attention to nutrition and enzyme replacement therapy and maximising compliance with a range of daily medications and exercise. Children and young people with CF are expected to adhere to a range of treatments and preventative therapies, including:

- routine clinic visits and physical examinations
- annual review including chest X-ray, blood tests, nutritional and gastrointestinal assessment, spirometry (from 5 years of age), sputum sample
- oral antibiotic therapy continuously or as needed
- pancreatic enzyme replacement
- nutritional and vitamin supplementation
- inhalations (bronchodilators, antibiotics, steroids)
- salt tablets
- oxygen.

In addition to exposure to normal childhood illnesses and injuries, children and young people with CF may also be hospitalised for a range of other complications associated with their disease. These include nasal surgery, procedures for more permanent intravenous access devices, insertion of gastrostomy for supplemental feeding or treatment for intestinal obstructions. Organ transplantation is an end-stage treatment for CF. In 2012, the Australian Cystic Fibrosis Data Registry reported 119 Australian patients who had received a transplanted organ. Bilateral lung transplant was the most common procedure (89 per cent); however, three patients received combined heart, lung and liver transplants, with five of seven single liver transplants performed on paediatric patients (CFA, 2013). Paediatric organ transplants must be conducted in specialist centres to ensure optimal treatment and survival.

Reflection points 10.2

- Chronic medical and genetic conditions require a daily, lifelong commitment to care. Investigate the research literature for studies on medication compliance in young people with chronic conditions as a way of informing your nursing care.
- The National Health and Medical Research Council (NHMRC) recently released a statement on DNA genetic testing in the Australian context. Genetic testing continues to present a range of challenges for health professionals and some tests are available for purchase via the internet (direct to consumer, or DTC). Think about some of the positive and negative outcomes of DTC testing and how you might discuss these with a family seeking your advice?

Transition to adult care

The range of chronic medical, metabolic and genetic conditions affecting children and young people is broad and, as we have seen, many will persist from childhood through adolescence and into adulthood. As such, individuals who experience these conditions and who survive to reach adulthood will face the important issue of **transitioning to adult care**. This process of transition involves the 'purposeful planned movement of adolescents and young adults with chronic physical and medical conditions from a child-centred to adult orientated health care system' (Blum et al., 1993; Bloom et al., 2012: 213).

> **Transition to adult care** The purposeful and planned movement of the care of adolescents and young people with chronic conditions from a child-centred to an adult health-care system

Transitioning from paediatric to adult care is a complex process, and often takes several years (Cystic Fibrosis Trust, 2014). The timing of the transition process is extremely important, but will likely be different for each young person. Transition will usually commence between the ages of 16 and 18 or when a young person leaves secondary school (Jermyn, 2013), but there is some variability around this, depending upon the organisation of the health-care service, the availability of resources in paediatric and adult care, the maturity and knowledge of the individual with the chronic condition, the nature of the condition, the country in which care is being delivered and personal preferences (Cystic Fibrosis Trust, 2014; Garvey et al., 2012; Jermyn, 2013; McInally, 2013; Tuchman & Schwartz, 2013). There is no 'right' time for transition, but setting a target transfer age helps with planning.

Successful transition of young adults to adult care must focus on both physical and psychosocial needs (for example, employment, housing, safety, driving, travel, sexual and reproductive health, alcohol, parenting, continued prescription of unsubsidised medications). As such, a transition process that focuses solely on the illness and medical treatment is unlikely to meet the needs of the young person (Fegran et al., 2014; Jermyn, 2013; Porter et al., 2014). Additionally, it is important to remember that the timing of most transition experiences will fall within a developmental stage in young people that is often associated with rebellion, non-compliance and sometimes frustration and anger, as the young person tries to make sense of the world and their place within it. For this reason, careful planning is needed to ensure a smooth and efficient transfer to adult care.

Important considerations during transition

Let's return to the situation of Ellen (Case Study 3.6), a 16-year-old young woman with CF. Ellen had graduated from the children's hospital transitional care program but held some reservations about moving to the adult hospital.

Ellen

Case study 10.2

Ellen is a 16-year-old young woman with CF. She has now transitioned to the adult CF clinic. Ellen was late for her first appointment because her mum couldn't work out where to park and Ellen had to walk a long way to the clinic, arriving exhausted and breathless. Ellen did not recognise any of the other patients in the waiting room, and some of them looked really sick. There was not a single staff member she recognised. She went to the coffee shop, but she missed seeing her friend Sharon behind the service counter. When her mother arrived, Ellen had been taken in to see the registrar, who was in process of asking her to recite her entire medical and surgical history from when she was a baby. Ellen said, 'Don't you have my notes from the other hospital? Can't you just read them?' The registrar then asked Ellen's mum to leave the room while she undertook a clinical examination. Ellen decided that she would not tell this stranger anything about her psychosocial history.

The move from paediatric to adult health-care services is characterised by a number of changes. Of particular importance is the assumption that, in adult services, the client will take a greater level of individual responsibility for managing their care (Begley, 2013; Chesshir et al., 2013; Fegran et al., 2014). Parents or caregivers who may previously have played a vital part in decision-making are designated to a more peripheral role (Jermyn, 2013). While this gives greater autonomy to the young person in making decisions about their care, some young people find this new responsibility intimidating or overwhelming. Some parents also find it difficult to disengage from a role they may have held for a long time. Appropriate support and advice during the transition process are therefore a major part of ensuring success (APA, 2009; Begley, 2013).

Second, a movement from paediatric to adult services requires getting used to a new health-care team and negotiating new relationships. The transition to adult care will often be accompanied by a move from specialist paediatric service providers (for instance, a paediatric endocrinologist, paediatric educator and dietitians for T1D patients) to adult service providers who may be based in a different hospital in a different region, and who also see many more patients with T2D. The young person will need (either in consultation with their paediatric team or independently) to find a suitable adult health-care provider, and work towards establishing rapport and understanding with the new health-care team, who often do not have the same extensive understanding of their previous care history (McInally, 2013; Oswald et al., 2013).

A third important change associated with the transition to adult care is the fact that this period will coincide with a number of other stage-of-life decisions. On reaching late adolescence, young people with a chronic disease may also seek to move out of the family home, go to university, start full-time work, embark on relationships or consider starting a family (Cystic Fibrosis Trust, 2014). These aspirations are often taken for granted by young people without chronic illness, but the outcome of these decisions can have a profound impact on the way a childhood chronic illness is managed in the young adult, and the kind of support required for continuation of comprehensive care.

Successful transition

A successful transition is promoted by health-care providers who listen to, and who are sensitive and supportive of, the needs of the transitioning clients. In their study of young people with T1D, Ritholz and colleagues (2014) reported that the transition process often raises a variety of emotions, including sadness and reluctance to separate from providers who have often been a part of the young person's life for a significant period of time. Consequently, it is important for adult providers to be aware of and sensitive to these emotions. Adult health-care providers also need to be cognisant that young people who are moving from a paediatric to adult service may have different needs from clients who have not previously been involved with health-care systems (Betz et al., 2013). Contrast the experience of Harriet (Case Study 10.1), for example, against that of a young adult presenting to an adult respiratory clinic for the first time. Throughout the transition process, young people may experience feelings of not belonging and of being redundant (Fegran et al., 2014). Adult health-care professionals need to understand, respect and actively acknowledge the knowledge and insight chronically ill young people have about their own bodies and own disease.

Another important factor in ensuring a successful transition is good preparation (Jermyn, 2013). The transition process may take a considerable amount of time, so it is recommended that the process starts early in the teenage years, progressing over the next few years with a view to moving to adult facilities around the age of 16–18 (Cystic Fibrosis Trust, 2014). Throughout, there must be active consultation between the young person, their family and both the paediatric and adult care facilities. Many health-care facilities have introduced formal transition programs to aid movement from paediatric to adult care, although there is a wide discrepancy in their availability across different conditions and across states and countries (McInally, 2013). Advance planning and encouraging young people to gradually take on more of the responsibility for health-care decision-making can also make the transition process smoother (Hilliard et al., 2014). Similarly, good relationships and clear communication between the paediatric, transition and adult health-care teams are vital (Kaufmann Rauen et al., 2013).

Standardising the content of transition preparation programs within a paediatric service improves program efficiency. Similarly, introducing transition-oriented clinics for late adolescents and young adults can also be effective in allaying common transition-related fears and establishing the young person's preferences for adult care (Hilliard et al., 2014). A carefully planned and well-executed transition process, with regular evaluations and reviews, will assist young people to maintain their health as they moved to adult care (Jermyn, 2013). Clear communication, early planning and the involvement of all stakeholders are just some of the defining features of successful transition programs.

Factors known to contribute to the successful transition of young people with chronic conditions to adult care are:

- a transition case manager for each individual
- planning the transition process over a period of time (years rather than months)
- involving the current main carer, GP and/or family in the process
- gradually encouraging more involvement of young person in health-care decision-making
- transition clinics (hybridisation of paediatric and adult service) and introduction to peers who have successfully made the transition
- clear communication between paediatric and adult health care providers at the transitioning institutions
- access to practical and online resources (checklists, maps, parking, names, contact details, who does what, chat rooms and blogs)
- flexibility and consideration of timing of other life events (such as final year at school)
- maintaining contact after the transition.

Sadly, however, the planning process for transition is often neglected (Fegran et al., 2014; Garvey et al., 2012; McManus et al., 2013). Gaps of six months or more are commonly reported between leaving the paediatric provider and establishing adult care (Garvey et al., 2012), especially when young people and their families are left to locate the adult service themselves (Fegran et al., 2014).

Ineffective transition and loss of young people to follow-up can be responsible for unnecessary morbidity, excess mortality, preventable emergency room attendances and expensive investigations. The flow-on effects for the young person are a potential loss of earnings, reduction in reproductive potential and impact on relationships. In one study of young people with T1D, fewer than half of the respondents reported receiving a recommendation for an adult provider, and fewer than 15 per cent reported having a transition preparation visit or receiving written transition materials (Garvey et al., 2012).

The health needs of young people with a chronic condition are multifaceted, and exist within a microsystem within which information flow, psychosocial support, models of transition, care and clinical expertise available from both adult and paediatric environments will directly affect ongoing care. Anticipated future needs include the establishment of specialist facilities and resources for transitioning groups, education and training for health-care professionals in the prevention and treatment of acquired complications associated with prolonged survival, and developing appropriate models of care for young adults surviving with these conditions. The lack of health-care professionals in the adult care sector who have specific experience in childhood chronic conditions, and problems finding an adult specialist, are understandable reasons for young people's dissatisfaction with transitioning (Hilliard et al., 2014; Oswald et al., 2013).

> *Reflection points 10.3*
>
> - In your work as a paediatric nurse, how have you contributed to preparing young people with chronic conditions for their transition to adult health care?
> - Do you know whether a transition to an adult health-care program is part of the service offered by the organisation for which you work. If so, what does the program comprise?
> - Parents and carers play a vital role in the planning of transition. What three things can you suggest to parents or carers to prepare their young person with a chronic condition for this process? (*Hint:* encourage the young person to keep a journal and write down questions.)

Summary

- Chronic conditions are those that cause a long-term (more than six months) functional limitation or health burden that requires care or services beyond

those regarded as routine. More than 35 per cent of children and young people in Australia have at least one long-term chronic condition.
- Asthma, diabetes and cancer are the most common chronic medical conditions affecting both adults and children in Australia. Collectively, these three conditions account for almost 20 per cent of the burden of disease among children aged 0–14 years. There are many other neurological, congenital and genetic conditions that significantly impact on the growth, ability and wellbeing of children.
- Asthma is the most common long-term chronic condition, affecting almost 10 per cent of all Australian children aged 0–14 years. It is likely that, rather than being a single condition, asthma represents a spectrum of conditions with different pathophysiology, and may place considerable burden on the child and family. While most often associated with hypersensitivity to allergens, environmental, lifestyle and genetic factors also contribute to the development of childhood asthma. Asthma can be managed effectively with appropriate preventer treatment, the avoidance or control of trigger factors, appropriate medication and an individualised asthma-management plan.
- Type 1 diabetes (T1D) is an autoimmune condition affecting approximately one in every 300 children and young people in Australia. Incidence increases with age, peaking during early adolescence. Likely to be caused by an interaction of genetic and environmental factors, damage to the insulin-producing (beta cells) of the pancreas causes blood glucose levels to become elevated. The incidence of Type 2 diabetes (T2D) may be increasing among children and young people due to increased levels of obesity and physical inactivity. The main aim of management of both T1D and T2D is the regular monitoring of blood glucose to achieve control of blood glucose levels with insulin treatment. Long-term glycaemic control will optimise the prognosis of the disease and maintain quality of life, normal growth and psychological wellbeing.
- There is limited reporting of the personal, social, community and economic costs of congenital, chromosomal and genetic conditions affecting Australian children and young people. Common congenital conditions include hypospadias, neural tube defects such as spina bifida, cleft lip or palate, intestinal atresia or stenosis, and limb-reduction deficits. The most common chromosomal birth defect is Trisomy 21, or Down syndrome.
- Cystic fibrosis (CF) is the most common life-limiting autosomal recessive genetic condition affecting people of European/Caucasian decent, with an

incidence of approximately one in every 2800 live births in Australia. More than 1500 different mutations of the gene responsible for the symptoms of CF have now been identified. The spectrum of illness is characterised by lung and gastrointestinal complications, but there is great variance in symptoms and the systems affected. Neonatal screening has contributed to improving the treatment of respiratory and nutritional symptoms, as have concurrent improvements in coordinated, multidisciplinary, CF centre-based care, availability of bacteria-specific antibiotics, improved physiotherapy techniques for chest clearance and maintenance of normal growth through nutritional support and pancreatic enzyme-replacement therapy.

- Children with chronic physical and medical conditions who survive to adulthood will need to make a transition to adult care at some time during their adolescence or early adulthood. Previously, many children with chronic congenital and genetic conditions died before reaching adulthood; therefore, few adult physicians are trained to care for the adult consequences of these disorders. There is no 'right' time for transition, but setting a target transfer age is known to assist planning and aid transfer. The transition process often raises a variety of emotions for the young person and their family, and it is important for adult care providers to be aware of these emotions. Clear communication, early planning and the involvement of all stakeholders are features of successful transition programs.
- The availability and accessibility of evidence-based recommendations for the care of children and young people with chronic conditions are variable. However, the children and young people living with these conditions, and their parents and carers, have great insight into what does and does not work for them. The nursing care of chronically ill children and young people therefore relies on a sophisticated and informed integration of the best available evidence from research, and careful listening and learning from the experience and needs of the whole family.

Learning activities

10.1 Using the resource link in the Further Reading section below, consult the *Australian Asthma Handbook* to write an asthma-management plan for Joel. Joel is 6 years old and has been hospitalised twice for acute asthma. His mother has recently remarried, and he has two siblings, aged 6 months and 2.5 years.

10.2 Smartphone applications, or 'apps', are being developed to greater levels of sophistication every day. Undertake an internet search of smartphone apps for managing T1D and T2D, and discuss what you find. Do you think smartphone apps make managing diabetes easier for children and young people? Is there any potential for harm?

10.3 Undertake an investigation at your workplace and report on the processes, plans and resources available for young people with chronic conditions transitioning to adult health care. If you work in an adult hospital, what processes, plans or resources are in place for the young person transitioning to the adult health-care environment?

Further reading

Asthma

- *The Australian asthma handbook* (2014) is the National Asthma Council Australia's flagship publication, providing national guidelines for asthma management and forming the foundation of all our health professional resources. See <www.nationalasthma.org.au/handbook>.
- The International Study of Asthma and Allergies in Childhood (ISAAC) has become the largest worldwide collaborative research project ever undertaken, involving more than 100 countries and nearly 2 million children. See <http://isaac.auckland.ac.nz>.
- The Global Asthma Network was established in 2012 to improve asthma care globally, with a focus on low- and middle-income countries, through enhanced surveillance, research collaboration, capacity-building and access to quality-assured essential medicines. See <www.globalasthmanetwork.org/publications/publications.php>.
- The Global Initiative for Asthma (GINA) works with health-care professionals and public health officials around the world to reduce asthma prevalence, morbidity and mortality. See <www.ginasthma.org>.

Diabetes

- *Diabetes Kids and Teens* is a website for children and teens with T1D. See <www.diabeteskidsandteens.com.au/parents_and_carers_1.html>.

- The *National Evidence-Based Clinical Care Guidelines for Type 1 Diabetes for Children, Adolescents and Adults* were developed by the Australasian Paediatric Endocrine Group and the Australian Diabetes Society. See <www.nhmrc.gov.au/guidelines/publications/ext4>.

Cystic fibrosis

- The Cystic fibrosis Standards of Care, Australia were developed collaboratively by Cystic Fibrosis Australia and the Thoracic Society of Australia and New Zealand. See <www.thoracic.org.au/imagesDB/wysiwyg/CF_standardsofcare_Australia_2008.pdf>.
- Cystic fibrosis support service organisations exist in every major jurisdiction of Australia, supporting research and lobbying for better health and wellbeing outcomes for those living with CF. See <www.cysticfibrosis.org.au>.

Transition to adult care

- The NSW Agency for Clinical Innovation (ACI)'s Transition Care Network is one example of a state-based organisation aiming to improve the continuity of care for young people with chronic health problems as they move from paediatric to adult health services. See <www.aci.health.nsw.gov.au/networks/transition-care>.

References

Abeywardana, A & Sullivan, E 2008, *Congenital anomalies in Australia 2002–2003*, AIHW, Sydney.

Australian Bureau of Statistics (ABS) 2009, *National Health Survey: Summary of results 2007–2008*, cat. no. 4430.0, ABS, Canberra.

Australian Diabetes Council (ADC) 2012, *Australian Diabetes Council Bariatric Surgery Position Statement*, http://www.australiandiabetescouncil.com/ADCCorporateSite/files/58/58103fe2-9871-4eda-842a-eb42151b2c61.pdf.

Australian Institute of Health and Welfare (AIHW) 2011, *Prevalence of type 1 diabetes in Australian children 2008*, AIHW, Canberra, viewed 20 March 2014, http://www.aihw.gov.au/publication-detail/?id=10737419239.

——2012, *A picture of Australia's children 2012*, AIHW, Canberra.

—— 2014a, *Incidence of insulin-treated diabetes in Australia 2000–2011*, AIHW, Canberra.

—— 2014b, *Type 2 diabetes in Australia's children and young people: A working paper*, AIHW, Canberra.

Australian Physiotherapy Association (APA) 2009, *Position statement: Transition of young people with a chronic health condition to adult health services*, APA, Melbourne.

Begley, T 2013, Transition to adult care for young people with long-term conditions, *British Journal of Nursing*, 22(9), pp. 506–11.

Bell, S, Robinson, P & Fitzgerald, D 2008, *Cystic fibrosis standards of care, Australia 2008*, Cystic Fibrosis Australia, Sydney.

Betz, CL, Lobo, ML, Nehring, WM & Bui, K 2013, Voices not heard: A systematic review of adolescents' and emerging adults' perspectives of health care transition, *Nursing Outlook*, 61(5), pp. 311–36.

Bloom, SR et al. 2012, Health care transition for youth with special health care needs, *Journal of Adolescent Health*, 51(3), pp. 213–19.

Blue, G, Kirk, E, Sholler, G, Harvey, R & Winlaw, D 2012, Congenital heart disease: Current knowledge about causes and inheritance, *Medical Journal of Australia*, 197, pp. 155–9.

Blum, RWM et al. 1993, Transition from child-centered to adult-health care systems for adolescents with chronic conditions, *Journal of Adolescent Health*, 14, pp. 570–6.

Catanzariti, L et al. 2009, Australia's national trends in the incidence of type 1 diabetes in 0–14-year-olds, 2000–2006, *Diabetic Medicine*, 26(6), pp. 596–601.

Chesshir, C, Brown, C, Byerley, A & Ward-Begnoche, WL 2013, Transition of health care from pediatric to adult care, *Journal of Pediatric Nursing*, 28(5), pp. 497–501.

Craig, M et al. 2011, *National evidence-based clinical care guidelines of type 1 diabetes in children, adolescents and adults*, AGPS, Canberra.

Cystic Fibrosis Australia (CFA) 2013, *Cystic fibrosis in Australia 2012: 15th Annual Report from the Australian Cystic Fibrosis Registry*, CFA, Sydney.

Cystic Fibrosis Trust 2014, Transition, viewed 17 April 2014, http://www.cysticfibrosis.org.uk/about-cf/living-with-cystic-fibrosis/transition.

Dijk, F, McKay, K, Barzi, F, Gaskin, K & Fitzgerald, D 2011, Improved survival in cystic fibrosis patients diagnosed by newborn screening compared to a historical cohort from the same centre, *Archives of Disease in Childhood*, 96(12), pp. 1118–23.

Ellwood, P et al. 2013, Do fast foods cause asthma, rhinoconjunctivitis and eczema? Global findings from the International Study of Asthma and Allergies in Childhood (ISAAC) Phase Three, *Thorax*, 68, pp. 351–60.

Fegran, L, Hall, EOC, Uhrenfeldt, L, Aagaard, H & Ludvigsen, MS 2014, Adolescents' and young adults' transition experiences when transferring from paediatric to adult care: A qualitative metasynthesis, *International Journal of Nursing Studies*, 51(1), pp. 123–35.

Garvey, KC et al. 2012, Health care transition in patients with type 1 diabetes: Young adult experiences and relationship to glycemic control, *Diabetes Care*, 35(8), pp. 1716–22.

Global Initiative for Asthma (GINA) 2012, *Global strategy for asthma management and prevention*, viewed 20 March 2014, http://www.ginasthma.org.

Hilliard, ME et al. 2014, Perspectives from before and after the pediatric to adult care transition: A mixed-methods study in type 1 diabetes, *Diabetes Care*, 37(2), pp. 346–54.

Jermyn, V 2013, 'You can't stay here!' Transition from paediatric to adult health care management for liver transplant recipients, *Transplant Journal of Australasia*, 22(3), pp. 15–18.

Kaufmann Rauen, K et al. 2013, Transitioning adolescents and young adults with a chronic health condition to adult health care – an exemplar program, *Rehabilitation Nursing*, 38(2), pp. 63–72.

Khairy, P et al. 2010, Changing mortality in congenital heart disease, *Journal of the American College of Cardiology*, 56(14), pp. 1149–57.

McDevitt, T & Ormrod, J 2007, *Common chromosomal and genetic disorders in children*, viewed 20 March 2014, http://www.education.com/reference/article/chromosomal-genetic-disorders.

McInally, W 2013, Lost in transition: Child to adult cancer services for young people, *British Journal of Nursing*, 22(22), pp. 1314–18.

McManus, MA et al. 2013, Current status of transition preparation among youth with special needs in the United States, *Pediatrics*, 131(6), pp. 1090–7.

Ministry of Health (NSW) 2012, *Infants and children – acute management of asthma*, NSW Ministry of Health, Sydney.

National Asthma Council of Australia (NACA) 2014, *Australian asthma handbook*, viewed 20 March 2014, http://www.asthmahandbook.org.au.

Oswald, DP et al. 2013, Youth with special health care needs: Transition to adult health care services. *Maternal & Child Health Journal*, 17(10), pp. 1744–52.

Porter, JS, Graff, JC, Lopez, AD & Hankins, JS 2014, Transition from pediatric to adult care in sickle cell disease: Perspectives on the family role, *Journal of Pediatric Nursing*, 29(2), pp. 158–67.

Reid, D et al. 2011, Changes in cystic fibrosis mortality in Australia, 1979–2005, *Medical Journal of Australia*, 195(7), pp. 392–5.

Riordan, J et al. 1989, Identification of the cystic fibrosis gene: Cloning and characterization of complementary DNA, *Science*, 245(4922), pp. 1066–73.

Ritholz, MD et al. 2014, Patient–provider relationships across the transition from pediatric to adult diabetes care: A qualitative study, *Diabetes Educator*, 40(1), pp. 40–7.

Tuchman, L & Schwartz, M 2013, Health outcomes associated with transition from pediatric to adult cystic fibrosis care, *Pediatrics*, 132(5), pp. 847–53.

11 Evidence-based nursing assessments and interventions: The family

Ibi Patane and Elizabeth Forster

Learning objectives

In this chapter you will:

- Gain an understanding that the focus of paediatric nursing care is both the child or young person and their family
- Explore contemporary family characteristics relevant to paediatric nursing
- Explore models of paediatric nursing care that promote family partnership and involvement
- Gain an understanding of family assessment and apply family assessment models to a case
- Gain an understanding of important considerations when conducting family assessment

Introduction

In paediatric nursing, families are central to the care of children – in fact, our patient is considered to be both the child and their whole family. In this chapter, you will explore what it means to be a family, models of paediatric nursing care that emphasise a focus on the child and family, and frameworks that can be used to assess families in paediatric nursing practice. You also will consider some of the tensions or challenges experienced by paediatric nurses when they care and advocate for children and families.

Families in contemporary Australian society

Families in Australia today are diverse in terms of their structure, membership and functions, and this makes the concept of 'family' quite challenging to define. It is perhaps useful to think of McCaffery's (1968) reference to pain as being 'whatever the patient says it is' and consider families to be defined by their members: even though members of a family may have no blood relation, they may consider themselves to be a family.

Contemporary Australian families may be:

- experiencing or adjusting to marital breakdown
- lone-parent households
- blended or step-families
- same-sex parents with children
- migrant and refugee families
- culturally and linguistically diverse
- experiencing domestic violence or coping with disability, injury or illness.
(Hayes et al., 2010; AIPC, 2012)

The nature of families has an impact on child health and wellbeing, and families are instrumental in ensuring that children's needs are met from birth through to adolescence and beyond. Families are the social connection between their members and the outside world, and are responsible for role modelling and socialisation. Negative or disruptive family functioning or environments in early childhood can have a lasting impact on a child's social, cognitive and emotional development, and these effects may be transferred to the next generation (Munns & Shields, 2013).

There are a variety of models that recognise and promote family involvement and participation in a child's care, and in this chapter we will look at two of these models: the Family Partnership Model and family-centred care.

Family Partnership Model

The Family Partnership Model was developed in the United Kingdom by the Centre for Parent and Child Support (Davis et al., 2002), and its original focus was to support early intervention in child mental health. It has been used internationally and within Australia, primarily within community child health practice. The principles, however, are relevant to any context where nurses are caring for children and their families. The Family Partnership Model aims to assist parents and children to:

- identify and build upon their strengths
- clarify and manage problems

- develop resilience and the ability to anticipate problems
- enhance/improve child development and wellbeing
- harness social support. (Davis et al., 2007)

The model also aims to foster community development and services development and improvement.

The model also outlines a variety of helper qualities, including respect, genuineness, empathy, humility, quiet enthusiasm, personal strength and integrity, as well as intellectual and emotional attunement (Davis et al., 2007). In addition, helpers use a variety of communication, problem-solving and negotiation skills in establishing an effective partnership with parents and implementing the helping process.

Child health nurses who have trained within the Family Partnership Model and used it in practice have described a shift in their practice so that they are moving away from telling parents what to do to solve a problem towards exploring and facilitating parent needs – that is, asking parents what the nurse could do to assist and what parents want from the nurse, which places greater emphasis on parent control during interactions (Fowler et al., 2012). Nurses also develop skills within the foundation of a trusting relationship with families to challenge negative constructions in order to 'develop different, more positive ways of thinking about issues' (Fowler et al., 2012).

Family-centred care

'Family-centred care' is a phrase that has had a variety of definitions and has been conceptualised in many ways. It is seen as a paradigm, a philosophy, a model of care and a practice theory (Mikkelsen & Frederiksen, 2011). For the purposes of this chapter, it will be seen as a model of paediatric nursing care, and will be defined using two definitions:

> A way of caring for children and their families within health services which ensures that care is planned around the whole family, not just the individual child/person, and in which all the family members are recognised as care recipients. (Shields et al., 2006)

> This support and care is delivered through a process of involvement, participation, and partnership underpinned by empowerment and negotiation. (Lambert et al., 2008)

Family-centred care is the most frequently used model to enhance the involvement of parents in their child's health care and, as seen in the above definitions, the focus for care is the child and all the family members (Coyne, 2013). Despite its widespread use in paediatric nursing care, there remains limited evidence that it impacts on outcomes despite a strong agreement among clinicians that it has benefits for both children and their families (Coyne, 2013; Shields, 2010).

Family-centred care has its challenges and, despite its popularity, its definition remains unclear in many settings, and its actual application in clinical practice has been questioned and scrutinised (Kuo et al., 2012). This may be because it contrasts with more traditional approaches to care, where responsibility and control rest with health-care professionals rather than parents (Kuo et al., 2012).

Some of the problems with its application in clinical settings are thought to be due to inadequacies in knowledge and skills, the increasing stress clinicians encounter in fulfilling their roles, problems with negotiation processes and power struggles between clinicians and parents, as well as insufficient organisational supports for its implementation (Coyne, 2013). Communication with families and the negotiation of care are sometimes challenging, and this is another reason for the problems that have emerged with the implementation of family-centred care, as reported by nurses (Coyne, 2013). Some clinicians may not like to relinquish control of certain aspects of care to parents, and this undermines the notion of partnership that is central to family-centred care (Coyne et al., 2011).

Reflection points 11.1

- Families may be quite diverse in terms of their composition and structure. In Australia, contemporary families may be adjusting to marital breakdown, be sole-parent, blended or same-sex parent families, be culturally and linguistically diverse, be experiencing stressors associated with domestic violence, have migration or refugee concerns, or be coping with a family member's disability, injury or illness.
- The Family Partnership Model can be used by nurses to enhance family strengths, problem-solving and resilience in order to optimise child development and wellbeing. It necessitates a shift away from traditional nurse-controlled way of approaching care towards care that explores and facilitates parents' preferences and needs.
- Family-centred care is a model of paediatric nursing care where the child and the whole family are the focus of care; it is underpinned by family involvement, participation and partnership in the child's care. Nurses caring

- for children continually negotiate with and empower parents to be involved in their child's care.
- Family assessment is integral to planning and providing family-centred care. All families have strengths that will assist them to develop resilience and adapt to stressors.

Family assessment

In order to provide a high standard of care to children and families, we need to understand the roles, functions, strengths and limitations, stressors and coping strategies that families engage in or experience. Family assessment is a way to ascertain information about each family and to explore how a health problem experienced by one of its members impacts upon the family.

A variety of family assessment models exist and are used by paediatric nurses – for example, the Calgary Family Assessment Model and the Friedman Family Assessment tool. Most assessment models will have a few elements of assessment in common, which usually include:

- a family genogram/ecomap or visual representation of the family structure
- assessment of the developmental stage of the family
- assessment of roles and functions within the family
- assessment of stressors experienced by the family
- assessment of coping strategies utilised by the family.

We will now discuss these elements of family assessment so that you have a good understanding of these in your paediatric nursing practice.

Family genogram/ecomap

The structure of the family is important to understand when considering family assessment. This can often be complex to explain, and **genograms** are a diagrammatic way to map the family structure and each person's relationship within the family unit in relation to the patient.

Figure 11.1 shows a simple genogram of a typical family, with both partners having remarried. The square shapes symbolise males and the circles females, with lines indicating relationships and crosses through lines indicating relationships that have ended (such as by death or divorce). The children are mapped and connected to their parents. The patient who is the focus of the genogram, Milly, is highlighted.

> **Genogram**
> A visual representation of a family's structure and relationships in respect to the patient of focus. Some may also include ages and health problems

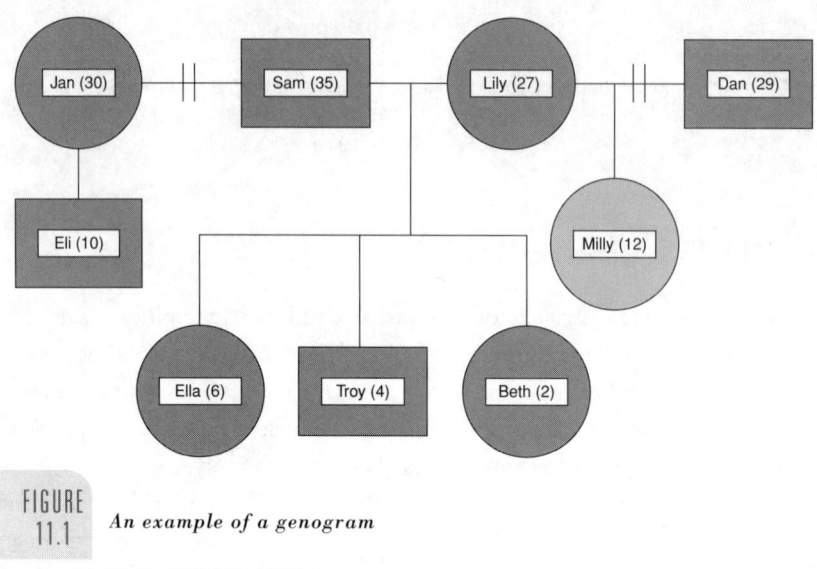

FIGURE 11.1 *An example of a genogram*

Further, the nurse can explore the family's interactions within their community and map these external interactions (Holtslander et al., 2013). These diagrams are called **ecomaps**, and can be useful when assisting families to draw on resources to assist them by identifying their current supports. The family is central in the ecomap, and the support systems are mapped, with the number and boldness of the connecting lines indicating the strength of the relationship and support (Neves et al., 2013). As shown in the ecomap in Figure 11.2, the couple report moderate support from each, and only one strong source of support from their community. One potential source of support is not linked at all; this could be family who may be geographically distant.

Ecomap A visual representation of the identified supports of the family unit

Family development

Family development can be understood from a variety of standpoints. Family developmental theory and family life-cycle stages (Carter & McGoldrick, 1999) are two ways of thinking about family development. Essentially, it is thought that family roles and tasks are influenced by the stage of the family. For example, a family with teenagers is likely to have different roles and focus from a beginning family experiencing the birth of their first child. Understanding the stages of development experienced by families over a lifetime can give

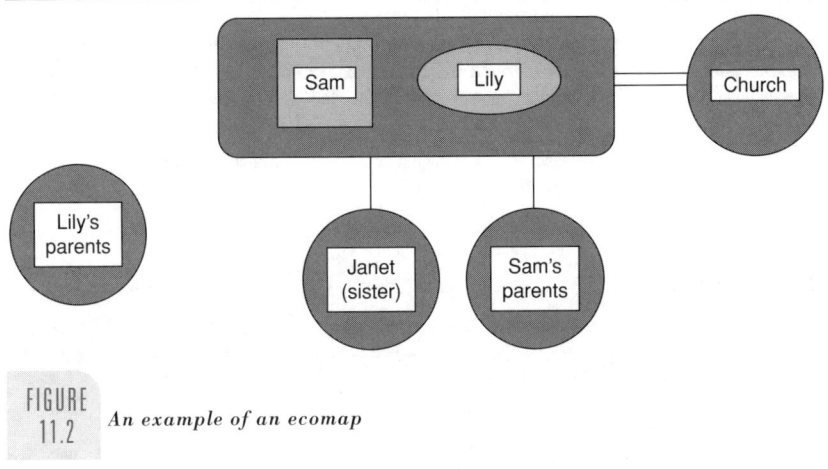

FIGURE 11.2 *An example of an ecomap*

paediatric nurses an understanding of significant events, challenges, roles and tasks that may occur during these times.

Carter and McGoldrick's (1999) family life-cycle stages include:

- leaving home: single young adults
- the joining of family through marriage: the new couple
- families with young children
- families with adolescents
- launching children and moving on
- families in later life.

One of the early criticisms of this model was that it was based on understandings of middle-class North American families, and therefore did not consider the dynamic and diverse nature of the families that exist in society today. Since it was first developed, a variety of other family life-cycle models have been developed and introduced, including family life-cycles for divorced and remarried, professional and low-income, adoptive and homosexual, bisexual and transgendered families (Wright & Leahey, 2009). The development of these family life-cycles reflects the limitations of a single model in terms of understanding family development across the lifespan, and acknowledges that families are diverse and constantly changing.

At each stage during the life-cycle, families have particular tasks to fulfil, and attachments between members form and change. Table 11.1 summarises some of the tasks and attachments that may be significant at each stage.

TABLE 11.1 *Family life-cycle stage tasks and attachments*

FAMILY LIFE-CYCLE STAGE	TASKS	ATTACHMENTS
Leaving home: single young adults	Differentiation of self in relation to family of origin	Attachment between young adults and their respective parents
	Development of intimate peer relationships	Attachment between parents
	Establishment of self in relation to work and financial independence	
The joining of family through marriage: the new couple	Establishment of couple identify	Attachments between spouses
	Realignment of relationships with extended families to include spouse	Attachments between each spouse and their respective families of origin
	Decisions about parenthood	Attachments with outside interests
Families with young children	Adjusting the marital system to make space for the child	Attachments between parents
	Joining in child-rearing, financial and household tasks	Attachments between parents and children
	Realignment of relationships with extended family to include parenting and grandparenting roles	Attachments between siblings
Families with adolescents	Adjusting parent–child relationships to allow adolescents to move in/out of the family system	Possible decrease in parental attachment for adolescent
	Mid-life marital and career issues	Adolescent attachment with peer group
	Beginning shift towards joint caring for the older generation	Attachment between family members
Launching children and moving on	Renegotiation of marital dyad	Attachments between family members
	Development of adult-to-adult relationships between parents and grown children	Attachments to outside interests
	Realignment of relationships to include in-laws and grown children	
	Dealing with disabilities and death of grandparents	
Families in later life	Maintaining own or couple functioning and interest in the face of physiological decline: exploration of new familial and social role options	Interdependence with the next generation
	Making room for the wisdom and experience of seniors	Intergenerational attachments, especially between daughters and parents
	Dealing with loss of spouse, siblings, peers and preparation for death	

Source: Adapted from Wright and Leahey (2009).

Family roles and functions

Families exist to meet the needs of the individuals within the family, and to expand through reproductive functions and ensure socialisation of new family members.

The main functions of the family can be summarised as follows:

- affective function – meeting psychological needs
- social function – meeting social needs and ensuring children become productive within their social group
- reproductive function
- economic function
- health-care function. (Friedman et al., 2003)

However, over time, traditional roles within the family have changed. Men were typically the 'breadwinners', who provided economic support, and women were the 'homemakers', who provided for the social and health needs of the family. Many families today choose not to have children or are non-traditional in the way they practise gender roles within the family. Families no longer live in extended groups, and form smaller, more isolated groups called 'nuclear families'. This limits support and impacts families in terms of economic, social and educative support. For example, previously new mothers experienced the support of older females in their family group with initiating and maintaining breastfeeding through the wisdom of experience, and received practical support in the care of their other children after birth. Today, families typically live in nuclear groups with often wide geographical distance between extended family members, and this support is often lacking.

Existing family-assessment frameworks have been criticised in terms of their use in Aboriginal and Torres Strait Islander families because of the diversity of family structure, geographical location and patterns of mobility among these families, as well as the limitations of these models in considering Aboriginal and Torres Strait Islander peoples' identity, spirituality and social and community lifestyle (Walker & Shepherd, 2008). Beween 2000 and 2002, a measure of Aboriginal family functioning was developed based on McCubbin & McCubbin's (1989) model of family protective factors and administered as part of the Western Australian Aboriginal Child Health Survey. This measure of Aboriginal family functioning was developed in collaboration with Aboriginal health professionals, and consisted of nine statements about family functioning to which family members can respond to in a five-point rating scale (based on the McMaster Family Assessment Device) from 'not at all' to 'very much'. The nine statements about family functioning include:

- The way we get together helps us to cope with the hard times.
- We like to remember people's birthdays and celebrate other special events.
- We find it easy to talk with each other about the things that really matter.
- We are always there for each other and know that the family will survive no matter what.
- When it comes to managing money we are careful and make good decisions.
- Our family has a lot in common in the interests we share and the things we do.
- People in our family are accepted for who they are.
- We have good support from our in-laws, relatives and friends.
- We have family traditions and customs we would like to pass on to our children. (Western Australian Aboriginal Child Health Survey, 2005: 602)

Stressors

Contemporary families cope with many day-to-day stressors. Common stressors for modern families are balancing a working life with the constant demands of raising children. However, there are more severe stressors that bring about change within a family unit. These can have a significant impact on children's development, and the family's strength and capacity to cope and develop resilience are important factors.

Such stressors can be major life events, such as death within the family or parental conflict, or they may be ongoing stressors, such as chronic disease and low socioeconomic status. High family stress correlates with a lower satisfaction with life in adolescents (Chappel et al., 2014). It is also known that accumulated stressors add to the burden. If children and their families do not adapt well to stress, this can lead to academic, interpersonal and emotional difficulties later in life

(Valdez et al., 2013). Therefore, it is important for nurses to guide families towards positive coping strategies, as discussed in the next section.

Coping strategies

Each family has its own culture, and will thus develop its own coping skills. When faced with stressors such as the experience of a severely or chronically ill child, family members may react in different ways. Coping is defined by Friedman and colleagues (2003: 466) as 'problem solving efforts by an individual'. These can be positive or negative. Coping was originally conceptualised as being either **emotion-focused coping** or **problem-focused coping**, with the first involving the regulation of negative emotions using strategies such as distancing, seeking emotional support or avoidance, and the second type involving a planned approach to addressing the problem using information-seeking and decision-making (Folkman, 2013). More recently, a third type of coping, known as **meaning-focused coping**, has been proposed, and includes drawing upon inner beliefs and values, revising goals, focusing on the strengths obtained through experience and reorganising priorities (Folkman, 2013).

Families have strengths that will enable them to develop coping skills when faced with stress. These are listed by Feeley and Gottlieb (2000) as their individual family traits, assets, capabilities and qualities such as motivation. Understanding the context of the family and the way each member of the family is situated in that family group (Jokinen, 2004) may assist you to identify and justify the coping strategies employed by that family and provide guidance towards positive coping strategies.

Gender is an important influence when it comes to coping, and mothers and fathers may have quite different coping styles (Brown et al., 2013). For example, in a study of parents whose child had been diagnosed with developmental delay, it was found that mothers tended to engage in emotion-focused coping whereas fathers used a more cognitive and logical style of coping (Barak-Levy & Atzaba-Poria, 2013).

Emotion-focused coping A style of coping where individuals use strategies such as distancing, seeking emotional support or avoidance in order to manage negative emotions

Problem-focused coping A style of coping where individuals use a planned approach to addressing problems, using strategies such as information-seeking and decision-making

Meaning-focused coping A style of coping often found among individuals encountering life-change events such as the critical illness or loss of a family member. Individuals draw upon their inner beliefs and values, revise goals, focus on the strengths gained from the life experience and reorganise their priorities

Families cope with stress in many ways. Table 11.2 summarises some of the coping strategies that can be seen in families that are experiencing stressful situations.

TABLE 11.2 *Family stress, coping and adaptation*

INTERNAL FAMILY COPING STRATEGIES	EXTERNAL FAMILY COPING STRATEGIES	DYSFUNCTIONAL FAMILY COPING STRATEGIES
Developing enhanced relationships within the family: • relying on each other • strengthening cohesion • developing flexible roles	Family social supports: • use of relatives and extended family as support • seeking advice from relatives • practical support from relatives	Denial of family problems and reactive behaviours such as: • emotional exploitation • blaming (scapegoating) • use of family myths that 'obscure reality and deny real issues' • triangulating of communication – using a third person to choose sides • authoritarianism
Cognitive strategies • being as 'normal' as possible • passive acceptance • 'reframing' expectations and maintain a positive outlook • joint problem-solving • being highly informed	Social support of friends: • seeking encouragement and support of friends • sharing concerns with friends • seeking information/ advice from friends, particularly those who have experienced similar problems	Family dissolution and addiction: • use of alcohol • use of drugs • use of gambling leading to family psychosocial issues of loss, abandonment, breakdown
Communication strategies: • honesty and openness • use of humour and laughter	Maintaining links in the community: • self-help groups • spiritual supports, including religious affiliations • more recently – social media networks	Family violence: • partner abuse • child abuse or neglect • sibling abuse or neglect • parent abuse

Source: Adapted from Friedman et al. (2003).

Clearly, families employ both positive and negative coping strategies when faced with stress. The serious or chronic illness of a child may cause families to react with guilt, fear, shock, uncertainty or grief (Jokinen, 2004), but then adaptive mechanisms will be employed to cope with the new 'normal'. It is important to identify a family's strengths and their available resources to guide them towards positive coping adaptation (Holtslander et al., 2013).

Case study 11.1 Audrey

You are working in a small hospital in a rural area. Audrey is an 8-year-old girl who has been brought to the hospital by ambulance following a severe asthma attack at her home during the night. This is her fourth admission for asthma in the last six months, and she has missed her last two scheduled outpatients appointments.

Audrey is not accompanied by her mother in the ambulance, and her mother, Conchetta, arrives about one-and-a-half hours later with her three younger children, all preschool-aged. Conchetta discloses that she could not come in the ambulance as her husband, Trevor, is a fly-in, fly-out mine worker who is currently away on a week-long shift.

Conchetta, 28, arrived in Australia six years ago from the Philippines with her daughter Audrey, and is now married to Trevor, 53. They have since had a further three children, now aged 3 years, 2 years and 6 months. They live in a rural area about 30 minutes' drive outside a small town, where they are renting a house on 2 hectares. Conchetta states that 'this always happens when Trevor is away. It is very difficult to cope with all the children when he's away, but he is very helpful when he is home. I don't know how I am going to spend time with Audrey this time in the hospital.' Conchetta has no other family in Australia, but reports a close relationship with her church, and says she has a friend 2 kilometres away, with whom she is quite friendly, and a sister-in-law who provides occasional help with the children.

Considerations and challenges in conducting family assessments

It is essential that nurses perform effective family assessments so they can plan and provide appropriate nursing care (Wright & Leahy, 2009). Family assessment is often complex, but it is fundamental if we are to provide family-centred care and meet the needs of the child and their family.

However, it is often difficult in practice to perform effective family assessment, and there can be many reasons for this. To perform a detailed effective assessment, time is required, and this is often difficult to achieve in a busy clinical day (Marron & Maginnis, 2009). It is also important that interruptions are minimised. As with any assessment process, the environment must be appropriate, with adequate privacy and comfort for the participants. The presence of the child or other children is often enough of a distractor, without the busy clinical environment also impinging on the process.

Kylie

Case study 11.2

Kylie is a 21-year-old mother to 6-month-old Skye, who has been admitted to the babies ward with severe diaper dermatitis. Kylie is a patient in a methadone program as she struggles to overcome her drug addictions. Her partner, Steve, is a recovering alcoholic and has sole custody of his 3-year-old son, Lucas. Skye has been seen by the Suspected Child Abuse and Neglect (SCAN) team on a previous admission at 1 month of age for failure to thrive. Kylie and Steve live in a caravan park an hour's drive from the hospital. In the few days since Skye's admission, you have heard other nurses making very critical and judgemental comments about Kylie and her parenting ability. You have noticed that Kylie hasn't been visiting as much during the day and did not stay overnight last night. When you ask Kylie how she's going, she bursts into tears and says, 'All you nurses are such bitches – you make out like I'm a bad mother and I don't need this crap. I'm taking Skye home right now. I don't care if it's against orders!'

When doing family assessments, it is necessary to form a therapeutic relationship with the family to encourage disclosure (Holtslander et al., 2013). Many nurses report discomfort with approaching more difficult topics such as child abuse or domestic violence, which may make them feel uncomfortable or challenged (Marron & Maginnis, 2009). This can be difficult for the family member to discuss, and may not be possible when the child or other family members are present. There can also be an emotional impact for you as the nurse, based on your own family experiences (Lee et al., 2012). Therefore, you need to be aware of your own feelings and prejudices when you are working with families, and be careful not to be judgemental or have preconceived ideas of what families should be or how they should behave.

When caring for children and families where domestic violence, substance abuse or child protection issues are present, it may be helpful to consider such parents as experiencing their own multi-faceted health problems, which are often the result of their own adverse life experiences. A study exploring parent perspectives of their experiences with child-protection services highlighted that many parents who are engaged with child-protection services have themselves been subjected to abuse or rejection as children, and are often marginalised as adults (Maiter et al., 2006). These experiences can undermine their ability to form effective relationships with others (Maiter et al., 2006). In addition, mothers who are struggling with substance abuse have often been subjected to previous trauma in their lives, or may have mental health problems such as anxiety or depression (Cleveland & Gill, 2013). When parents are being investigated in relation to child protection, they often feel extremely vulnerable and have the greatest need for support (Maiter et al., 2006). Such mothers feel that they are constantly being watched and their parenting judged, with the possibility of their children being removed an ongoing threat (Reid et al., 2008). If, at these times, they are met with a lack of care or judgemental attitudes by health-care professionals, this can worsen their vulnerability and sense of isolation. Sadly, health-care professionals working with these families have been found to be judgemental and uncaring, and have labelled parents unfairly (Maiter et al., 2006).

The relationship between nurses and mothers can have a powerful effect on the mother–child relationship and engender greater confidence and assertiveness in the mothering role (Cleveland & Gill, 2013). Nurses who express caring towards both mother and baby, and who engage mothers in the care of their infant, are valued by mothers who are struggling with drug addiction. Conversely, nonverbal behaviours such as eye-rolling, obvious surveillance and judgemental conversations among staff are a heavy burden for mothers, who perceive that nurses fail to see the person behind the drug addiction and don't notice their efforts to be a good mother (Cleveland & Gill, 2013).

Nurse can empower mothers by ensuring they collaborate with mothers, rather than treating them as if they are inferior. Reducing real or perceived power differentials is essential for an effective helping relationship (Maiter et al., 2006; Carter, 2002). Some nurses working with mothers experiencing drug addiction and their babies describe working in parallel rather than in partnership with these families and, rather than embodying a family-centred care approach, consider the baby to be the focus of care (Fraser et al., 2007). Nurses can speak out against unprofessional care and encourage mothers to make formal complaints if they receive such care. They can role-model their regard and respect for the dignity of mothers like Kylie in Case Study 11.2. Placing mothers like Kylie in touch with supports to continue with her recovery from drug addiction, and giving praise for positive interactions with her baby and good parenting are also important. Parents appreciate health-care professionals who are genuine, empathetic, helpful, willing to listen, non-judgemental and accepting (Maiter et al., 2006).

Cultural safety Awareness of one's own cultural identity and attitudes, and how these might influence patient care; implementing care that is acceptable to and promotes a sense of safety among patients and their families regardless of background or cultural identity

When approaching any family, the concept of **cultural safety** should be considered. Cultural safety was first introduced in the

1980s, and encourages nurses to reflect upon their own cultural identities and attitudes, and how these might influence the way they interact with others (De & Richardson, 2008). We need to be open and accepting in our communication with others.

Nurses should not make assumptions about families based on gender, culture, ethnic, political or religious background, since these groups may not be homogeneous (Manchester, 2013). However, these considerations can be incorporated into your family assessment. It is important to remember that culture is not necessarily linked to ethnicity, although this is a common belief (Manchester, 2013; De & Richardson, 2008). We are all members of many cultures, and this will change as we move through life stages and our needs alter (Friedman et al., 2003). For example, as a nursing student, you are part of the university culture and way of life, and you will move into the workplace culture when you graduate. You will move through many different cultures in your personal and professional life.

Developing an understanding of the individual family's cultural, ethnic and spiritual perspective will assist you to understand the family and their needs, which contributes to care planning. Asking open-ended questions can lead to deeper exploration of these topics. This will help you understand the family's needs and their basis for decision-making in order to provide culturally safe, sensitive and individualised care (McEvoy, 2003).

These are some of the reasons why, in practice, a detailed family assessment is often not performed or is ineffective. As a nurse, you need to identify those children and families who require detailed family assessment – and this may involve referral to other health professionals, particularly social workers, who are experts in interviewing and family assessment.

Summary

- Within paediatric nursing, the patient is considered to be both the child and all members of their family. Nurses need to assess, plan, implement and evaluate care in conjunction with the child and family.
- The Family Partnership Model and family-centred care are two models that recognise the centrality of families in paediatric nursing and encourage nurses to work in partnership with families to ensure optimal health outcomes for the child and their family.
- Family assessment is integral to the effective care of children and families, and incorporates consideration of family composition, structure, family

development/life-cycle stage, roles and functioning, stressors and coping strategies.
- When conducting family assessments, nurses need to be mindful of their verbal and nonverbal communication skills, the environment, and their own influences and perceptions, which may consciously or unconsciously impact on communication with and assumptions about families.

Learning activities

11.1 Re-read Case Study 11.1. Draw a genogram of this family's structure. Try drawing an ecomap of Conchetta's support system.

11.2 Based on your reading so far, what life-cycle stage is this family in?

11.3 Some aspects of this case study may challenge your belief system. Consider these and explain why this may be so.

11.4 What are the stressors for both Audrey and Conchetta? Write these down and then consider how these could be useful when planning care for Audrey in the context of her family.

11.5 What are some of the risks you can identify for this family? What are some positive coping strategies with which you could assist Conchetta?

Further reading

Holtslander, L, Solar, J & Smith, NR 2013, The 15-minute family interview as a learning strategy for senior undergraduate nursing students, *Journal of Family Nursing*, 19(2), pp. 230–48. This article provides a concise overview of, and guide for conducting, documenting and reflecting upon, a short family-assessment interview. It is a useful reading to prepare for conducting a family assessment interview.

References

Australian Institute of Professional Counsellors (AIPC) 2012, Trends and statistics of the contemporary family, viewed 24 March 2014, http://www.aipc.net.au/articles/trends-and-statistics-of-the-contemporary-family.

Barak-Levy, Y & Atzaba-Poria, N 2013, Paternal versus maternal coping styles with child diagnosis of developmental delay, *Research in Developmental Disabilities*, 34(6), pp. 2040–6.

Brown, F, Whittingham, K, Boyd R & Sofronoff, K 2013, Parenting a child with traumatic brain injury: Experiences of parents and health professionals, *Brain Injury*, 27(13–14), pp. 1570–82.

Carter, CS 2002, Perinatal care for women who are addicted: Implications for empowerment, *Health & Social Work*, 27(3), pp. 166–74.

Carter, EA & McGoldrick, M 1999, *The expanded family life cycle: Individual, family, and social perspectives*, Allyn and Bacon, Boston.

Chappel, AM, Suldo, S & Ogg, JA 2014, Association between adolescents' family stressors and life satisfaction, *Journal of Child & Family Studies*, 23, pp. 76–84.

Cleveland, L & Gill, S 2013, Try not to judge: Mothers of substance-exposed infants, *American Journal of Maternal Child Nursing*, 38(4), pp. 200–5.

Coyne, I 2013, Families and health-care professionals' perspectives and expectations of family-centred care: Hidden expectations and unclear roles, *Health Expectations*, doi: 10.1111/hex.12104.

Coyne, I, O'Neill, C, Murphy, M, Costello, T & O'Shea, R 2011, What does family-centred care mean to nurses and how do they think it could be enhanced in practice? *Journal of Advanced Nursing*, 67(12), pp. 2561–73.

Davis, H, Day, C & Bidmead, C 2002, *Working in partnership with parents: The parent advisor model*, Psychological Corporation, London.

Davis, H, Day, C, Bidmead, C, MacGrath, M & Ellis, M 2007, Current family partnership model, Centre for Parent and Child Support, viewed 25 March 2014, http://www.cpcs.org.uk/uploads/downloads/family%20partnership%20model/Current%20FPM%20Framework.pdf.

De, D & Richardson, J 2008, Cultural safety: An introduction, *Paediatric Nursing*, 20(2), pp. 39–43.

Feeley, N & Gottlieb, LN 2000, Nursing approaches for working with family strengths and resources, *Journal of Family Nursing*, 6, pp. 9–24.

Folkman, S 2013, Stress, coping and hope, in BI Carr & J Steel (eds), *Psychological aspects of cancer*, Springer, Berkeley, CA, pp. 119–127.

Fowler, C et al. 2012, Working in partnership with parents: The experience and challenge of practice innovation in child and family health nursing, *Journal of Clinical Nursing*, 21, pp. 3306–14.

Fraser, JA, Barnes, M, Biggs, HC & Kain, VJ 2007, Caring, chaos and the vulnerable family: Experiences in caring for newborns of drug-dependent parents, *International Journal of Nursing Studies*, 44(8), pp. 1363–70.

Friedman, MM, Bowden, VR & Jones, EG 2003, Family stress, coping and adaptation. In MM Friedman, VR Bowden & EG Jones, *Family Nursing. Research, Theory and Practice*, Pearson Education, Englewood Cliffs, NJ, pp. 463–510.

Hayes, A, Weston, R, Qu, L & Gray, M 2010, *Families then and now 1980–2010*, Australian Institute of Family Studies, Melbourne.

Holtslander, L, Solar, J & Smith, NR 2013, The 15-minute interview as a learning strategy for senior undergraduate nursing students, *Journal of Family Nursing*, 19(2), pp. 230–48.

Jokinen, P 2004, The family life-path theory: A tool for nurses working in partnership with families, *Journal of Child Health Care*, 8(2), pp. 124–33.

Kuo, DZ et al. 2012, Family-centred care: Current applications and future directions in pediatric health care, *Maternal Child Health Journal*, 16, pp. 297–305.

Lambert, V, Glacken, M & McCarron, M 2008, 'Visible-ness': The nature of communication for children admitted to a specialist children's hospital in the Republic of Ireland, *Journal of Clinical Nursing*, 17(23), pp. 3092–102.

Lee, ACK, Leung, SSK & Mak, YW 2012, The application of family-nursing assessment skills: From classroom to hospital ward among final-year nursing undergraduates in Hong Kong, *Nurse Education Today*, 32, pp. 78–84.

Maiter. S, Palmer, S & Manji, S 2006, Strengthening social worker–client relationships in child protective services: Addressing power imbalances and 'ruptured' relationships, *Qualitative Social Work: Research and Practice*, 5(2), pp. 167–86.

Manchester, A 2013, Cultural safety should be reviewed, *Kai Tiaki Nursing New Zealand*, 19(9), p. 14.

Marron, CA & Maginnis, C 2009, Implementing family health assessment: Experiences of child health nurses, *Neonatal, Paediatric and Child Health Nursing*, 12(1), pp. 3–8.

McCaffery, M 1968, Nursing practice theories related to cognition, bodily pain and man–environment interactions, UCLA Student Store, Los Angeles, CA.

McCubbin, HI & McCubbin, MA 1989, Families coping with illness: The resiliency model of family stress, adjustment and adaptation. In CB Danielson, B Hansel-Bissel & P Winstead-Fry (eds), *Families, health, & illness: Perspectives on coping and interventions*, Mosby, St Louis, MO.

McEvoy, M 2003, Culture and spirituality as an integrated concept in pediatric care, *American Journal of Maternal Child Nursing*, 28(1), pp. 39–43.

Mikkelsen, G & Frederiksen, K 2011, Family-centred care of children in hospital: A concept analysis, *Journal of Advanced Nursing*, 67(5), pp. 1152–62.

Munns, A & Shields, L 2013, Indigenous families' use of a tertiary paediatric hospital in Australia, *Nursing Children and Young People*, 25(7), pp. 16–23.

Neves, ET, Cabral, IE & da Silveira, A 2013, Family network of children with special needs: Implications for nursing. *Review Latino-Am Emfermagem*, 21(2), pp. 562–70.

Reid, C, Greaves, L & Poole, N 2008, Good, bad, thwarted or addicted? Discourses of substance-abusing mothers, *Critical Social Policy*, 28(2), pp. 211–34.

Shields, L 2010, Questioning family centred care, *Journal of Clinical Nursing*, 7(18), pp. 2629–38.

Shields, L, Pratt, J & Hunter, J 2006, Family centred care: A review of qualitative studies, *Journal of Clinical Nursing*, 15(10), pp. 1317–23.

Valdez, CR, Chavez, T & Woulfe, J 2013, Emerging adults' lived experience of formative family stress: The family's lasting influence, *Qualitative Health Research*, 23(8), pp. 1089–1102.

Walker, R & Shepherd, C 2008, Strengthening Aboriginal family functioning: What works and why? *Australian Family Relationships Clearinghouse Briefing*, 7, pp. 1–11.

Western Australian Aboriginal Child Health Survey 2005, viewed 15 June 2014, http://aboriginal.telethonkids.org.au/media/399793/measuring_social_and_emotional_wellbeing.pdf.

Wright, LM and Leahey, M 2009, *Nurses and families: A guide to family assessment and intervention*, 5th edn, FA Davis, Philadelphia.

12 Evidence-based care of children with complex medical needs

Nicola Brown

Learning objectives

In this chapter you will:

- Develop your understanding of evidence-based nursing assessments and interventions used in the care of infants, children and young people with complex medical needs

- Explore causes of complex medical health problems in children and young people

- Appreciate the critical role of families in the care of children with complex medical needs

- Consider resources and services available to families of children and young people with complex medical needs

Introduction

Children with complex medical needs and their families are important and frequent consumers of paediatric health-care services (Burns et al., 2011); however, their needs are not always met (Kirk & Glendinning, 2004; Noyes et al., 2014). These children are most frequently cared for at home, with parents primarily responsible for their day-to-day care. Children and young people with such needs are likely to require multidisciplinary team management, frequent use of out-patient and in-patient services, psychosocial and socioeconomic support, and resources to maintain health and enable participation in school and other activities of daily living (Burns et al., 2011). The care parents may be required to provide at home is likely to include procedural care such as suctioning or medication administration, and physical care such as manual handling, feeding and toileting (Rehm, 2013).

Children and young people who are dependent on medical technology have a higher risk of severe acute illness and are more likely to require admission to an intensive-care unit (Burns et al., 2011; Rehm, 2013). Furthermore, some illness may be life-limiting, resulting in premature death in childhood, adolescence or early adulthood. As a result, some children and young people may require palliative care services towards the end of their illness.

It can be difficult to determine when a child with a chronic condition can be defined as having complex medical needs. What one family finds complex, another family may adapt to more easily. One child with a particular condition may have less severity and more function than another child with the same or a similar condition. Furthermore, the discussion around the care of children with complex medical needs has often used different terms for similar things – care that is 'medically complex', or children who are 'technology dependent' or 'medically frail'. For the purposes of this chapter, children with complex medical needs are defined as those children with substantial family-identified needs, characteristic complex and/or chronic conditions, functional limitations and high health-care use (Cohen et al., 2011).

In this chapter, we will explore some of the causes of complex medical needs in children and young people, and discuss related nursing care and interventions. The important and central role of parents, caregivers and families in the care of children with complex medical needs will also be considered.

Types of conditions associated with complex medical needs

Max, Jamie and Caleb

Case study 12.1

Max and Jamie are new friends – 6-year-old boys who have recently started school. Each boy has complex medical needs. The school that Max and Jamie attend is a school for children with high-support needs, with teachers who specialise in the education of children with special needs and additional support staff to assist with the care needs of the children. Caleb is an older boy, aged 10 years, attending a mainstream public primary school, with support from a teacher's aide.

Max has a rare protein metabolism condition, and requires feeding with a specialised formula via a gastrostomy button. In early infancy, Max began to have seizures, and in later infancy, his parents noticed that he was not developing as quickly as his older siblings had done. He was slower to sit, crawl and walk. At 6 years of age, Max has difficulty standing and walking, and has begun to use a walker to assist with mobility. Jo, Max's mother, is his full-time carer, and a single mother since Theo, Max's dad, left. Theo has little subsequent contact with the family.

Jamie has cerebral palsy. Jamie was born prematurely at 32 weeks and required admission to a special care nursery. One of the earliest indicators that Jamie may have had a physical disability was identified by the child and family health nurse, when Jamie still had problems with head control at 4 months. Now Jamie uses a wheelchair for mobility as he has a significant motor impairment due to bilateral spastic quadriplegia. The level of motor impairment means that Jamie needs considerable physical care, including urinary catheterisation, gastrostomy feeding, transferring and hygiene care. Jamie has difficulties communicating, and is using a picture board to assist with this. Jamie lives at home with his parents, Ruth and Adrian, and two older siblings.

Caleb was diagnosed with Duchenne muscular dystrophy at 4 years of age. Caleb's parents had noticed that he took longer to start walking than other children, and at age 4, Caleb could not run well, jump or ride a tricycle. As his dystrophy progressed, Caleb needed to start wearing orthotic braces and began using a motor scooter at school and home. At age 10, Caleb is using a wheelchair to mobilise, but can still stand and weight-bear for short periods, transferring himself with support from chair to bed. He is able to feed himself, and can write and communicate independently. Caleb's parents have decided not to have any more children. They do not wish to risk having another child with muscular dystrophy and want to devote their efforts to caring for Caleb.

Each boy has required admissions to hospital for acute illness in the past. Most recently, Max suffered a fall during a seizure, and sustained a mild concussion when his head hit the kerb. Both Caleb and Jamie have had admissions to hospital for respiratory distress due to pneumonia after upper respiratory tract infections.

Diseases that might result in a child with complex medical needs are generally rare; however, the range of diseases defined as 'rare' is vast. There are approximately 8000 rare diseases, which affect 6–10 per cent of the population (Zurynski et al., 2008), and these rare disorders may be evident at birth or emerge during childhood. Children with such diseases may have mild to profound disability, and may have complex medical needs. It is beyond the scope of this chapter to explore all conditions that might require a child and family to receive complex medical care. Instead, some examples are provided to highlight the more 'common' of the 'rare' conditions.

Cerebral palsy (CP) is the most common physical disability in childhood, with a prevalence of 2.1 children with CP per 1000 live births (Australian Cerebral Palsy Register Group, 2013). Cerebral palsy is an umbrella term for non-progressive but often changing motor impairment that occurs before or soon after birth (Eunson, 2012). For the majority of children, the brain injury associated with CP is most likely to have occurred during prenatal and perinatal development (Australian Cerebral Palsy Register Group, 2013; Eunson, 2012). No two children or young people with CP are the same. CP can impact on an

Cerebral palsy (CP) An umbrella term for non-progressive but often changing motor impairment that occurs before or soon after birth

individual's physical or intellectual function, activities of daily living and participation in community life (Novak et al., 2013).

As the standard of antenatal and perinatal care improved significantly over recent decades, it was anticipated that the prevalence of cerebral palsy might decline (Mutch et al., 1992). However, the survival rates of children with more severe types of CP has improved as medical interventions for children born prematurely or disabled have improved (Eunson, 2012). Current risk factors associated with CP include prematurity, low weight for gestational age, multiple pregnancy and maternal genitourinary infections (Australian Cerebral Palsy Register Group, 2013; Eunson, 2012). The majority of children (including Jamie) have spasticity (86.6 per cent), and may have other impairments in addition to motor impairment, including epilepsy or intellectual, speech, visual or hearing problems (Australian Cerebral Palsy Register Group, 2013).

Muscular dystrophies are a group of neuromuscular genetic disorders that result in the progressive deterioration of muscle strength and function, another significant cause of physical disability in children and young people. The most serious impacts of this deterioration include diminished respiratory function and immobility (Wang et al., 2010). Most forms occur in children, although some children are not diagnosed until later in life.

> **Muscular dystrophies** A group of neuromuscular genetic disorders that result in the progressive deterioration of muscle strength and function

Detection and diagnosis of muscular dystrophy can take some time. Usually parents detect some delay in motor milestones and seek advice during the toddler and preschool years. A combination of clinical signs such as motor delay, serum creatinine kinase, muscle biopsy and genetic screening are used to determine the presence and type of dystrophy (Mercuri & Muntoni, 2013).

The most common form of muscular dystrophy in children is Duchenne muscular dystrophy, an X-linked recessive gene affecting male children like Caleb. Duchenne dystrophy is a life-limiting condition; however, survival into early adulthood has improved with increasing access to mechanical ventilation and use of antibiotics to treat respiratory infections (Mercuri & Muntoni, 2013). As a result, the number of adolescents with Duchenne dystrophy who require support during transition from paediatric to adult services has increased. Longer survival is associated with increased likelihood of cardiac muscle involvement. Severe ventricular arrhythmia may eventuate and sudden death may be the first indication of this (Mercuri & Muntoni, 2013; Wang et al., 2010).

There are many different types of metabolic conditions, some of which result in developmental disability and may also require specialist care and alternative nutrition. Many of these conditions are detected soon after birth through the newborn screening program (Wilcken, 2006). All infants born in Australia have a heel-prick blood sample taken and tested for the presence of a number of metabolic and genetic conditions, including inborn errors of metabolism such as **phenylketonuria (PKU)**, hypothyroidism and CF (NHMRC, 2002). For some children, like Max, the metabolic condition may not detected until after birth. Metabolic and genetic conditions may be detected by parents and health-care professionals when there are concerns about delays in development or regressed development, or idiopathic seizures.

Some children may have complex, chronic respiratory conditions, often associated with **premature birth** or respiratory complications in the neonatal period. Examples include chronic neonatal lung disease or subglottic stenosis. The impact of these respiratory conditions may lessen as the child develops and the respiratory tract becomes larger. Depending on the nature of the condition, these children may require an artificial airway (usually a tracheostomy) and/or oxygen therapy in the early years of life.

> **Phenylketonuria (PKU)**
> A metabolic disorder that is present at birth and caused by an autosomal recessive gene. Essentially, the condition results in a failure to metabolise phenylalanine, an amino acid found in proteins and some artificial sweeteners. If PKU is undetected and not treated, it can cause a range of serious health effects, including intellectual disability and seizures. It is important that it is detected early in life to prevent these complications
>
> **Premature birth** The live birth of an infant before 37 weeks' gestation

Families and children with complex medical needs

In most situations, children with complex medical needs are ultimately cared for by parents and family members at home. However, in many cases, infants and children are cared for a prolonged period of time in hospital prior to discharge into the care of their family (Elias et al., 2012; Noyes et al., 2014). Prior to discharge, parents and caregivers often need to learn new skills and gain new knowledge in order to care for their child at home, and integrate the care into the day-to-day life of the family.

Children are now frequently sent home with the ongoing need for interventions such as oxygen, tracheostomies, ventilation, enteral feeding, care of intravenous devices and complex medication regimes (to name just a few) that previously would have occurred in hospital (Elias et al., 2012). It is important to remember that not every child who requires complex medical care will end up at home with their family. Different families have different levels of capacity to support a child with complex medical needs. Some children may eventually live in out-of-home care, either in a foster family or in a long-term care unit.

When children with complex needs become acutely unwell and need admission to hospital, it is critical to remember that the parents or the child's primary caregiver(s) are often the experts in the care of their child. They know their child best, and often detect subtle changes in the child's behaviour or response before expert clinicians would. Parents may have had many years of experience in continuously caring for a child with a particular condition. If their child is dependent on technology, they often have a very good understanding of that technology, and have developed practical 'know-how' about the finer nuances of their child's equipment. In these situations, health-care professionals can be somewhat intimidated by parents' expertise! The best thing we can do is acknowledge and draw on that expertise, to provide the best possible care for the child in partnership with the parents or caregiver(s).

Caring for a child with complex medical needs increases the burden of care for parents and family members. It can be difficult to assess the extent of the burden of care for a family. Each family has different capacity for function, and each child has different characteristics as an individual that can make caring for that child at home easier or more difficult (Eddy & Engel, 2008; Pangilinan & Hornyak, 2013; Toly et al., 2012a). Depending on the nature of the child's needs, there may be considerable time requirements for care and the need to learn a range of new skills and areas of knowledge (Kuo et al., 2011). To some extent, it is likely to be easier for families to adapt to managing a child's illness at home when there are less demanding levels of care, skill or technology required, or the condition is non-life-threatening.

Depending on the level of care required, parents may need to reconsider their commitments outside the home, and this can result in increased social isolation, potential decrease in income and increased costs for the care of their child (Cockett, 2012; Kuo et al., 2011). Mothers are often the primary caregivers of children with complex needs, and as such may be at a higher risk of depression due to the burden of care (Toly et al., 2012b). The nature of the child's condition may also mean that the child requires frequent hospitalisation, out-patient appointments and/or invasive procedures that may be intrusive on family life, cause pain and suffering for the child and increase the stress on parents and families (Kuo et al., 2011). Wherever possible, it is best to provide services to support children to remain at home with their family and within their community, to enhance their opportunity to participate in normal, day-to-day life, for example, school, leisure activities and family life (WHO, 2012). While it may be ideal to discharge a child with complex needs to their own home as soon as possible, social, financial and environmental issues can delay discharge and prolong hospitalisation (Graf et al., 2008).

Caring for a child with complex needs can be demanding on parents, and some families may choose to take a break from the demands of caring for a child with complex needs. **Respite care** may be provided for brief periods of time at home, or overnight – either within the home or in another venue – by extended family, trained carers in the home or specific respite care organisations (MacDonald & Callery, 2004). Some parents may view an admission to hospital as a form of respite. Parents of children with complex needs can find it difficult to access community-based respite care that meets the needs and expectations of the child and the family (Dybwik et al., 2011; Ling, 2012; MacDonald & Callery, 2004; Murray, 2007).

> **Respite care** Temporary care provided to children with complex needs by another, to provide parent(s) or primary caregiver(s) with the opportunity for a break from the demands of care

Many children with complex health needs will have life-limiting conditions. For example, children like Caleb, with Duchenne's muscular dystrophy, may die in adolescence or early adulthood. Families such as Caleb's will know this soon after a diagnosis is made, and will experience feelings of sadness and grief before Caleb passes away. **Anticipatory grief** can help parents, siblings and other loved family and friends to prepare and adjust for the time when their child is gone. For further discussion about palliative care, end-of-life care and grieving, see Chapter 6.

> **Anticipatory grief** The experience of the grief response, when the child or person is expected to die at some point in the future as a result of illness or disability

---

Reflection points 12.1

The proportion of children who survive childhood and adolescence with complex health-care problems is increasing due to advances in medical treatments and technologies. What are the implications of this trend for:
- families
- paediatric health-care professionals
- community health-care services for children
- school and education services?

Nursing assessment and interventions

A broad scope of conditions is associated with complex medical needs, and therefore the discussion of the range of likely nursing interventions is considerable and beyond the scope of this chapter. Instead, the more common nursing assessment and care issues are discussed, including respiration, mobility, nutrition and communication.

Respiration

Some children will require respiratory support as part of their condition, or as their condition progresses. This can take several forms, depending on the nature of the respiratory impairment, including the need for a tracheostomy, ventilation and/or oxygen therapy.

Children with chronic lung disease as a result of prematurity or disease may require long-term oxygen therapy (Balfour-Lynn et al., 2009). Sometimes children with neuromuscular conditions – even non-progressive conditions such as cerebral palsy – can develop chronic lung disease as a result of aspiration or reflux, and may require oxygen therapy (Kontorinis et al., 2013). Children who are on long-term oxygen as a result of prematurity may eventually 'outgrow' their need for it. Children in this situation often require weaning from oxygen therapy under supervision in hospital.

Some children may require creation of a tracheostomy and insertion of a tracheostomy tube to maintain a patent airway. Indications for a tracheostomy may include airway obstruction, difficulty maintaining a patent airway or the need for long-term ventilation (Bassham et al., 2012).

One of the issues with the creation of a tracheostomy is that the insertion of an airway into the trachea bypasses the upper airway. In normal respiration, the upper airway humidifies and filtrates the air before it reaches the lower airway, reducing the risk of infection. As a result, children with a tracheostomy tube would usually have a 'Swedish nose', or heat moisture exchanger, in place to help humidify and filter air.

Caleb will eventually require ventilation support as his respiratory muscles weaken. Initially, Caleb may only require non-invasive ventilation such as continuous positive airway pressure (CPAP) at night, to reduce the likelihood of nocturnal hypoventilation (Wang et al., 2010). As his condition deteriorates, he may require insertion of a tracheostomy tube and continuous long-term ventilation. An increasing number of children requiring long-term ventilation are cared for in the community (Australasian Paediatric Respiratory Group, 2008). In order to care for children who require ventilation at home, families often require assistance from community-based carers, trained in the care of people who are medically stable, but dependent on ventilation for survival (Lewarski & Gay, 2007).

Children like Caleb and Jamie with impaired respiratory function are at higher risk of respiratory infections, and are more likely to require hospitalisation when unwell. It is essential that parents and health-care professionals know the child's baseline parameters when they are well, are attuned to the signs of increasing respiratory effort and infection, and are trained in cardiopulmonary resuscitation. Additionally, parents and families need a clear plan for managing illness at home, and should know when and where to seek help from acute health-care services, including the ambulance service. For further information on physical assessment and the deteriorating child, see Chapter 8.

Mobility

Children who have motor impairment may have difficulty with mobility. It is important to bear in mind that the extent of motor impairment associated with different conditions can vary. For example, although Jamie requires a wheelchair, not all children with CP will. On the other hand, motor impairment will get worse over time in some children with progressive conditions, as it has done for Caleb with muscular dystrophy. Regardless of the condition or prognosis, the main aim for children with motor impairment is to maintain function and independence where possible, for as long as possible.

The care that a child with motor impairment needs includes several priorities and a range of nursing interventions. One of the most important priorities is the prevention or delay of contractures and maintaining posture, as these factors are key to maintaining current level of motor function (Eddy, 2013). Physical therapy is an important intervention in maintaining function, and requires a multidisciplinary approach from a range of health-care practitioners, including physiotherapists, occupational therapists and orthopaedic specialists (Pangilinan & Hornyak, 2013). Nurses and parents may be required to assist children in passive range of motion exercises, the application of splints, positioning to promote best posture and prevention or delay of scoliosis, which can result in difficulties with respiration as well as problems with mobility (Eddy, 2013). Depending on the extent of the impairment, children may require assistance with transferring or use of walkers, wheelchairs or standing boards. Any child with impaired mobility is at risk of skin breakdown and has a higher risk of falls. Nursing staff need to assess the level of risk for both skin breakdown and falls, and institute appropriate nursing interventions (Crisp et al., 2013).

Children with impaired mobility may require nursing assistance or have specialist intervention to meet their hygiene and elimination needs. Some children may not have bladder or bowel control, and may use nappies or incontinence pads, or need assistance to use a toilet or commode. Others may require intermittent urinary catheterisation or have an indwelling urinary or suprapubic catheter.

Whether nurses, other health-care professionals or parents are assisting children with mobility problems, it is important to adhere to the principles of manual handling. Carers can often become quite fatigued by the physical demands of lifting and transferring children, and time should be made for rest.

Nutrition and hydration

Some children are unable to meet their hydration and nutritional needs due to difficulties with oral feeding, and may require enteral feeding via a nasogastric, nasojeujunal tube or via gastrostomy. Nasogastric tubes are usually used as a short-term form of enteral feeding. Children who require long-term or permanent enteral feeding are more likely to have a gastrostomy created and a gastrostomy tube or button inserted.

A gastrostomy is created via a surgical procedure under general anaesthetic. A puncture site (stoma) is inserted through the abdomen and into the stomach. Either a tube or button device is inserted into the stoma and may be secured with a suture. The tube or button device maintains patency of the stoma and acts as a conduit for fluid and formula. Similar to a nasogastric tube, the position of the tube or device is confirmed by aspirating gastric fluid and testing with litmus paper. There are several risks with the formation of a gastrostomy. The tube can migrate through the stomach and into the bowel, causing obstruction. Gastric secretions can ooze around the site, causing skin irritation.

Depending on the reason for enteral feeding, children may require bolus feeding during the day and continuous overnight feeds. In order to meet their metabolic needs for growth, children may have high-calorie feeds. Some children may require different types of formula, depending on their conditions.

Some children with complex medical conditions of the gastrointestinal tract may not be able to digest or absorb food and fluids. For these children, nutrition may need to provided intravenously (parenteral nutrition), usually via a central venous access device (CVAD). Their need for parenteral nutrition may be temporary or permanent.

Ideally, it is better for children to maintain hydration and nutrition by feeding orally. Eating is a pleasurable experience, and an important milestone in language development. Some children may be able to take oral food and fluids, but may require assistance with drinking and feeding. Other children may have difficulty with swallowing, and may require pureed or mashed foods. In each of these instances, children should be supervised during meals to monitor for any signs of choking or aspiration.

When children are dependent on others for their nutrition, it is essential that their level of nutrition and hydration is monitored – both by regular measurements of height and weight to monitor growth, and by observing for signs of inadequate nutrition and hydration such as constipation and decreased urine output.

Communication

Some children with complex medical needs may have problems with speech, language or intellectual capacity. Any of these problems can reduce or interfere with their communication and understanding. Children with impairment in speech may use a variety of devices in order to communicate with others, from simple pictures to sophisticated computer-assisted devices.

Developing skills in communication with children who are well and developing normally can be challenging for health-care professionals – it can be more complex when the child has difficulty communicating. The principles of interpersonal communication that we use for all peoples are equally important for children with difficulty in communication. Our body language, the way we position ourselves to communicate, the tone of voice we use, the simplicity of the language we use – all of these are valuable ways in which we can enhance communication with children.

Again, parents are often a very good source of advice, as they understand the special ways in which their individual child communicates their needs to the world. This can be particularly important when caring for children with communication impairment when they are unwell. Parents are often able to interpret their child's unique ways of communicating pain, fear or distress (Burkitt et al., 2011; Solodiuk et al., 2010).

Summary

- Children with complex needs and their families are frequent consumers of acute paediatric health-care services due to higher risk of acute illness.
- Although different types of conditions that result in complex medical needs are 'rare', they are 'common' in the children requiring acute paediatric health care.
- The impact of complex medical needs on day-to-day life for children and families is individual and complex.
- Parents and primary caregivers of children with complex health-care needs have special expertise in their child, and specialist knowledge of the condition as it relates to their child.
- There is considerable variation between individual children and their individual nursing needs; however, nursing interventions for issues associated with impairment of respiration, mobility, nutrition and communication may be required.

Learning activity

The nature of health-care funding in Australia means that there is often some variation between local areas in the provision of resources to support the care of children with complex needs, depending on whether the funding is provided at a state or territory, or Commonwealth level. It is useful for nurses and other health-care professionals who care for children with complex needs to have an understanding of the availability of resources and funding for families, and to know where to locate this information.

In this activity, use the internet to undertake a search of resources in your area for children with a specific complex medical need and their families. Use Table 12.1 as a template to begin with, but you may have additional information that you may want to add to your search. An example (based on Carer's Allowance) is provided to help you get started.

TABLE 12.1 *Resources for children with complex medical needs*

RESOURCE	FUNDING SOURCE	DETAILS	SOURCE/LINK
Carer's allowance	Commonwealth government	The carer must be caring for one or more dependant children under 16 years with a recognised disability or medical condition lasting 12 months or longer and receiving care in home or hospital	<www.humanservices.gov.au/customer/enablers/centrelink/carer-allowance/eligibility>
Pharmaceutical cost assistance			
Equipment supplies			
Respite care			
School information			
Disease/condition support network			
Costs associated with hospital admissions			

Further reading

Parent resource: InterACT 2007, *There's no such thing as a silly question: A practical guide for families living with a child with chronic illness, disability, mental illness or a life-threatening condition*, InterACT, Canberra. Given the relative rarity of the individual conditions, it can be difficult to develop resources for parents that are specific to their condition. In recognition that some of the information that parents need is common, irrespective of the type of illness or condition, a group of Australian parents developed a book resource for parents and families caring for children with additional needs. This book is available online at <www.respitesouth.org.au/library/theres-no-such-thing-silly-question-practical-guide>.

References

Australasian Paediatric Respiratory Group 2008, *Ventilatory support at home for children*, viewed 3 April 2014, http://www.thoracic.org.au/documents/papers/aprghomeventilationguideline.pdf.

Australian Cerebral Palsy Register Group 2013, *Australian Cerebral Palsy Register: Report 2013*, viewed 20 March 2014, https://www.cerebralpalsy.org.au/wp-content/uploads/2013/04/ACPR-Report_Web_2013.pdf.

Balfour-Lynn, IM et al. 2009, BTS guidelines for home oxygen in children, *Thorax*, 64 (Suppl. 2), pp. 1–26.

Bassham, BS et al. 2012, Difficult airways, difficult physiology and difficult technology: Respiratory treatment of the special needs child, *Clinical Pediatric Emergency Medicine*, 13(2), pp. 81–90.

Burkitt, CC, Breau, LM & Zabalia, M 2011, Parental assessment of pain coping in individuals with intellectual and developmental disabilities, *Research in Developmental Disabilities*, 32(5), pp. 1564–71.

Burns, K et al. 2011, Increasing prevalence of medically complex children in US hospitals, *Pediatrics*, 126(4), 638–46.

Cockett, A 2012, Technology dependence and children: A review of the evidence, *Nursing Children and Young People*, 24(1), 32–5.

Cohen, E et al. 2011, Children with medical complexity: An emerging population for clinical and research initiatives, *Pediatrics*, 127(3), pp. 529–38.

Crisp, J, Taylor, C, Douglas, C & Rebeiro, G (eds) 2013, *Potter & Perry's fundementals of nursing*, Elsevier, Sydney.

Dybwik, K, Tollali, T, Nielsen, EW & Brinchmann, BS 2011, 'Fighting the system': Families caring for ventilator-dependent children and adults with complex health care needs at home, *BMC Health Services Research*, 11, p. 156.

Eddy, LL (ed.) 2013, *Caring for children with special healthcare needs and their families: A handbook for healthcare professionals*, Wiley-Blackwell, Malden, MA.

Eddy, LL & Engel, JM 2008, The impact of child disability type on the family, *Rehabilitation Nursing Journal*, 33(3), pp. 98–103.

Elias, ER, Murphy, NA & Council on Children with Disabilities 2012, Home care of children and youth with complex health care needs and technology dependencies, *Pediatrics*, 129(5), pp. 996–1005.

Eunson, P 2012, Aetiology and epidemiology of cerebral palsy, *Paediatrics and Child Health*, 22(9), pp. 361–6.

Graf, JM, Montagnino, BA, Hueckel, R & McPherson, ML 2008, Children with new tracheostomies: Planning for family education and common impediments to discharge, *Pediatric Pulmonology*, 43(8), pp. 788–94.

Kirk, S & Glendinning, C 2004, Developing services to support parents caring for a technology-dependent child at home, *Child: Care, Health and Development*, 30(3), pp. 209–18.

Kontorinis, G, Thevasagayam, MS & Bateman, ND 2013, Airway obstruction in children with cerebral palsy: Need for tracheostomy? *International Journal of Pediatric Otorhinolaryngology*, 77(10), pp. 1647–50.

Kuo, DZ, Cohen, E, Agrawal, R, Berry, JG & Casey, PH 2011, A national profile of caregiver challenges among more medically complex children with special health care needs, *Archives of Pediatrics & Adolescent Medicine*, 165(11), pp. 1020–6.

Lewarski, JS & Gay, PC 2007, Current issues in home mechanical ventilation, *Chest*, 132(2), pp. 671–6.

Ling, J 2012, Respite support for children with a life-limiting condition and their parents: A literature review, *International Journal of Palliative Nursing*, 18(3), pp. 129134.

MacDonald, H & Callery, P 2004, Different meanings of respite: a study of parents, nurses and social workers caring for children with complex needs, *Child: Care, Health and Development*, 30(3), pp. 279–88.

Mercuri, E & Muntoni, F 2013, Muscular dystrophies, *The Lancet*, 381(9869), pp. 845–60.

Murray, S 2007, Families' care of their children with severe disabilities in Australia: Social policy and support, *Community, Work & Family*, 10(2), pp. 215–30.

Mutch, L, Alberman, E, Hagberg, B, Kodama, K & Perat, MV 1992, Cerebral palsy epidemiology: Where are we now and where are we going? *Developmental Medicine & Child Neurology*, 34(6), pp. 547–51.

National Health and Medical Research Council (NHMRC) 2002, *Child health screening and surveillance: A critical review of the evidence*, viewed 20 March 2014, http://www.nhmrc.gov.au/_files_nhmrc/publications/attachments/ch42.pdf.

Novak, I et al. 2013, A systematic review of interventions for children with cerebral palsy: State of the evidence, *Developmental Medicine & Child Neurology*, 55(10), pp. 885–910.

Noyes, J, Brenner, M, Fox, P & Guerin, A 2014, Reconceptualizing children's complex discharge with health systems theory: Novel integrative review with embedded expert consultation and theory development, *Journal of Advanced Nursing*, 70(5), pp. 975–96.

Pangilinan, PH & Hornyak, JE 2013, Rehabilitation of the muscular dystrophies, *Handbook of Clinical Neurology*, 110, pp. 471–81.

Rehm, RS 2013, Nursing's contribution to research about parenting children with complex chronic conditions: An integrative review, 2002 to 2012, *Nursing Outlook*, 61(5), pp. 266–90.

Solodiuk, JC et al. 2010, Validation of the Individualized Numeric Rating Scale (INRS): A pain assessment tool for nonverbal children with intellectual disability, *Pain*, 150 (2), pp. 231–6.

Toly, VB, Musil, CM & Carl, JC 2012a, Families with children who are technology dependent: Normalization and family functioning, *Western Journal of Nursing Research*, 34(1), pp. 52–71.

—— 2012b, A longitudinal study of families with technology-dependent children, *Research in Nursing & Health*, 35(1), pp. 40–54.

Wang, CH et al. (2010). Consensus statement on standard of care for congenital muscular dystrophies, *Journal of Child Neurology*, 25(12), pp. 1559–81.

Wilcken, B 2006, Newborn screening for inborn errors of metabolism. In J Fernandes, J Saudubray, G van den Berghe & JH Walter (eds), *Inborn metabolic diseases*, Springer, Heidelberg, Germany, pp. 49–57.

World Health Organization (WHO) 2012, *Early childhood development and disability: A discussion paper*, viewed 22 April 2014, http://apps.who.int/iris/bitstream/10665/75355/1/9789241504065_eng.pdf?ua=1.

—— 2013, Preterm birth, World Health Organization fact sheet, viewed 22 April 2014, http://www.who.int/mediacentre/factsheets/fs363/en.

Zurynski, Y, Frith, K, Leonard, H & Elliott, E 2008, Rare childhood diseases: How should we respond? *Archives of Disease in Childhood*, 93(12), pp. 1071–4.

Index

abdominal pain 220–2
  analgesic relief 221
  appendicitis 221–2
  case study 220
abnormal posturing 124
Aboriginal people, health/welfare
  over-representation 61–3
abrasions 217
Acute Lymphoblastic Leukaemia
  (ALL) 16–17
acute otitis media (AOM)
  199–200
  case study 199
  earaches 200
  signs 199–200
acute respiratory illness 202–6
  case study 202
  characterised by airway
    obstruction 203
adolescence 3, 13, 212
  Gillick test, *Gillick*
    competence 38–9
  identity versus identity
    confusion 65–9
  peers, sense of difference
    from 66
  see also Australia's children
    and young people;
    young people
adolescents
  behavioural and mental
    problems, prevalence
    of 22–3
  with chronic conditions
    246–51
  communication with 153–4
  depression and 214
  development 213
  discussion regarding death/
    end-of-life care 153–4
  families with 266
  fatigue, descriptions of 148
  hospitalisation 22–3
  life, satisfaction with 268
  mental health
    determinants 177–8
    promoting strategies 182
  mental illness/illness 162–84
  promoting resilience/positive
    adaptive responses
    178–82
  risk-taking behaviours 21, 23
  self-harm and 214
  specific age-related needs
    213
  transitioning to adult care
    246–51
adrenaline nebulisers 129
adults
  adult depression 175
  adult health burden 20
  common chronic medical
    conditions 230
  single young adults 266
advanced life support
  basic life support–advanced life
    support distinction 132–3
  paediatric 132–3
age 21
  Australian age-of-majority
    legislation 37–9
  children's age and
    development 192
  chronological age and pain
    assessment measures 200
air filtration 286
airways 128–30
  A–airway (Primary Assessment
    Framework) 115–16
  airway obstruction 115
    children at risk of 129
    extent 204
    upper or lower 203
  airway patency and speech 115
  blockage by secretions 128
  C–circulation (Primary
    Assessment
    Framework) 118–23
  clear airways 224
  compromised airways risk 115
  oropharyngeal airways 129–30
  positioning of the head, neural
    position/'sniffing' 128–9
alcohol
  alcohol abuse, psychosocial
    issues 225
  alcohol poisoning 224–5
    case study 224
    risks 224
  binge drinking 224
  CNS depressant 224
  consumption 224
  sedative effects 224
algorithms 194
altruism 95
anaesthesia 196–7
analgesia 218
  abdominal pain relief 221
  patient-controlled
    analgesia 223
  sedative effect 217
  use in postoperative care
    223
  WHO analgesic ladder
    143–4
Angelman syndrome 242
answerable research
  questions 79–80
antenatal period 180
antibiotic therapy 200
antipyretic medications
  191–2
  risk 191–2
anxiety 21, 23, 152–3, 174–6
  maternal anxiety 57
    nursing interventions 58
  peer group non-
    conformance 66
  persisting 72
  separation anxiety 54, 175
appendicitis 221–2
  acute appendicitis, causes
    221
  appendix perforation 221
  diagnosing, laparoscopy 221
  symptoms 221–2
  sexual history and 222
art therapy 153
aspirin 191
assessment
  accurate assessment data 53
  capillary refill assessment
    220
  of dehydration 194–5
  family assessment 263–74
    frameworks 267–8
  fatigue assessment tools/
    scales 147–8
  of head injuries 215–17
  neurological assessment,
    rapid 215–17
  neurovascular assessment,
    components 220
  nursing assessment 56, 212–
    25, 233–5, 237–9, 240–1,
    243–6, 286–90
    for ADHD 167–9
    for ASD 170–1
    evidence-based care
      and 189–206, 212–25,
      229–51
  parent–infant
    attachment 54–5
  Paediatric Assessment
    Triangle 111–13

assessment (cont.)
  pain assessment/
    management 143–7,
    200–2, 218, 220, 223
  observational and
    behavioural pain-
    assessment tools 201
  postoperative assessment 223
  Primary Assessment
    Framework 111
  sedation assessment 217
  structured assessment
    (paediatric patients) 111–
    14
  symptoms, assessment and
    management 142
asthma 14–15, 230, 232–5
  asthma management
    plans 233, 235
  case study 234
  characterised 232
  childhood asthma patterns 232
  clinical examination and
    medical history 233
  deaths due to 15
  good asthma control, NACA
    definition 235
  hospital rates for 15
  indicators 15
  management 232
  NACA description 232
  nursing assessments and
    interventions 233–5
  poor asthma control 235
  prevalence 14–15
  severity of 233–5
  symptoms 233
    pattern and severity 234–5
  treatment 234
    bronchodilators 234
    corticosteroids 234
    preventer medication 234–5
    symptom-control
      medication 234
  treatment protocols 232
  unstable ('brittle') asthma 235
asylum seekers
  case study 64–5
  determination process 65
attachment theory 51–2
  parent–infant attachment 52–4
  case studies 52–3
Attention Deficit Hyperactivity
  Disorder (ADHD) 22,
  166–9

case study 166–7
comorbidities 167
non-stimulant drugs/long-
  acting medications 168
nursing assessment 167–9
nursing interventions 167–9
sub-types 167
Australia 36–7
  age-of-majority legislation
    37–9
  Australian children 49–72
    mental health disorders
      affecting 165–6
  Australian communities 49–72
  Australian families 8–10,
    49–72, 267–8
  child mortality 141
  child rights in 29–44
  'lucky country' case study 4
  political orientation 4
  population 4
  regional areas
    hospitalisation rates 17
    tooth decay levels 21
  rural/remote areas
    cancer survival rates 17
    case study – Aboriginal
      families in 62–3
    coordinated care in 237
    head injuries incurred in
      217
    hospitalisation 214
    tooth decay levels 21
Australian Aboriginal people 4
  families 267–8
    family functioning 267–8
    health determinants 61–3
    inter-professional
      connections 63
    psychological and family
      issues 62–3
  population age distribution
    comparison 8
  Western Australian Aboriginal
    Child Health Survey 267
Australian Bureau of Statistics
  (ABS) 3, 5
chronic condition,
  definition 229
Australian Cystic Fibrosis Data
  Registry (ACFDR)
  243–4
Australian Institute of Health
  and Welfare (AIHW) 5,
  162–3, 177–8

Australian Research Alliance
  for Children & Youth
  (ARACY) 177–8
  research 179–82
    Nest action agenda 179–82
Australia's children and young
  people 3–24, 229–51
  health of 10–18
    dental health 20–1
    indicator measurement 4–6
    health and wellbeing 5–6
    key national health
      indicators 7
    rate-based calculations 5
  infants 11–12
  mental health of 22–4
    determinants 21, 23
  mortality 10, 11
  mothers and babies 6–7
Autism Spectrum Disorder
  (ASD) 169–71
  case study 170
  characterisation 169–70
  diagnosis 170
  nursing assessment and
    interventions 170–1
  transition to high school 170
autonomy principle 37–9, 86,
  88–9, 95
  versus shame and doubt 55–6
AVPU (alert, verbal, responsive to
  pain, unconscious) 125

Baby Boomer generation 8
bacteria 190
basic life support
  basic life support–advanced
    life support distinction
    132–3
  paediatric 132–3
behaviour
  behavioural disorders
    Attention Deficit
      Hyperactivity
      Disorder (ADHD) 22
    causes of 22
    hospitalisation rates 22
    Obsessive Compulsive
      Disorder (OCD) 22
    prevalence 22–3
  behavioural responses, to
    acute/chronic illness 49
  behaviour-modification
    programs 173
  Child Behaviour Checklist 165

COMFORT behaviour
    scale 201
  repetitive behaviour 169–70
beneficence 87–8, 95
  benefit versus harm
    case study 79
  in paediatric research 91–4
  risk of 91–4
best interest 36, 38, 39, 92
beta cells 236
bipolar disorder (BD), 22, 164
blood glucose 237
  stabilisation 241
blood pressure 119–20
  blood pressure cuff size 120–1
body language 154
body mass index (BMI) 19
body surface area (BSA) 192
  BSA–mass ratio 198
bolus 131–2
  bolus feeding 288
bradycardia 119
brain
  chemoreceptor trigger zone
    (CTZ) 151
  hippocampus, alcohol damage,
    susceptibility to 224
  medulla oblongata 151
breastfeeding 10
breathing 128–30
Bristol Stool Form Scale 151
bronchiolitis 204–5
bronchodilators 234

cachexia 151
cancer 16–18, 230
  Acute Lymphoblastic
    Leukaemia (ALL) 16–17
  childhood cancer 17
    new cases 17
    survival 17
  five-year survival rates 17
  treatment, services and early
    detection 17
cannulation (intravenous)
    196–8
  preparing child and family
    for 197
  reducing pain, topical
    anaesthetics to 197
  topical anaesthetics 196–7
capillary refill 121–2
  capillary refill assessment 220
    sites 122
  factors affecting 121–2

cardiopulmonary arrest 111
cardiopulmonary resuscitation
    (paediatric)
  paediatric self-inflating
    bag 133
  parental presence during
    133–5
cardiovascular compromise 110
care
  adult care 246–51
  advanced care planning 153–4
    models 153
  continuity of care 237
  coordinated care in 237
  end-of-life care 141–56
  evidence-based care, 279–93
  family-centred care 36,
    261–3
  individual holistic care 142
  individual responsibility
    for 248
  nursing care 203
  paediatric care 141–56, 261–3
  palliative care 141–56
  physical care 279
  planning and delivery,
    stakeholder engagement
    in 34
  postoperative care 223
  preoperative care 222–3
  primary health care services,
    access strategies 237
  transition to adult care 246–51
  unprofessional care 273
caregivers
  children's health decisions/
    behaviours 59
  infant attachment to 51–2
  information provision 124–5
  knowledge of children's mood
    and behaviour 58
  primary caregivers
    caregiver expertise 284
    mothers as 284–5
catecholamines 118
central nervous system
    (CNS) 224
central venous access device
    (CVAD) 289
cerebral palsy (CP) 281–2
  prevalence and survival
    rates 282
  risk factors 282
champions 99
chest recession/retraction 116

child abuse and neglect 39–40,
    179–80
  injury presentations 42
  notification 39–40
    substantiation 40
  recognition of 40
  reporting
    compromised legislative
      compliance 41–2
    health professionals' role
      in 40
    mandatory reporting 40
  risk of 59
child maltreatment 41–4
child protection 32, 272–3
  child-protection registrar 42
  legislation 39–40
  multidisciplinary response
    to 43
child rights
  in Australia 29–44
  legislation 30–5
  practice implications 35–44
  priorities 39–40
childhood 3
  assumptions regarding 29–30
  childhood asthma patterns 232
  childhood cancer, Australian
    rates 17
  childhood growth 230–1
  childhood obesity 20
  emotional maturation 230–1
  mental illness/illness 162–84
  middle/late childhood 60–5
  morbidity and mortality
    patterns in 21, 23
  social development 230–1
children
  acute otitis media
    (AOM) 199–200
  acute respiratory illness
    202–6
  acutely ill child 189–206
  age 192
  anxiety 57
  with breathing difficulties
    149–50
    case study 152
  with CF 244–5
    hospitalisation with system
      complications 246
    management plan 245–6
    respiratory infections 245
    treatment and preventative
      therapies 245–6

children (cont.)
  Child Behaviour Checklist 165
  child behaviour management 168
  child depression 175
  children's choices, acknowledging 36
  children's health care, parental involvement in 262
    model 260–1
  child's best interest 36, 38, 92
  child-specific treaties 33
  with chronic illness 50, 229–51
    common chronic medical conditions 230
    and their families 230
  communication with 153–4
  and their communities 49–72
  with complex medical needs 283–5
    admission to hospital 284
    burden of care 284
    communication 289–90
    evidence-based care 279–90
    nutrition and hydration 288–9
  consent circumstances 90
  death rate 12
  dehydration 193–5
  dental health 20–1
  development 192
    developmental achievements 58
    developmental regression 58
    dynamic process 164–5
    psychological development 50–1
  emerging health priorities 18–23
  families
    burden of care of children 284
    family nature, impact of 260
    'launching' children by 266
    siblings 135, 155–6
    with young children 266
  fatigue, descriptions of 148
  fever in children 190–3
  gastroenteritis 195–6
  health and wellbeing 260
  health disruptions 50–1
  holders of rights view 30
  hospitalisation 246
    developmental limiting 50

Indigenous children 12, 17, 199
intervention, ongoing need for 283–4
intravenous site/infusion 198
intravenous therapy 196–8
mental health
  case study 176
  case study resolution 184
  determinants 177–8
  promoting 176–84
  promoting strategies 182
  services 164
mobility 198
mood and behaviour 58
mother–child relationship 273
needs 260
pain assessment 200–2
parent–child conflict 32–3
participation in research
  assent 91
  risk associated with 93
peers, sense of difference from 50
play and art therapy 153
promoting resilience/positive adaptive responses 178–82
research, participation in 38
researching with 84
the sick child
  normal fluid/electrolyte balance restoration 196–8
  recognising and responding to 109–35
  successful engagement (research) 100
  with T1D 237
  T2D management 240–1
  wellbeing 231
  worries and fears 153
  see also Australia's children and young people
child-specific treaties 33
'chin lifts' 129
chromosomal birth defects 241
chromosomal disorders 241–6
chronic conditions 241–6
chronic illness/conditions 13–14, 229–51, 268
  ABS definition 229
  asthma 232–5
  chronic lung disease 286
  chronically ill children and their families 230

common conditions 230
congenital, chromosomal and genetic disorders 241–6
diagnosis and treatment 55–6
management 231
predictors of adjustment to 59–60
risk of abuse and 59
transition to adult care 246–51
variations in/between conditions 230
circulation 194–5
  circulatory compromise *case study* 123
  circulatory support 130–2
  circulatory system 11
Clinical Dehydration Scale (CDS) 194
clinical examination 233
clinical practice *see* practice
coercion 89
cognition
  cognitive function 237
  cognitive impairment, treatment preferences 32–3
  skills 53
colour (skin) 194–5, 220
COMFORT behaviour scale 201
communication 53, 289–90
  with children and adolescents 153–4
  communication facilitation 142
  and the family in paediatric end-of-life care 154–6
  interpersonal communication principles 288, 289
  poor/inadequate communication 128
  reducing anxiety 152
  social communication deficits, ADHD and 169–70
communities 10, 49–72
  community-based early intervention 175
comorbidities 12, 167, 175, 240
compensatory mechanisms 118
complaints 273
complex medical needs 279–90
  case study 280–1
  conditions associated with 280–3
  diseases resulting in 281–3
  families and children with 283–5

computerised tomography scan (CT) 215–17
conceptual thinking 60–1
Conduct Disorder (CD)
   case study 171–2
   Oppositional Defiant Disorder (ODD) and 171–3
confidentiality 88
conflict 32–3
   autonomy versus shame and doubt 55–6
   conflicting values 85
   identity versus identity confusion 65–9
   initiative versus guilt 56–60
   intimacy versus isolation 69–72
   trust versus mistrust 51–5
congenital disorders 241–6
consciousness
   AVPU assessment 215
   level of 124, 129
   monitoring 224
consent
   ethical review bodies and 90–1
   Gillick test 38
   Gillick competence 38–9
   implied consent, opting in/out 85
   informed consent 223
   to medical treatment 38
      court-given consent 38
   minor's consent capacity 90
   in paediatric research 89–91
   voluntary consent 86
   from young people/children 90
continuous positive airway pressure (CPAP) 286
Convention on the Rights of the Child 31–2
   Article 19 31–2
   children's rights categories 31–2
   ratification 31
coping
   coping strategies 269–71
      for anxiety 152
      case study 271
      positive and negative 270–1
   gender influence 269
   types 269
corticosteroids 203, 204, 234

croup 203–4
   extent of airway obstruction 204
   medications for 204
cues 52–3
culture
   cultural considerations 64–5
   cultural identities and attitudes 273–4
   cultural safety 273–4
   family's cultural perspective 274
   fostering a positive sense of culture and identity 181–4
cystic fibrosis (CF) 242–6, 283
   Australian Cystic Fibrosis Data Registry (ACFDR) 243, 246
   case study 248
   CFTR protein ΔF508 242
   clinic/hospital setting 244–5
   cystic fibrosis transmembrane regulator (CFTR) protein gene 242
   epithelial cells, channelling across 242
   establishing treatment 244
   improved survival, contributing factors 243
   incidence 242
   management 244, 245–6
   mean age of death from 243
   medical complications 245
   newborn screening programs 243–4
   nursing assessments and interventions 243–6
   treatment and preventative therapies 245–6
   organ transplantation end-stage treatment 246

death
   asthma, attributable to 15, 232
   causes of 214
   child mortality 12, 141
   conversations about dying 153–4
   discussion regarding 153–4
   Sudden Infant Death Syndrome (SIDS) 11, 12
decision-making
   responsibility 250
   health-care decisions 36

   medical decisions, autonomy and 37–9
Declaration of Helsinki 86
Declaration of the Rights of the Child 30–1
   general principles 30–1
dehydration 123, 193–5
   assessment 194–5
   scales/algorithms 194
demographics 8–10
dental health 20–1
   dental/gum problems, pain from 21
   disparities across age and population groups 21
   fluoridated water 21
   indicators 20
   oral examinations 20
depression 21, 23, 174–6
   adolescent issue 214
   child and adult depression 175
   paternal and maternal depression 174
   persisting 72
deterioration (clinical) 111, 114–25
diabetes 15–16, 230
   comorbidities 240
   hospital rates for 15
   International Diabetes Federation (IDF) 16
   Living with Diabetes blog 238
   National Evidence-based Guidelines for Type 1 Diabetes in Children, Adolescents and Adults 238
   Type 1 diabetes 15, 236–9
   Type 2 diabetes 15–16, 239–41
   incidence and indicator 16
Diagnostic and Statistical Manual of Mental Disorders (DSM) 164, 169
diet 195–6
disability 14, 230
   D–disability (Primary Assessment Framework) 124–5
   developmental disability 283
   physical disability
      cerebral palsy 281–2
      muscular dystrophies 282
   risk of abuse and 59
disclosure 272

INDEX

discomfort 92
diseases 286
  burden of disease 230
    mental health disorders 21, 23
  chronic disease 268
  complex medical needs, resulting in 281–3
  rare disease 281–3
disorders
  behavioural disorders 22
    ADHD 22
    OCD 22
  chromosomal disorders 241–6
  congenital disorders 241–6
  externalising disorders 60
    conduct disorders 171–3
  genetic disorders 241–6
  internalising disorders, anxiety and depression 174–6
  mental health disorders 21, 23
    bipolar disorder 22, 164
    schizophrenia 22
  neuromuscular genetic disorders 282
  psychological disorders, T1D concurrence 237
  separation anxiety disorder 54, 175
domestic violence 272–3
Down syndrome 241–2
Duchenne muscular dystrophy 282
dyspnoea 149–50
  cognitive and affective relationship with 149–50
  dyspnoea–physiological processes relationship 149–50
  management 149
    opioid use 150
    parental perceptions 150
    non-pharmacological and pharmacological relief strategies 150

earaches 200
early adulthood 69–72
  developmental regression 71–2
  intimacy versus isolation, sick young adult and 69–72
  case study 70–1
early childhood 3
  initiative versus guilt 56–60
ecomaps 263–4

showing family support systems 264
educational performance 237
electrolyte balance 196–8
elimination 288
emergencies
  case study 224
  children aged 0–4 189
  emergency procedures 222
EMLA (topical anaesthetic) 196–7
emotions 249
  emotional abuse 42
  emotional confidence 22
  emotional health 21–3
  emotional reactions 152–3
  emotional responses to acute/chronic illness 49
  siblings of dying child 155
  emotion-focused coping 269
end-of-life care
  Australian paediatric care settings 141–56
  decreased nutritional intake 151–2
  discussion regarding 153–4
  paediatric end-of-life care 142
  children, breathing difficulties and 149–50, 152
enteral feeding 289–90
equity 94–6
ethics
  ethical review bodies and consent 90–1
  human research ethics 84–9
    committees 88, 93, 96–101
    future perspectives 85
  principles 94
  research ethics 85–7
  unethical practice 87
ethnicity 274
ethnography 36–7
Eustachian tubes 199
evidence
  basing practice on 83
  as contextualised knowledge 82–4
  evidence implementation 98–9
  external and internal evidence 78, 82
  from research 77–8
  possibilities from delivery/demand side 81–2

evidence-based care
  acutely ill young person 212–25
  care of children with complex medical needs 279–90
  childhood/adolescent mental illness and illness 162–84
  complex medical needs, children with 279–90
  end-of-life and palliative care–Australian settings 141–56
  nursing assessments and interventions 189–206, 212–25, 229–51, 259–74
  the sick child, recognising and responding to 109–35
evidence-based practice
  definition 80–4
  five As of 82
  recommendations 82
  research process and 83
externalising disorders 60

face masks 205–6
FACES pain scale 202, 223
FACE-TC 153
fairness 94–6
  burden of research and 95
families
  Aboriginal and Torres Strait Islander families 267–8
  access to 36–7
  with adolescents 266
  assessment of 263–74
    family-assessment frameworks 267–8
    nursing assessments and interventions 259–74
  assumptions regarding 274
  Australian Aboriginal families 61–3
  Australian families in contemporary society 259–60
  demographic characteristics 8–10
children
  burden of care 284
  chronically ill children and their families 230
  'launching' and moving on 266
  siblings of dying child 155–6
  and their communities 49–72

INDEX

complex medical needs
  and 283–5
coping strategies 269–71
  positive and negative 270–1
cultural, ethnic and spiritual
  perspectives 274
development 264–6
  life-cycle stages 265–6
discussion regarding death/
  end-of-life care 153–4
economic and social
  situations 10
external interactions,
  ecomaps 263–4
family environment 59–60
family functioning 267–8
  economic and social 231
  statements 268
Family Partnership
  Model 260–1
family-centred care 36, 261–3
grandparents 156
information provided to
  154–5
in later life 266
marriage, joining through 266
nature of 260
  dynamic and diverse 265
nuclear families 267
in paediatric end-of-life
  care 154–6
  communication with 154–6
principle of family unity 33
roles and functions 267–8
  changing roles 267
  gender roles 267
single young adults leaving
  home 266
strengths 269
stressors 268–9
structure, genograms 263–4
support for 264
  limits on 267
tasks and attachments (life-
  cycle model) 265–6
with young children 266
young people, individuals
  within 213–14
family assessment 263–74
  considerations and
    challenges 271–4
  case study 272
  minimising
    interruptions 271
  elements 263–74

family genogram/
  ecomap 263–4
family-assessment frameworks,
  criticisms 267–8
nursing assessments and
  interventions 259–74
therapeutic relationship,
  encouraging
  disclosure 272
Family-Centred (FACE)
  Advanced Care
  Planning 153
Family Law Act 1975 38
Family Partnership Model 260–1
  child health nurses – shift in
    practice 261
  helpers, qualities and skills 261
family-centred care 261–3
  clinical practice
    application 262
  focus for care 262
  implementation 262
fatigue 147–9
  assessment tools/scales 147–8
  child and adolescent
    descriptions 148
  Fatigue Scale – Child 147–8
  other symptoms, association
    with 147
  pain/dyspnoea treatment side-
    effects link 147
  treatment and management
    strategies 148–9
  exercise 148
  nutrition promotion and
    energy conservation 148
febrile seizures 193
fever 190–3
  case study 190
  febrile seizures 193
    prophylactic treatment 193
  infection, response to 190
  intervention 191
  monitoring and
    management 190–1
fine motor coordination 60
five Ps 220
fixated interests 169–70
FLACC scale 201
fluid balance 196–8
  charts 198
fontanel 124
Footprints 153
fracture 218–20
  incomplete fractures 218

management 218–20
  infection control 218
  pain assessment/
    management 218
  plaster casts 220
  stabilising 218
  types of bone fractures 219

gastroenteritis 195–6
  acute gastroenteritis, hydration
    and diet for 195–6
gastrointestinal (GI)
  disturbances 150–2
  Bristol Stool Form Scale 151
  nausea and vomiting 151
  opioid administration
    link 150–1
gastronomy 288, 289
gender
  coping, gender influence
    on 269
  gender-biased research 172
  gender roles 267
general anaesthetics 218
genetic disorders 241–6
genetics
  CF 242–6
  chromosomal birth defects 241
  genetic conditions 14
  low-risk human leukocyte
    antigen (HLA)
    genotypes 236
  single gene defects 242
    neurofibromatosis 242
    X-linked recessive gene 282
genograms 263–4
Glasgow Coma Scale
  (GCS) 125–6, 215
glucagon 239
  glucagon-producing cells 236
glucose 195–6
glycaemic control 237, 238, 239
Gorelick Scale 194
government, Australian
  government, health
    conditions 13–14
grandparents 156
grief 154
  anticipatory grief 285
  threefold layers 156

harm
  harm versus benefit *case
    study* 79
  risk of 91–4

head injuries 214–16
 assessment 215–17
  case study 214
  injury/risk category 215
 discharge preparation 217
 injury history 217
 internal/external
  categorisation 215
 monitoring 215
 risk groups 216
 rural area, incurred in 217
 severity of 215–17
  history, accord with 217
  initial response 215
  risk factors estimation 215
headbox oxygen 205
health
 adult health burden 20
 of Australian children and
  young people 5–6, 10–18
 family nature impact 260
 emerging health priorities 18–23
  dental health 20–1
  overweight and obesity
   18–20
  social and emotional
   health 21–3
 guidelines for ethical conduct
  of health/biomedical
  research 86
 health determinants 61–3
  social determinants 61–3
 health indicators 4–6
  variations 10
 mental health 66
 Ottawa Declaration on the
  Rights of the Child to
  Health Care 91
health-care professionals
 adolescent development,
  knowledge of 213
 child abuse and neglect,
  reporting 40
 information provision to
  families 154–5
 transition–new health-
  care team/new
  relationships 248
heart conditions 11
heart rate
 bradycardia 119
 parameters 119
 rhythm and 118–19
 stroke volume 118, 119, 121
heat moisture exchanger 286

history
 head injuries and 216
 injury history 217
  correlation 218
 medical history – asthma 233,
  234
 sexual history 222
hormones 118
hospitalisation
 of adolescents 22–3
 airway obstruction and 203
 hospitalisation with system
  complications (CF) 246
 Indigenous people, rates of
  17
 key issues 213–14
 leading causes
  congenital anomalies 241–6
  injury 214
  poor social development
   and 60
  quality of attachment, risk
   to 52
  reactions to 54
   exacerbating factors 54
  reasons for children
   requiring 189–206
  in remote areas 214
  for rotavirus 195
hospitals
 admissions
  of children 284–5, 287
  to ICU 280
  related to alcohol abuse 225
  of young people 213–14
 adolescent unit 213
 clinic/hospital setting for
  CF 244–5
 discharge from 220
  preparation for 217
 emergency departments,
  children aged 0–4,
  presenting 189
 hospital experiences 69
 hospital separation rates 14
 in-patient setting
  ambulatory care section
   237
  critical ethnography
   studies 36–7
 regional hospitals 217
Hudson masks 130
human research
 ethics and 84–9
 future perspectives 85

human research ethics
 committees (HRECs) 88,
  93, 96–101
 review of research 96–7
humidification 206, 286
hydration 225, 288–9
 for acute gastroenteritis 195–6
 artificial hydration 151
 feeding orally 289
 monitoring 289
 normal fluid/electrolyte
  balance restoration 196–8
 status 122
hygiene 288
hyperactivity 166
hypertonia 124
hypoglycaemia 124
 insulin treatment 237
 self-management 239
hypospadias 11, 241
hypothyroidism 283
hypotonia 124
hypovolaemia 120, 123, 131–2

identity
 cultural identities and
  attitudes 273–4
 fostering a positive sense of
  culture and identity
  181–4
 identity versus identity
  confusion 65–9
 sense of identity, achieving
  66
illness
 acute respiratory illness
  202–6
 childhood/adolescence
  mental illness and illness
  162–84
 chronic illness 229–51
  quality of attachment, risk
   to 52
 severe acute illness 279
 severity and chronicity 59–60
 terminal illness, emotional
  reactions 152–3
immobility 282
immunisation
 national immunisation
  schedules 12
 rates 10
Implementation of International
 Rights of the Child 33–5
 child-specific treaties 33

INDEX **303**

indicators
  asthma indicators 15
  health and wellbeing
      indicators 4–6
  key national health indicators 7
      cancer 17
      Type 2 diabetes
          indicators 16
      variations 10
  measurement 4–6
  Type 2 diabetes indicators 16
Indigenous people
  Indigenous children
      death rates 12
      five-year survival rates 17
      hospitalisation rates 17
      otitis media incidences 199
industry versus inferiority 60–5
infancy 3, 11–12
  growth and psychosocial
      development 53, 55–6
  infants
      hospitalised infants 53
      infant mortality 10, 11
      infant mortality rates 12
      respiratory distress *case
          study* 114
      parent–infant attachment 52–4
      the sick infant 51–5
      the sick toddler 55–6
infarction 221
infection
  fever, response to infection 190
  infection control 218
inflammation 199
informed consent 223
initiative versus guilt 56–60
  case study 57
injuries 214–20
  acceleration–deceleration
      injuries 42
  head injuries 214–16
  injury presentations–child
      abuse and neglect 42
  injury–history correlation 218
  musculoskeletal injuries
      218–20
  trauma from 214
in-patients 279
institutionalisation 173
insulin 236
  insulin production failure and
      insulin resistance 240
  insulin treatment 237
      subcutaneous injections 238

intensive care unit 280
internalising conditions 60
International Covenant on
    Economic, Social and
    Cultural Rights, Article
    12(1) 31
interventions
  for CF 243–6
  children, ongoing need
      for 283–4
  community-based early
      intervention 175
  evidence-based care 189–206,
      212–25, 229–51
  acutely ill young
      person 212–25
  for fever 191
  medical interventions 282
  nursing interventions 56,
      286–90
      for ADHD 167–9
      for ASD 170–1
      for asthma 233–5
      to meet hygiene and
          elimination needs 288
      parent–infant
          attachment 54–5
      physical therapy 287–8
      for T1D 237–9
      for T2D 240–1
      targeting maternal
          anxiety 58
      timing of 53
  parenting interventions for
      ADHD 168
intimacy versus isolation 69–72
intraosseous needles 131–2
intravenous access 131
intravenous therapy 196–8
  intravenous cannulation 196–8
  intravenous fluids – types and
      volumes 198
  site
      location of 198
      monitoring site/
          infusion 198
ischaemia 221

'jaw thrusts' 129
justice 87–8
  in paediatric research 94–6

Klinefelter syndrome 242
knowledge
  contextualised knowledge 82–3

evidence as 82–4
generating through
    research 79–80
Knowledge to Action (KTA)
    framework 98–9

lacerations 217
laparoscopy 221
laryngotracheo-bronchitis
    see croup
legislation
  Australian age-of-majority
      legislation 37–9
  medical treatment consent
      to 38
  child-protection legislation,
      priorities 39–40
  child rights legislation
      Australian 33–5
      international 30–3
  state/territory legislation–
      minor's consent
      capacity 90
life
  life-limiting conditions 285
  lifespan 177
  quality of life 151
  satisfaction with
      (adolescents) 268
life-cycles
  family life-cycle stages
      model 265–6
      criticisms 265
      tasks and attachments 265–6
liminality state 71–2
long-acting methylphenidate/
    amphetamine
    medications 168

mandatory reporting 40–4
  case study 43–4
  resolution 43–4
manual handling principles 288
marriage 266
maternal depression 174
mean number of decayed,
    missing or filled teeth
    (DMFT) 20, 21
meaning-focused coping 269
medical interventions 282
medical treatment 38
medications
  administration 279
  anti-pyretic medications 191–2
  for croup 204

medications (cont.)
  medical identification bracelet 192
  oral medications, administering 192–3
  right medication, right dose, right route, right time, right person 192
  usual medications doses 144–5
mental health 21, 22–4, 66
  antenatal period, developing during 180
  defining 163, 177
  determinants 177–8
  promoting in children and young people 176–84
mental health disorders 21, 23, 163–5
  adverse outcomes, children 175
  affecting Australian children 165–6
  causes of 22
  children scoring 'of concern' 166
  defining 163
  Diagnostic and Statistical Manual of Mental Disorders 164, 169
  hospitalisation rates 22
  paternal and maternal depression, influence of 174
  prevalence 22–3
mental health problems 163–5
  risk and protective factors 173–4
mental illness
  childhood/adolescence mental illness and illness 162–84
  prevalence 22
metabolic conditions 283
  phenylketonuria 283
methodological approaches 79–80
middle/late childhood 60–5
migration 8
Mind Matters program 180
Minimum Standard for Nurses Caring for Children and Young People 34–5
  extract 34–5
minors 90
Mission Australia Youth Survey 178

mistrust versus trust 51–5
mobility 287–8
monitoring
  for adverse effects (surgery) 223
  consciousness level 224
  fever 190–1
  of head injuries 215
  of height and weight 237
  intravenous site/infusion 198
  of nutrition and hydration 289
  of research 96–101
morbidity 16–18
  patterns in teenage years 21, 23
mortality
  child mortality 141
  infant mortality 10, 11, 16–18
    rates variance 12
  patterns in teenage years 21, 23
  rates 11
    children 12
    Indigenous children 12
mothers
  maternal anxiety and child's anxiety 57
  mothers and babies 6–7
  nurses, empowerment by 273
  as primary caregivers 284–5
  relationships
    mother–child relationship 273
    nurse–mother relationship 273
    power differentials, reducing 273
motor impairment 281–2
  contractures, prevention or delay of 287
  function and independence, maintaining 287
muscle/limb tone 124
muscular dystrophies 282
  detection and diagnosis 282
  Duchenne muscular dystrophy 282
musculoskeletal injuries 218–20
  fracture 218
music therapy 152
myoclonus 144

nasal prongs 130, 206
nasogastric tubes 289–90

National Aboriginal and Torres Strait Islander Health Plan 2013–2023 61–3
National Asthma Council of Australia (NACA) 232, 235
National Statement on Ethical Conduct in Human Research 85, 87, 89, 91, 96–7
  contribution to research 97–8
  'over-researching' of specific paediatric groups 98
  participating for success 100–1
  partnering
    in evidence implementation 98–9
    in research 99–100
  representative laypersons 97–9
  ward-based 'patient committees' 97–8
nausea 151
needs
  of children 260
  complex medical needs 279–90
  hygiene and elimination needs 288
  needs focus of transition (to adult care) 247
  specific age-related needs 213
  of young people with chronic illness 251
neglect 39–40
  child maltreatment form 42
neonates 6
Nest action agenda 179–82
  being loved and safe 179–82
  fostering a positive sense of culture and identity 181–4
  promoting positive participation 181
neural tube defects 241
neurocognitive deficits 224
neurological assessment 124–5
  frequency of 215–17
  level of consciousness, using AVPU 215–17
  paediatric neurological assessment tools 125–7
neurological compromise *case study* 127
neurological congenital anomalies 14

neuromuscular conditions 286
neuromuscular genetic disorders 282
neurovascular impairment 220
neurovascular observations 218–20
nocturnal hyperventilation 286
non-discrimination rights 31
non-maleficence 92
non-pharmacological pain relief 146–7
  cognitive and behavioural techniques 146
  massage 146
non-pharmacological strategies 150
non-steroidal anti-inflammatory drugs (NSAIDs) 143–4
non-stimulant drugs 168
non-verbal behaviours 273
norovirus 195–6
NSW Ministry of Health Clinical Practice Guideline for Acute Management of Asthma 232
nuclear families 267
numerical rating scores (NRS) 202, 223
Nuremberg Code (1947) 86
nurses
  adolescent development, knowledge of 213
  assumptions regarding families 274
  child health nurses – shift in practice 261
  cultural identities and attitudes 273–4
  feelings and prejudices 272
  general paediatric nurses, mental disorders, understanding of 164
mothers
  empowering 273
  encouraging to make complaints 273
  nurse–mother relationship 273
  power differentials, reducing 273
  negotiating parent–child conflict (treatment preferences) 32–3
nurse–child relationship 173

role-modelling 273
state and territory mandated reporting (child maltreatment) 41–4
  case study 43–4
support for siblings of dying child 155–6
thoughts and feelings, engaging with parents regarding 154
unprofessional care, speaking out against 273
nursing assessment 259–74, 286–90
  for CF 243–6
  evidence-based care 189–206, 229–51
  acutely ill young people 212–25
nursing assistance 288
nutrition 288–9
  artificial nutrition 151
  decreased nutritional intake 151–2
  dental/gum problems, pain impact 21
  feeding orally 289
  monitoring 289
  'obesity epidemic' 19, 20

obesity 18–20, 240
  body mass index (BMI) 19
  childhood obesity prevalence 20
  'obesity epidemic' 19, 20
  socioeconomic areas 19–20
observation
  close observation 53, 215–17
  neurovascular observations 218–20
Obsessive Compulsive Disorder (OCD) 22
operations
  preoperative care 222–3
  preparations for 222–3
    preoperative sedation 223
  procedures
    elective procedures 222
    emergency procedures 222
opioids 217
  dyspnoea management 150
  opioid administration–GI link 150–1
  sedative effects 148
  side effects 144–5

myoclonus 144
  strategies to address 145
  weak opioids 144
Oppositional Defiant Disorder (ODD) 171–3
oral antibiotics 200
oral corticosteroids 203
oral examinations 20
oral medications 192–3
  administering 192–3
  body surface area 192
  liquid preparation 192
oral rehydration therapy (ORT) 195–6
organ transplantation 246
Organization for Economic Cooperation and Development (OECD) 5–6
oropharyngeal airways 129–30
out-patients 279
overweight 18–20
  BMI 19
  socioeconomic areas 19–20
oxygen saturation 117
  pulse oximeters 117
oxygen therapy 205–6
  face masks 205–6
  headbox oxygen 205
  humidification 206
  long-term oxygen therapy 286
  nasal prongs 206
oxygenation 130

Paediatric Assessment Triangle 111–13
  child's appearance 112
  child's circulation 113
  child's work of breathing 112–13
paediatric care
  Australian settings for 141–56
  paediatric setting, research in 77–102
paediatric end-of-life care
  central tenets 142
  context 142
  families in 154–6
  paediatric palliative care, distinction 142
paediatric health-care services 279–90
  children's choices, acknowledging 36

paediatric multidisciplinary
    team 142, 237, 279
paediatric nursing
  Australian context 1–24,
    29–44, 49–72, 77–102
  family-centred care 261–3
paediatric palliative care
  case study 152
  paediatric end-of-life care,
    distinction 142
  usual medications doses 144–5
  weight loss and cachexia 151
paediatric patients
  cardiopulmonary arrest 111
  clinical signs 111
  deterioration 116
    causes 111
    recognition using
      Primary Assessment
      Framework 114–25
  paediatric early warning
    tools 109
  respiratory and cardiovascular
    differences 110
  structured assessment 111–14
paediatric research
  beneficence in 91–4
  consent in 89–91
  justice in 94–6
pain 220
  abdominal pain 220–2
  analgesia use 217, 223
  from dental/gum problems 21
  distraction 197
  earaches 200
  from inflammation 199
  non-pharmacological pain
    relief 146–7
  pain assessment/
    management 143–7,
    200–2, 218, 220
    assessment tools 223
    postoperative
      management 223
    recommended procedures
      for procedural/
      postoperative pain
      assessment 200
  pain scales 223
  reducing cannulation pain 197
  a subjective experience 200–2
  WHO analgesic ladder 143–4
palliative care
  Australian paediatric care
    settings 141–56

paediatric palliative care 142
  team support for siblings of
    dying child 155–6
pallor 220
pancreas 236
paralysis 220
parents
  authoritative parenting style
    61
  burden of care (children) 284
  children's conduct problems,
    behaviour associated
    with 172
  children's health decisions/
    behaviours 59
  commitments outside
    home 284
  coping styles 269
  dyspnoea, parental perceptions
    of 150
  hospital discharge
    preparation 217
  information provision 124–5
  involvement in children's
    health care 262
  model 260–1
  knowledge of children's mood
    and behaviour 58
  multi-faceted health problems
    272
  parental expertise 284
  parent–child conflict 32–3
  parent–infant attachment
    52–4
  parenting interventions for
    ADHD 168
  parent's role, assumptions
    regarding 29–30
  resuscitation, parental presence
    during 133–5
  standing parental consent 91
  support for
    death and end-of-life
      care 154
    during investigation 273
    thoughts and nurses
      engagement regarding
      feelings 154
    wellbeing of 180
paresthesia 220
PARIHS model 98–9
participation
  participation rights 32
  positive participation 181
  through technology 181

paternal depression 174
patient-controlled analgesia 223
peers 21
  sense of difference from 50, 66
    case study 67–8
perceptual thinking 60–1
perforation 221
perfusion 120–1
peripheral vasoconstriction 121
pharmacological strategies 150
phenylketonuria (PKU) 283
physical abuse 59
physical care 279
physical inactivity 240
physical therapy 287–8
PICO(T) format 80
play 153
poisoning 224–5
population
  census 7–8
  dental health disparities
    across 21
  Indigenous–non-Indigenous
    population age
    distribution comparison 8
  infant mortality rates across 12
positive adaptive responses
  promotion 178–82
Post-Traumatic Stress Disorder
  (PTSD) 65
postoperative care 223
  adverse effects monitoring 223
  pain management 223
  postoperative assessment 223
power
  disparity in relationships 30
  power differentials 273
practice
  applying new knowledge
    to 22–4, 101–2
  basing on evidence 83
  evidence-based practice 80–4
  family-centred care
    application 262
  practice implications – child
    rights 35–44
  translation of hospital
    experiences to 69
  unethical practice 87
Prader-Willi syndrome 242
premature birth 283
prematurity 286
premorbid function 58
preoperative care 222–3
preventer medication 234–5

INDEX **307**

Primary Assessment Framework (ABCD assessment) 111–13, 128
  A–airway 115–16
  B–breathing 116–17
  C–circulation 118–23
  D–disability 124–5
  case study 114
principle of family unity 33
privacy 88
problem-focused coping 269
protection rights 32
psychosocial development (Erikson) 51
  developmental stages 51
pulse 220
  carotid pulse 121
  peripheral pulses and perfusion 120–1
pupil size/reactivity 125
pyrogenic cytokines 190

rate-based statistics 5
recovery position 224
relationships
  disparity in 30
  dyspnoea and 149–50
  intimate relationships 69–70
  mother–child relationship 273
  new health-care team/new relationships 248
  nurse–child relationship 173
  nurse–mother relationship 273
  power differentials in 273
  therapeutic relationship 272
  transition to new health-care team/new relationships 248
research
  Australian Code for the Responsible Conduct of Research 88
  burden of research 95
  children and young people, researching with 84
  definition 79–80
  evidence-based practice and 83
  gender-biased research 172
  generating knowledge through 79–80
  guidelines for ethical conduct of health/biomedical research 86

  human research 84–9
  Involving People in Research 99
  merit and integrity 87–8
  monitoring and participation 96–101
  National Statement on Ethical Conduct in Human Research 85, 87, 89, 96–7
  standing parental consent 91
  new knowledge to practice, application 101–2
  paediatric research 89–91
  paediatric setting 77–102
  participation in research assent 91
  inconvenience associated with 92
  research design 80
  research ethics 85–7
  research evidence 77–8
  possibilities from delivery/demand side 81–2
  research governance 88
  principles 88
research ethics
  Belmont Report 86, 87
  core principles 87–9
  experiments
    Tuskagee Experiment 86
    unethical experiments 85
  fundamental principles 85
resilience 177
  promoting 178–82
resources 279
respect (for persons) 87–8
respiration 286–7
  B–breathing (Primary Assessment Framework) 116–17
  breath sounds and air entry 117
  chronic respiratory conditions 283
  grunting 117
  nursing care 203
  respiratory compromise 110
  respiratory function 282
  respiratory infections 203, 287
    CF and 245
  respiratory rate parameters 117
  respiratory support 128–32
  respiratory syncytial virus (RSV) 204–5

respite care 285
Reyes syndrome 191
rights
  Australian legislation 33–5
  Ottawa Declaration on the Rights of the Child to Health Care 91
  UN Convention rights
    non-discrimination rights 31
    participation rights 32
    protection rights 32
    survival and development rights 31–2
risk
  airway obstruction, children at risk of 129
  of anti-pyretic medications 191–2
  associated with alcohol poisoning 224
  to benefits and harm 91–4
  of cardiovascular compromise 110
  cerebral palsy risk factors 282
  of coercion 89
  of compromised airways 115
  discomfort 92
  of disease/mental illness 65
  head injuries
    injury/risk category 215
    risk groups 216
  levels 96–7
  of mental health problems 173–4
  of physical abuse – children with disability/chronic illness 59
  to quality of attachment 52
  for research participants 88
  of respiratory compromise 110
  risk categories 93
  risk-taking behaviours 21, 23
  for T2D 240
rotavirus 195–6

scales 194
  Bristol Stool Form Scale 151
  Clinical Dehydration Scale (CDS) 194
  COMFORT behaviour scale 201
  FACES pain scale 202, 223
  fatigue assessment tools/scales 147–8
  Fatigue Scale–Child 147–8

scales (cont.)
   FLACC scale 201
   Glasgow Coma Scale
      (GCS) 215
   Gorelick Scale 194
   numerical rating scales 202, 223
   pain scales 223
   scales/algorithms
      (dehydration) 194
   visual analogue scales 202
   (WHO) Scale 194
schizophrenia 22
school attendance 21
sedation 217, 218
   preoperative sedation 223
   sedative effects
      of alcohol 224
      of analgesics 217
      of opioids 148
   see also analgesia
self-harm 214
self-report tools 202
sensation 220
separation anxiety 54, 175
sepsis 221
'serve and return interactions' 180
services
   in-patient services 279
   mental health services 164
   out-patient services 279
   paediatric health-care
      services 279–90
sexual history 222
Shaken baby syndrome 42
siblings 135, 155–6
   emotional responses 155
skin
   colour 194–5, 220
   condition of 198
   skin mottling 121
social confidence 22
social development 60
social health 21–3
social health determinants 61–3
   inequities 62
social interactions 21, 169–70
socioeconomic status 268
sodium solutions 195–6, 198
spirituality 274
Standards for the Care of
      Children and Adolescents
      in Health Services 34
stress/stressors 268–9
   chronic conditions, diagnosis
      and treatment 55–6

   ongoing stressors 268
   regression of developmental
      gains reaction 56
   stress response 53
   toxic stress 177
   see also coping strategies
stridor 203–4
substance abuse 272–3
suctioning 279
Sudden Infant Death Syndrome
      (SIDS) 11
   prevention of 12
support
   circulatory support 130–2
   for families 264, 267
      from grandparents 156
   psychological and
      socioeconomic
      support 279
   respiratory support 128–32
   for siblings of dying child
      155–6
      from nurses/palliative care
      team 155–6
   ventilation support 286–7
surgery
   elective surgery 222
   emergency surgery 222
survival and development
      rights 31–2
Swedish nose 286
symptom-control
      medication 234

teams
   multidisciplinary team
      management 142, 155–6,
      237, 279
   team support for siblings of
      dying child 155–6
technology
   improved technology 85
   medical technology 279
   parental expertise 284
   participation through 181
temperature
   body temperature
      level 191
      mean range 190–1
tetanus boosters 218
therapeutic relationship 272
tooth decay 20
topical anaesthetics 196–7
   EMLA 196–7
   to reduce cannulation pain 197

Torres Strait Islander peoples
   families 267–8
   health/welfare over-
      representation 61–3
   population age distribution
      comparison 8
toxic stress 177
tracheostomy 286
   tracheostomy tubes 130
transitioning to adult care 246–51
   case study 248
   characterised by changes
      248–9
   decision-making
      responsibility 250
   important considerations 247–9
   individual responsibility for
      care 248
   new health-care team/new
      relationships 248
   planning process 250–1
   stage-of-life decisions,
      coinciding with 249
   standardising program
      content 250
   successful transitions 249–51
      contributing factors 250
      emotional factors 249
      good preparation 249–50
   transition, needs focus 247
   transition commencement
      247
Trisomy 21 241–2
trust versus mistrust 51–5
   nursing assessment and
      interventions 54–5
   resolution 51–2
Turner syndrome 242
Type 1 diabetes (T1D) 15, 236–9
   common acute and chronic
      complications 239
   essential care aspects 238
   hypoglycaemia
      complication 237
   insulin treatment 237, 238
   management, blood glucose
      control–insulin treatment
      balance 237
   nursing assessments and
      interventions 237–9
   presentation and
      symptoms 236–7
   prevalence 236
   rising incidence 236
   T1D–T2D distinction 236

Type 2 diabetes (T2D) 15–16,
    239–41
  characteristics 240
  complications prevention 241
  management strategies 240–1
  national incidence 239–40
  obesity and physical
    inactivity and 240
  nursing assessments and
    interventions 240–1
  prevalence 239–40
  risk factors 240
  self-management 240
  T1D–T2D distinction 236
  treatment aim 241

Universal Declaration of the
    Rights of the Child
    (Article 3) 31
urine output 122–3
  colour and concentration 122

values 85
vascular access 130–2
venepuncture 196
  see also cannulation
    (intravenous);
    intravenous therapy
ventilation support 286–7
violence 272–3
viruses 190, 195–6
  respiratory infections caused
    by 203–4
visual analogue scales (VAS) 202
vomiting 151

weight
  at birth 10

overweight 18–20
  see also obesity
weight loss 151
wellbeing
  of Australian children and
    young people 5–6, 231
  family nature impact 260
  defining 163
  indicators of 4–6
  measurements 177–8
  of parents 180
whistleblowing 82
World Health Organization
    (WHO)
  palliative care definition 142
  WHO analgesic ladder 143–4
    adaptation 143–4
    criticisms 143
    NSAIDs 143–4
    weak opioids 144
  (WHO) Scale 194

young people 13
  acutely ill young people
    212–25
  best interest 92
  with CF 244–5
    hospitalisation with system
      complications 246
    management plan 245–6
    treatment and preventative
      therapies 245–6
  with chronic illness 50,
    229–51
    health needs 251
    mental health of 66
    optimal independent
      functioning 66

consent circumstances 90
death, causes of 214
dental health 20–1
development
  environment, translation to
    practice 69
  psychological
    development 50–1
emerging health priorities
  18–23
families, individuals
  within 213–14
health disruptions 50–1
hospitalisation 213–14
  developmental limiting 50
  discharge preparation 217
  injuries 214
marginalised and
  disengaged 181
mental health
  case study 176
  case study resolution 184
  promoting 176–84
  services 164
participation in research
  assent 91
  risk associated with 93
peers, sense of difference
  from 50
researching with 84
with T1D 237
with T2D 240–1
transitioning to adult care 246–51
  decision-making
    responsibility 250
  see also adolescence;
    Australia's children and
    young people